# The CRA's Guide to
# **Monitoring Clinical Research**

Second Edition

Karen E. Woodin, Ph.D. & John C. Schneider

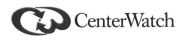

100 North Washington Street, Suite 301
Boston, MA 02114
www.centerwatch.com

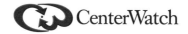

**The CRA's Guide to Monitoring Clinical Research, Second Edition**
by Karen E. Woodin, Ph.D., and John C. Schneider

**Editors**            **Design**
Sara Gambrill         Paul Gualdoni
Steve Zisson          Todd E. Casselman

# TABLE OF CONTENTS

CRAs must be a "Jack or Jill of all trades" because there are so many activities and tasks that they will be involved in if doing this job for any length of time.

**The Mindset of a Concierge**

*During a recent teaching assignment, I stopped by the concierge desk at the hotel to check on activities and restaurants in the area. The concierge was a delightful person, who was able to tell me everything I wanted to know and who obviously enjoyed her work. Not only did the experience leave me with the knowledge I sought, but I also felt good as a result of my interaction with this personable individual. As I walked out the door with all the maps and instructions I had been given, I was pondering my experience with the concierge and thought, "that is what a good CRA should be."*

*As you prepare for your site visits, try putting yourself in the mindset of a concierge, providing investigators and their staffs with the information and knowledge needed to do a good clinical study, while leaving them feeling good about you and the sponsor, both throughout and after the trial. Having a site's good feelings extend after the completion of a study makes it easier for a CRA to enlist the site for future studies, just as a good concierge generates repeat business for the hotel.*

*—JC*

## CRA Tasks

CRAs are involved in a variety of research-related activities. Some of these are listed in Table 1. You may be able to add other activities to the list. This table provides graphic proof that a good, experienced CRA has a wealth of knowledge and skills.

CRAs must also be able to work under adverse conditions, think on their feet and be away from home for days at a time. Travel today is strenuous, time-consuming, frustrating and stressful. Being alone under conditions and in places unfamiliar to you may be unsettling.

**The Two Sides of Being a CRA**

*Before I accepted a job as a CRA, my future boss gave me the opportunity of going out to the field and working for a week with two senior CRAs in the group. Monday morning I flew to New Orleans and met with one of the senior CRAs, Phil. He picked me up in the rental car, and since he rents so frequently, they always save him a Cadillac. He then drove me* to the hotel, where he is always given a wonderful room on the concierge level since he stays there so frequently.

The following two days convinced me there was no job on earth better than that of a CRA. At every investigative site we visited, the investigators and coordinators were waiting to meet with us—the materials were all out and ready, the case report forms completed and done well, everything running as smooth as silk. And the final touch—at every restaurant, Phil was greeted by name, asked after his welfare, and seated at a choice table. I thought to myself, "It can't get much better than this!"

Late Wednesday afternoon, Phil put me on the plane to Washington National to meet the second CRA, Ron. He picked me up about 10:30 at night in the dim, almost deserted terminal. Outside, it was dark, cold, and a light rain was falling as we hiked to the far end of a huge parking lot to retrieve Ron's car for the 50-mile drive to the Holiday Inn (clean, basic, no frills). Dinner was a quick run through McDonald's drive-in for a hamburger, since there was no meal on the plane.

Ron retrieved me at 6 the next morning for the trek to our 7 a.m. appointment. We were there on time, but no one else was. We waited for 45 minutes until the study coordinator showed up, apologetic but late. Nothing was ready for our visit. This set the tone for the next two days—everything that could have gone wrong did. Sites were unprepared, forgot about the appointment, had emergencies come up so they couldn't meet with us. We experienced an unusual string of bad luck for two entire days.

When Ron put me on the plane bound for home, I realized how lucky I'd been to see both the good and the difficult aspects of the CRA job. Things never go smoothly all the time (even for Phil), and a good CRA can roll with the punches and fix things for the next time. I learned a great deal from both of them, and was able to start my career with a good, solid base of knowledge about working in the field.

—Karen

In addition to the stress of travel and working conditions at sites that are often less than ideal, medical institutions and private practice facilities rarely have enough room because clinical studies usually don't enjoy a very high priority with regard to space. Consequently, you might well be doing your various monitoring tasks in some pretty uncomfortable places. It's hard to work when you're balancing everything on your knees or leaning over an exam table in between patient visits.

## Career Preparation

How does someone prepare for this complex, challenging career? Today, most CRAs have a bachelor's degree in nursing or in one of the natural or medical sciences. There appears to be a growing trend toward the advent of a Physician's Assistant (PA) degree or Pharm. D. degree as an excellent background for becoming a CRA. There are no undergraduate programs that specifically train for this career. However, many universities are now offering postgraduate courses in clinical research (some are web-based) that are comprehensive and provide excellent training (See Appendix D). There are also courses taught by professional societies such as the Drug Information Association (DIA)[1] and the Association of Clinical Research Professionals (ACRP).[2]

People trying to get that first CRA position often feel as though they're caught in a "catch-22." Employers want to hire someone with experience, but how can you get experience without being able to get a job? Unfortunately, there is no easy answer. Generally speaking, CROs tend to hire more "first-timers" than the large pharmaceutical houses. However, don't exclude the pharmaceutical companies from your list when you send out your resume. Once you get your first CRA position, give it everything you have. A good track record is the greatest asset in furthering your career.

As you gain more experience, you will be able to register with a job listing service. CenterWatch's JobWatch service has job listings available online. New positions are posted on the web site at www.centerwatch.com/jobwatch. Resumes can be submitted online for free, where employers and recruiters can search them. Monitorforhire.com, another job listing service, places blinded profiles of monitors on its site at www.monitorforhire.com. Listed monitors need at least two years of field monitoring experience and must go through a qualification and verification process. ACRP and DIA also list job postings on their websites.

Most sponsor companies have from two to four levels of CRA positions in their career path. The differences are primarily related to experience. One key difference is the CRA's ability to evaluate a potential study site and determine whether that site has the expertise, experience, resources and patients to do a particular study well. A CRA who can consistently find good investigators who can generate accurate, timely data with a minimum of enrollment problems is a valuable asset to a sponsor company or contract organization.

The more experienced CRAs will also have a better understanding of the scientific method, which enables them to recognize actions and procedures that could bias the study and invalidate the data. Expertise in these key areas is developed only over time, which is why experience and proven performance are of such high value. Generic job descriptions for two levels of CRAs, plus a job summary comparing tasks for entry level and advanced CRAs are included in Appendix D.

Once on the job, knowledge, networking and common sense are your best weapons. You never outgrow your need to learn. Be prepared to read quite a bit. At the top of your reading list should be the federal regulations that govern the conduct of clinical research. (These are included in Appendix G.) All CRAs should read the regulations periodically and must also be aware of changes in the regulations. Don't rely too heavily on the advice of colleagues because they may not have read the regulations recently either. The ICH Guidelines and the Belmont Report should also be on your list of required reading.

Standard operating procedures (SOPs) are an important tool for CRAs and should be used to help manage their work and as overall guidance. This means that the CRA does not always have to rely on intuition or ethical standards; the SOPs will provide a basic level from which to approach both tasks and problems. Sponsors and CROs will almost always have a complete set of SOPs that govern monitoring activities, including:

- Investigator selection
- Clinical trial agreements
- Collection and maintenance of study documents
- Initiation of a clinical trial
- Routine monitoring of a clinical trial
- Source data verification
- Investigational product handling and accountability
- Site visit monitoring reports
- Reporting noncompliance
- Study closeout
- Audits of clinical sites
- Serious adverse event (SAE) reporting

The CRA should develop a large network of peers and colleagues. One of the best ways to do this is through membership in professional associations. ACRP (www.acrpnet.org) and DIA (www.diahome.org) are the two largest associations. It's a good idea to join at least one of these organizations. Both have journals, provide training and offer information, sponsor meetings and workshops. Try to attend at least one professional meeting each year as these are great learning opportunities, as well as perfect networking events. Check out the web sites and talk with current members to get a feel for which organization best meets your particular needs. You will want to maintain a list of colleagues you feel comfortable calling when you have a problem, or have an idea you want advice on.

Finally, rely on your common sense as well as your business sense. The people doing your studies are your customers; you are out of work without them. Treat them accordingly. Be polite, courteous and kind. Return calls promptly and tell them what you will be doing during the visit, who you wish to have available and how long you plan to be there in advance of scheduled visits. A detailed discussion of the business approach to monitoring is covered in Chapter 10.

## In the Future

What's coming in the future? Some industry watchers believe that, with the advent of electronic clinical trials (eClinical trials), the role of the CRA may be changing to include a greater computer component. CRAs will need to be well versed in a variety of data entry and management programs, on-line editing capabilities, and may, in fact, actually perform direct data entry and/or cleanup at sites. Be ready and prepared for change, as change always occurs over time.

There is a trend toward certification for CRAs. Currently, both ACRP and the Society of Clinical Research Associate (SoCRA)[3] offer certification programs for CRAs; both programs require experience and passing a written examination. Although it is not necessary, at this point, for a CRA to be certified, it does add to a person's credentials and credibility. In the future, it may well become standard practice for CRAs to be certified. At some point in his or her career, the CRA should investigate and work toward achieving certification. A certified CRA may have an edge when it comes to being hired or promoted.

## Your Value

The importance of the CRA role in clinical research cannot be over-emphasized. CRAs are on the front line and play a major role in study conduct and quality. Bad studies are not usually the fault of site personnel; they result from poor planning and study design, and from improper selection, preparation and training of the study site. A CRA may not be involved in planning and study design, but the last three are usually CRA responsibilities.

Few people on the drug development team have as much direct impact on study quality and timeliness as the CRA.

The CRA also has an influence on the bottom line for a drug program. The CRA is the main defense against data errors during clinical trials, which cost millions of dollars to correct. In addition, based on the annual sales of an average performing drug, the cost for each day's delay in getting the drug approved is more than a million dollars.[4] The CRA has a major impact on the timely completion of trials, assuring that company development timelines are realistic and are met or exceeded. It's not hard to understand the value of a good CRA in terms of program quality and cost.

# Key Takeaways

- CRAs are paramedical personnel who perform a variety of clinical research monitoring activities in support of a drug development program.
- CRAs must be self-starters, with excellent interpersonal relationship skills, who are detail-oriented and have excellent written and oral communication skills.
- CRAs must possess a breadth of clinical knowledge that enables them to provide investigative site personnel with the information they need to perform good clinical trials.
- CRAs need to be adaptable and have the ability to work under a wide variety of conditions.
- CRAs must keep learning and should develop a large network of peers and colleagues.
- CRAs play a major role in the conduct quality and timeliness of clinical trials.

### References
1. www.diahome.org
2. www.acrpnet.org
3. www.socra.org
4. "Losing Ground in the Battle Against Development Delays," CenterWatch, December 1998, Vol. 5, Issue 12, CenterWatch Editorial, p.1.1.

CHAPTER 2

# The History Behind
# the Regulations

Good Clinical Practices (GCPs) are the accepted procedures for conducting clinical trials.

GCP is defined as: an international ethical and scientific quality standard for designing, conducting, recording and reporting trials that involve the participation of human subjects. Compliance with this standard provides public assurance that the rights, safety and well-being of trial subjects are protected, consistent with the principles that have their origin in the Declaration of Helsinki, and that the clinical trial data are credible.*

GCPs are derived from federal regulations, ethical codes, ICH guidelines and official guidance documents. They evolved because of concerns about the treatment of human research subjects around the world, and about the reliability of the data and conclusions from trials. Concern about data and conclusions goes beyond the need to protect subjects in clinical trials, extending to the greater goal of protecting all patients who use pharmaceutical products. There are serious consequences for not following the GCPs, including loss of revenue and loss of reputation. Also, not following GCPs can expose sponsors and investigative sites to legal liability, not only from study subjects, but from future users of the medication (class action suits, for example).

---

* According to the International Conference on Harmonisation of Technical Requirements for Registration of Pharmaceuticals for Human Use (ICH) Guideline for Good Clinical Practice, as published in the Federal Register, May 9, 1997.

Understanding why the regulations were developed, and some of the factors that will undoubtedly lead to additional regulations in the future, will help you become a better CRA.

Just in the past few years, several large institutional review boards (IRBs) have had their activities curtailed by the U.S. Food and Drug Administration (FDA) and the Office for Human Research Protection (OHRP) because of serious problems and deficiencies found during inspections. Because of these findings, clinical trials at some of these institutions had enrollment halted, or were closed completely. Sponsor companies suffered because they were counting on the data to support their new drug applications (NDAs), and the respective institutions suffered because of the loss of study revenues and the intangible loss of their status in the clinical trials community. The discovery of serious problems at a handful of IRBs has already resulted in increased government surveillance, primarily by increasing the number of IRB inspections, and a reorganization within the U.S. Department of Health and Human Services (HHS) to better handle the need for this increased surveillance.

There have also been concerns raised about the potential problems inherent in genomics research, both from an ethical viewpoint and because genomics involves new and untried research techniques. As we watch these trends, it is not unlikely to expect changes in federal regulations that further tighten the requirements for doing research. CRAs should be aware of these changes and be prepared to make appropriate adjustments in the way they work with investigative sites and clinical trials. It is wise to be cognizant of the current research environment and to be prepared for impending changes. You will be a better CRA by having an understanding of why the pharmaceutical industry is so highly regulated, and why the primary vehicles for human subject protection, institutional review boards and informed consents, are so important.

Crisis is an impetus for change. Crises breed controversy, leading to the involvement of Congress, which then enacts legislation. Some of the major milestones in the regulations and in human subject protection and the crises that spurred them, where appropriate, are discussed below.

# Regulation and Human Subject Protection Milestones

### 1848: Drug Importation Act

The first regulatory action regarding drugs came in 1848, when Congress enacted a law requiring the United States Customs Service to stop the importing of adulterated drugs from outside the country. It took another fifty-plus years for the next major piece of legislation to come about.

## 1862: Bureau of Chemistry

In 1862, President Abraham Lincoln appointed Dr. Charles M. Wetherill, a chemist, to serve in the new Department of Agriculture. This was the beginning of the Bureau of Chemistry, which in 1927 became the Food, Drug and Insecticide Administration. The name was changed to Food and Drug Administration (FDA) in 1930.

## 1906: Food and Drugs Act

Until the Food and Drugs Act was signed by President Theodore Roosevelt in 1906, there was no comprehensive statute regulating drugs. Before this, standard medical practice consisted of activities such as purges and bloodletting. There were very few effective drugs on the market (opium, cocaine). All products could be freely advertised and sold and were readily available without need for any prescription. Then along came Dr. Wiley.

Dr. Harvey W. Wiley was the Chief Chemist at the Department of Agriculture from 1883 to 1912. He had a driving interest in the adulteration of food and drugs, and set up a plan to investigate food preservatives. In 1902, Dr. Wiley set up his "poison squad"—a group of young, unmarried men who had volunteered to test foods Dr. Wiley thought might contain unhealthy preservatives or coloring agents. The squad lunched together, trying out the various substances that Dr. Wiley wanted to test. Judgment on the degree of harm the substances caused was based on how sick these men got after eating them. Over the course of the five years these experiments were carried out, they proved conclusively that many preservatives were harmful to health.

It was at least in part because of Dr. Wiley's work that Congress passed the 1906 Pure Food and Drugs Act, which prohibited the interstate transportation of adulterated and misbranded foods, drinks and drugs. It didn't limit companies from producing the items, but it cut down on their ability to widely market them, as these items could not be taken across state lines.

## 1938: Food, Drug, and Cosmetic Act

The next major crisis was precipitated by the use of Elixir of Sulfanilamide. Sulfanilamide was a tablet—a very large tablet—used to treat infections. The manufacturer wanted to use it in children, but the tablet was too big for them to swallow, so the company decided to make it into a liquid by adding diethylene glycol, the principal ingredient of antifreeze. The company was able to get a liquid form and tested it for flavor—it tasted just fine. Unfortunately, it never tested the resulting liquid for toxicity. It was very toxic, causing the deaths of more than a hundred people, many of them children.

The FDA had no authority to withdraw this product from the market for safety reasons, as there were no regulations regarding safety. The agency could, however, remove it for mislabeling. It was called an elixir, and elixirs had to contain alcohol, which Elixir of Sulfanilamide did not. Based only on this, the FDA was able to have this unsafe product removed from the market.

As a direct result of this tragedy, Congress passed the 1938 Food, Drug and Cosmetic Act. For the first time, a pre-market approval of "new drugs" was required for safety. "New drugs" meant new chemical entities or combinations. Drugs marketed prior to 1938 were specifically exempted ("grandfathered" in) as long as their labeling didn't change. There was no definition of safety in the act; however, the general understanding was that the benefits must outweigh the risk. The act also did not require active approval by the FDA. Unless the FDA objected within sixty days of the NDA (New Drug Application) being filed, the manufacturer could automatically begin marketing. No proof of efficacy was required. Between 1938 and 1962, most NDAs filed were essentially just testimonials from physicians.

## 1947: Nuremberg Code

After the initial Nuremberg Trial of Nazi leaders, a series of supplemental trials were held. The trial, officially known as United States v. Karl Brandt et al. and commonly referred to as "The Nazi Doctors Trial," was held from December 9, 1946, to July 19, 1947. As the title indicates, the judges and prosecutors in this court trial were all from the United States. The 23 defendants (including 20 physicians)—all members of the Nazi Party—were charged with murder, torture and other atrocities committed in the name of medical science.

When the final judgment in the Nazi Doctors Trial was delivered on July 19, 1947, 15 of the 23 defendants were found guilty. Seven were sentenced to death. Four American judges presiding issued a ten-point code that described basic principles of ethical behavior in the conduct of human experimentation. This ten-point code is known as the Nuremberg Code. Although the Code focuses on the ethical treatment of humans in non-therapeutic research (research not intended to result in a cure for a condition), the elements described form the cornerstone for the guidelines and regulations we have today and reflects the modern thinking that:

- Informed consent should be obtained without coercion.
- The experiment should be useful and necessary.
- Human experiments should be based on previous experiments with animals.
- Physical and mental suffering should be avoided.
- Death and disability should not be expected outcomes of an experiment.
- The degree of risk taken should not exceed the humanitarian importance of solving the problem.
- Human subjects should be protected against even remote possibilities of harm.
- Only qualified scientists should conduct medical research.
- Human subjects should be free to end an experiment at any time.
- The scientist in charge must be prepared to end an experiment at any stage.

## 1962: Kefauver-Harris Amendments (Drug Amendments of 1962)

In the late 1950s, thalidomide was being tested extensively in Europe, and to some degree in the United States. It was a sleeping pill, and pregnant women were included in the testing groups. Unfortunately, it had a terrible effect on the fetus if taken during the first trimester, and many children born to women who had taken thalidomide suffered from phocomelia, a shortening of the limbs resulting in arms that looked like flippers. Dr. Francis Kelsey at the FDA was responsible for much of the research that defined the link between phocomelia and thalidomide use in pregnancy.

The Kefauver-Harris amendments, passed in part due to the aroused public support for stronger drug regulation because of the thalidomide tragedy, form the basis of the current IND (Investigational New Drug) Application regulations. For the first time, drugs were required to have proven efficacy, as well as safety. Also for the first time, an active FDA approval was required, not just the review and 60-day waiting time. In addition, this law required mandated reporting of adverse events and disclosure of risks in advertisements.

Much to the chagrin of pharmaceutical manufacturers, as part of this regulation, the FDA also had to re-review all the NDAs submitted between 1938 and 1962 to see if these products met the new efficacy standard. There were numerous lawsuits over the definition of substantial evidence of efficacy, including the Pharmaceutical Manufacturers Association vs. the FDA,[1] and suits by almost all major pharmaceutical manufacturers. This controversy led to the definitions of "adequate and well-controlled" clinical investigations required today.

## 1964: Declaration of Helsinki

The World Health Organization spent more than ten years working on the statement of ethical principles that became known as the Declaration of Helsinki. This document defined rules for "therapeutic" and "non-therapeutic" research. It repeated the Nuremberg Code requirement for consent for non-therapeutic research but allowed for enrolling certain patients in therapeutic research without consent. The Declaration of Helsinki also allowed legal guardians to grant permission to enroll subjects in research, both therapeutic and non-therapeutic, and recommended written consent—an issue not addressed in the Nuremberg Code. In addition, the Declaration of Helsinki requires review and prior approval of a protocol by an IRB. Several revisions have been made to this document, including a Clarification.

## 1979: The Belmont Report

The National Research Act, passed by Congress in 1974, created the National Commission for the Protection of Human Subjects of Biomedical and Behavioral Research. This commission wrote a document entitled Ethical Principles and Guidelines for the Protection of Human Subjects of Research, which became known as the Belmont Report when it was published in 1979. The three basic principles of the Belmont Report are respect for persons, beneficence, and justice.

1.  Respect for persons is manifested by the informed consent process, as well as in safeguards for vulnerable populations, such as children, pregnant women, mentally disabled adults, and prisoners. Other important concerns of respect for persons are privacy and confidentiality.
2.  Beneficence has two general characteristics: do no harm, and maximize benefit while minimizing risk. Beneficence is manifested in the use of good research design, competent investigators, and a favorable risk/benefit ratio.
3.  Justice implies fairness, and is manifested in the equitable selection of subjects for research, ensuring that no group of people is "selected in" or "selected out" unfairly based on factors unrelated to the research. This means that there must be appropriate inclusion/exclusion criteria and a fair system of recruitment.

The Belmont Report forms the cornerstone for the ethical treatment of human subjects of research.

## 1987: IND Rewrite Regulations

Additional regulation was enacted after three extreme examples of abuse illustrated the need for further protection of human subjects:

- **Tuskegee Syphilis Study[1]**
  In this study, which began in 1932 and extended for more than forty years, several hundred black males with syphilis were enrolled. They were not informed about the purpose of the study, but were told that government doctors were examining people for "bad blood." Even after penicillin became available and was known to be effective for syphilis (1943), the males in this study were not treated with it. This study was not stopped until 1973, when treatment was given as needed. In 1997, President Clinton made a formal apology to study subjects and their families.

- **Jewish Chronic Disease Hospital Study[2]**
  In 1963, physicians at this hospital were interested in studying the nature of human transplant rejection. To do this, they injected live cancer cells into indigent, elderly patients suffering from a variety of chronic debilitating diseases without their consent. The subjects were not told about the live cancer cells because the physicians thought the cells would be rejected anyway, and they didn't want to alarm the subjects.

"non-clinical" can be used interchangeably, but in this book, we use the term pre-clinical.

The purpose of pre-clinical studies is to provide information on safety and, if possible, efficacy in order to begin conducting clinical studies in humans. The information gathered from pre-clinical studies provides the pharmaceutical company, the FDA and the IRB with enough evidence to make reasonable decisions about exposing humans to the compound. The information from pre-clinical studies includes: data on acute toxicity; the kinetics and metabolism of the drug; and organ sensitivity. But most importantly, these studies determine a starting dose with an acceptable margin of safety so that there is minimal chance of endangerment to human study subjects.

## Drug Discovery

The discovery of new substances, which subsequently become marketed drugs or biologics, occurs in a number of ways. There is direct research, during which medicinal chemists create compounds with structures likely to evoke the kind of physiological effect they are looking for. Another approach is to change the molecular structure of known compounds in hopes of improving safety or efficacy, while creating a new chemical entity that is sufficiently different from the parent compound to allow for the filing of a new patent.

In addition to classical chemistry, there are many new laboratory tools for developing viable drug substances. Computer technology provides many methods for molecular structuring. There are also computer-readable chemical libraries, which may contain several hundred thousand molecular structures. Many pharmaceutical companies have contracts with firms that provide these libraries; the companies take these chemical structures from the database and perform structure/function/activity computations and computer modeling to look for a hit on a potential compound. Pharmaceutical companies can also perform high throughput screening and other computer-related inquiries to look for hits. Other methods include gene sequencing, gene vector delivery and recombinant DNA.

Naturally occurring compounds are another source of potential pharmaceuticals. A number of drugs originated from soil samples (antibiotics), plants (digitalis) and other natural materials such as coral (prostaglandins).

Serendipity plays a role in any research program. Some very exciting compounds have been discovered by accident. Many drugs are marketed for an indication that was discovered by accident during studies for the primary indication. One example is Rogaine®. This compound, minoxidil, was originally developed as an antihypertensive (Loniten®). Its hair-growing capability wasn't known until subjects enrolled in the hypertension studies began exhibiting accelerated hair growth—in all the wrong places. Women weren't thrilled with their new mustaches and bushy eyebrows that grew together in the middle. Based on this unwanted side effect, the company eventually developed a topical formulation of minoxidil as a hair growth product.

## Pre-clinical Studies of Product Candidates

Once a compound appears to be a viable product candidate, it must be determined if the compound is reasonably safe for initial testing in humans and exhibits pharmacological activity that might justify developing it commercially. This pre-clinical work will focus on collecting data and information to establish that humans will not be exposed to unreasonable risks in early phase clinical studies. This evidence will be presented to the FDA in an IND application.

The first step is to determine the basic physical, chemical and biological characteristics of a new compound:

- Preliminary analytical methods and release criteria must be defined prior to beginning toxicology studies. Methodology and release criteria will change and become better defined as more work is completed and additional information becomes available.
- Data must be developed that will provide evidence of the stability of the compound for the duration of the toxicology studies and the clinical trials.
- A formulation of the compound for use in animals and humans must be developed.
- Bioavailability studies must be done to demonstrate equivalence each time the formulation is changed.
- For biologics (monoclonal antibodies, vaccines, etc.), steps such as the identification of adventitious agents and the characterization of cell lines must be completed. (Adventitious agents are impurities or contaminates; for example, all vaccines that are bovine-based must now be checked for "mad cow disease.")

The outcomes for these parameters change as the pre-clinical studies progress. They may even change as phase I and phase II studies in humans are carried out. This ongoing process will result in a final formulation by the time phase III studies begin.

There will be a final collection of analytical methods, release criteria and formulation prior to beginning phase III studies, and all excipients must be identified both quantitatively and qualitatively. (An excipient is an inert substance that forms part of the vehicle for delivering a drug, e.g., gum arabic or starch.)

Once a compound is characterized and satisfactory stability data are in hand, pre-clinical studies can be initiated. The type of studies and their design will vary depending on the intended use of the drug or biologic being developed. The purpose of pre-clinical studies is to characterize the toxic effects of the compound with respect to target organs dose dependence and relationship to exposure. The studies must normally be conducted using two routes of administration: the route intended for human administration—oral, nasal, topical, etc.—and intravenous (IV). If only the IV route will be used in humans, then no other route needs to be studied in pre-clinical investigations.

These pre-clinical studies will establish a number of different things, including:

- The highest dose of the compound that can be tolerated, as well as a low dose that evokes no overt toxicity, in order to determine initial dosing in humans and to characterize potential organ-specific adverse events.
- Proposed dosing, route of administration and duration of treatment for phase I studies.
- Whether the observed adverse effects are reversible.

The recommended pre-clinical safety studies necessary to obtain marketing approval for a pharmaceutical include: genotoxicity studies, single and multiple (repeated) dose toxicology studies, local tolerance studies, and teratology or reproductive studies.

Other pre-clinical studies that must be completed are pharmacology studies for safety and pharmacokinetic studies that identify absorption, distribution, metabolism and excretion of the compound (ADME studies).

Following are brief descriptions of the different types of pre-clinical studies that are required to support clinical trials for a pharmaceutical product.

### Single Dose Toxicity Studies

Often referred to as acute toxicity studies, single dose toxicity studies should be done in at least two non-human mammalian species. An acceptable alternative is dose escalation studies. Acute toxicology studies examine the toxicity produced by one or more doses of the compound during a period of 24 hours or less, followed by a 14-day non-treatment observation period. The observation period is used to look for delayed toxicity and recovery from overt toxicity. Information from these studies is useful in choosing the doses for repeated dose studies.

### Repeated Dose Studies

Sometimes referred to as sub-chronic and chronic toxicology studies, repeated dose studies should be conducted for a period of time consistent with the therapeutic indication and the length of the proposed clinical program. In general, the duration of these studies, which must be conducted in two non-human mammalian species (one rodent and one non-rodent species), should equal or exceed the length of the clinical trials. The longest chronic toxicity study duration is nine to twelve months.

### Safety Pharmacology Studies

These studies assess the effect of the drug on vital functions, such as respiratory, central nervous and cardiovascular systems in animals. Safety pharmacology studies may be conducted separately or with toxicology studies. In general, these studies look at what the drug does to the body at pharmacological (intended) doses and should be completed prior to human exposure in phase I.

### Pharmacokinetic Studies

Pharmacokinetic studies (PK studies) look at what the body does to the drug in animals. They are also known as ADME studies because they answer questions related to the absorption, distribution, metabolism and excretion of the test substance. Note that the pharmacokinetic (PK) studies in animals are the counterpart to phase I clinical trials in humans.

### Genotoxicity Studies

Genotoxicity studies are done to determine if mutations or chromosomal damage occur when exposed to the drug. These *in vitro* tests (*in vitro* means "in glass," as opposed to *in vivo*, which means in living organisms) must be completed prior to human exposure. Positive findings dictate additional testing and may be an indication for carcinogenicity testing.

### Carcinogenicity Studies

These studies in animals are required for compounds that are expected to be used continuously for six months or longer or intermittently for periods that, when combined, equal six or more months of continuous use. These studies do not need to be done in advance of clinical trials unless there is cause for concern. Carcinogenicity studies are generally not required for drugs intended to treat subjects with life expectancy of less than two to three years (e.g., anti-cancer drugs) or if treatment is for short duration (e.g., anesthetics). These studies are typically performed in rats and mice and involve daily dosing of the animals for two consecutive years (approximately 90% of the rodent's life span) to determine if the drugs, when used for a lifetime, elicit cancer in the animals.

### Reproductive Toxicity Studies

Reproductive toxicology studies involve the administration of multiple doses of the drug before, during and after the gestational period in animals to assess the drug's effect on fertility, reproduction and fetal toxicity. There are three segments in this testing.

- Segment I is the general study of fertility and reproductive performance in one non-human species, usually the rat.
- Segment II evaluates the effect on the fetus (teratology) and is done in two non-human species, usually the rat and rabbit.
- Segment III is the peri- and postnatal portion assessing the effect on the unborn or litters. This testing is also done in two non-human species.

Male fertility studies in animals should be done prior to initiation of phase III trials. Women who are unable to bear children (permanently sterilized or postmenopausal) may be enrolled in clinical trials without any

both. Their purpose is to determine whether or not the investigational drug demonstrates efficacy for the proposed indication within the safe dose range established in phase I. Short-term adverse effects and risks are also assessed. While the focus of phase II studies is primarily efficacy, they also assess safety. Dose range finding, e.g., establishing a minimum and maximum effective dose, and pharmacokinetic (PK) data correlating blood levels of the investigational drug with pharmacological effect (also known as the pharmacokinetic/pharmacodynamic relationship) are also studied during phase II.

Near the end of phase II, most sponsors will meet with the FDA to review the results obtained to date and present their plans for phase III. This is called the end-of-phase II meeting. The FDA views these meetings as being of considerable assistance to both themselves and the sponsor for planning later studies of the compound. Pursuant to the provisions of PDUFA, agreements reached at these meetings are binding on the FDA and sponsor.

Remember that there are pre-clinical studies that may have been active during phase I, but must be completed before phase II can start. This requirement is shown in Table 2.

---

**Table 2**

Pre-clinical requirements before initiating phase II studies in the U.S.:
- Repeated dose toxicity studies in two species (one non-rodent) for a period of time equivalent to the length of the phase II studies. Six-month rodent and chronic non-rodent studies will support clinical trials of six months' duration in the U.S. Studies of longer treatment duration are supported by nine- to twelve-month long pre-clinical studies.

Source: Safety Studies for the Conduct of Human Clinical Trials for Pharmaceuticals, U.S. Department of Health and Human Services and the FDA (CDER and CBER), July 1997, ICH

---

## Phase III Clinical Trials

Phase III studies are only initiated if the data generated in phase I and II have a satisfactory safety profile and there is sufficient evidence of efficacy. The purpose of phase III studies is to demonstrate the safety and efficacy needed to assess the risk/benefit relationship for the intended use of the investigational drug and to provide adequate data for the product package insert.

Phase III studies are expanded, controlled studies in large patient populations (often thousands of patients) that represent the types of patients the compound is intended to treat after it is marketed. They may extend over several years. The development plan for the compound usually includes many different studies, including more than one multicenter study using the same or similar protocols. Multicenter studies are those for which multiple investigative sites all follow the same protocol, and for which the data are pooled together in one group for analysis.

The FDA requirement for registration of a drug is two "adequate and well-controlled" (primary efficacy) studies. However, under the FDAMA legislation of 1997, the FDA may allow one study instead of two for a product where it is determined (by FDA) that "data from one adequate and well-controlled clinical investigation and confirmatory evidence (obtained prior to or after such investigation) are sufficient to establish effectiveness."[3] The decision to do one, rather than two, adequate and well-controlled studies is not one that a sponsor will make on its own. This decision will be made after consultation with and the support of the FDA.

As is the case for phases I and II, there are a number of pre-clinical studies that must be completed before or during the phase III program. The completion of these studies is required before a sponsor can file the NDA with the FDA (See Table 3). We will discuss the NDA in more detail later in the chapter.

**Table 3**

Pre-clinical requirements for initiation of phase III studies in the U.S.:
- Repeated dose toxicity studies in two species (one non-rodent) for a period of time equivalent to the length of the phase III studies. Six-month rodent and chronic non-rodent studies would support clinical trials exceeding six months.
- Carcinogenicity studies if the duration of treatment of the drug is expected to be six months or longer or if intermittent exposure is equal to six months of continuous exposure, or if there is cause for concern. Carcinogenicity studies are not required if the patients receiving the drug have a life expectancy of less than two years.
- Fertility studies in males.
- Repeated dose toxicology studies that include an evaluation of female reproductive organs must be done if women of non-childbearing potential are used.
- Assessment of female fertility and embryo-fetal development if women of childbearing potential will be included.
- All reproduction toxicity studies and the standard genotoxicity tests should be completed if pregnant women will be included.

Source: Safety Studies for the Conduct of Human Clinical Trials for Pharmaceuticals, U.S. Department of Health and Human Services and the FDA (CDER and CBER), July 1997, ICH

## The NDA (New Drug Application)

The NDA is a formal request to be allowed to market a drug. The sponsor submits the NDA to the FDA at the time that the primary efficacy studies (phase III) are complete. The company is essentially telling the FDA that it has completed the necessary safety and efficacy requirements needed for approval. This signals the end of phase III, although there are likely to be some studies still in progress.

In the NDA, as in the IND, the sponsor is informing the FDA of everything that is known about the drug to date. This includes copies of all protocols and case report forms from studies. (These applications can be enormous.) The regulations for NDAs are found in 21 CFR 314. They delineate the particular information that must be included.

Field-based CRAs are unlikely to be involved in helping put together an NDA submission. However, CRAs who are based in-house may well be involved in helping to assemble the clinical section. Often CRAs are involved in a last-minute push to retrieve and/or clean up data that are needed for the NDA; it seems that there are always some outstanding data that need to be collected and entered into the database very quickly in order to process material for the NDA. CRAs may also be asked to re-verify information from sites when questions arise during the NDA writing process.

Part of the NDA is the proposed package insert that the sponsor would like to use with the drug. This is the information that goes with the drug that tells physicians abut the drug and how it should be used. The package insert negotiations between the sponsor and the FDA can be extensive.

There is an active approval process for an NDA (as opposed to the passive 30-day wait for an IND). The sponsor must receive a formal approval letter from the FDA before marketing of the drug can begin.

## Phase IIIb Clinical Studies

A sponsor will frequently have some studies that are still active at the time they file the NDA for a new compound. There are also studies that may be initiated and conducted while the NDA is pending approval. These studies are known as phase IIIb studies. The purpose of these studies may be to gather additional safety data, or to gather information on additional indications for the drug, or to assess its use in special patient populations such as geriatric patients.

## Phase IV Clinical Studies

Phase IV studies are those done after the approval of the NDA, often to determine additional information about the safety or efficacy profile of the compound. They consist of studies:

- Required as a condition of approval by the FDA
- Long-term safety studies required by the FDA
- Conducted to study the compound in comparison with other marketed products
- Designed to familiarize physicians with the compound

If the sponsor was allowed to file the NDA with one, rather than two, adequate and well-controlled studies, the FDA may require that one or more additional confirmatory studies be completed within a certain time period of the approval. This is a condition of the approval; if it is not met, the approval may be withdrawn.

The FDA may also require that a sponsor do a long-term safety study as a condition of approval. These studies are often referred to as epidemiologic or post-marketing surveillance studies. These may be required because the FDA has seen problems with similar compounds, or because the compound is novel and the FDA thinks additional safety information will be beneficial.

---

**Table 4: Notes on Studies in Women and Children**

The past few years have seen greater emphasis on studying new compounds in women and children. This is due to the fact that these populations were understudied and that many compounds do not work the same in women or children as they do in men. Consequently, the FDA determined that studies should include women and children if the compounds would be used to treat them after marketing. The rationale is that it is preferable to determine the effects of the compound under the controlled conditions in clinical trials as opposed to uncontrolled use of the drug after marketing.

CRAs should know some basic things about the testing of compounds in women of childbearing potential, pregnant women, and children.

Women of childbearing potential are a major concern in clinical trials because of the possibility of unintentional exposure of an embryo/fetus before data are available relative to potential risk. Some teratology work (segments I and II) is usually done before entering women of childbearing potential in a clinical trial, although this is not essential.

In the United States, women of childbearing potential may be included in early studies prior to completion of reproductive toxicology studies, providing that the studies are carefully monitored and all precautions are taken to minimize exposure *in utero*. This generally involves pregnancy testing and establishment of highly effective methods of birth control. Continued monitoring and testing should continue throughout the trial to ensure compliance with all measures intended to prevent pregnancy.

If women of childbearing potential are used in a clinical trial prior to completion of the teratology studies, the informed consent process should clearly indicate the possible risk associated with taking the investigational drug since effects on the embryo/fetus are unknown.

If pregnant women are to be enrolled in clinical trials, all reproductive toxicity studies and genotoxicity tests must be completed. Data from any previous experience in humans will also be needed.

If children are to be included in clinical trials, repeated dose toxicity studies and all reproductive toxicity and genotoxicity studies should have been completed. In addition, safety data from previous studies in human adult populations should be available.

In conclusion, there are many sources of information available to CRAs that will help them ensure compliance when working with investigative sites on clinical trials. CRAs should utilize these resources when doing their job.

## Key Takeaways

- The FDA regulations pertaining to clinical trials are found in 21 CFR Parts 11, 50, 54, 56, 312 and 314.
- The ICH Guidelines for Good Clinical Practice should be followed in clinical trials.
- The FDA publishes many guidelines and information sheets pertaining to the appropriate conduct of clinical trials.
- Good clinical practices are the ethical and clinical standard for designing, conducting, analyzing, monitoring and reporting on clinical trials.
- There are differences between FDA and HHS rules for doing research in human subjects.
- CRAs should read and be familiar with the regulations that pertain to clinical trials and the ICH guidelines.

### References
1. ICH Guideline for Good Clinical Practice as published in the Federal Register May 9, 1997.
2. Information Sheets for IRBs and Investigators, Appendix 11. www.fda.gov/oc/ohrt/irbs.

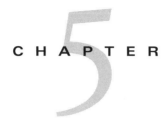

# Institutional Review Boards

When conducting clinical trials, the safety of human subjects comes first. The two main safeguards for human subjects are Institutional Review Boards (IRBs) and the informed consent process. In this chapter, we'll discuss IRBs—what they are, their purpose and how they function.

The regulatory definition of an IRB is: "any board, committee or group formally designated by an institution to review, approve the initiation of and to conduct periodic review of biomedical research involving human subjects. The primary purpose of such review is to assure the protection of the rights and welfare of the human subjects."[1] Notice that an IRB must approve a study before it can start. All research done in humans in the United States must be approved by an IRB. (21 CFR Part 56 contains the regulations that pertain to IRBs.)

Since many companies do research globally, a CRA should be aware that ethical reviews of protocols are conducted outside the United States. The Independent Ethics Committee (IEC) is the body analogous to an IRB in countries outside the United States. The IEC is an independent body, the responsibility of which is to ensure the protection of the rights, safety and well-being of human subjects involved in a trial by reviewing and approving/providing a favorable opinion on the trial protocol and informed consent. Both IRBs and IECs have one fundamental purpose: to protect the rights, safety and welfare of human subjects in research. In general, IECs give a favorable opinion about the research, rather than an actual approval; this difference in wording is the main difference between the two groups. For all practical purposes, the favorable opinion of an IEC carries the same weight and is just as binding as the approval of an IRB; it is especially viewed as such for any studies that will be submitted to the FDA for registration purposes.

Our discussion, however, will focus on IRBs and the U.S. regulations for IRBs and investigators.

An investigator who is planning to conduct a trial must contact an IRB, submit the appropriate materials, including the proposed protocol and consent form, and wait for formal approval from the IRB before he or she may initiate the trial. (Details about this process will appear later in this chapter.) Interacting with and asking an IRB for approval are the responsibilities of the clinical investigator, not the pharmaceutical company that is sponsoring the research. (Note: Occasionally a sponsor may submit documents to the IRB on behalf of investigators.) However, the CRA will verify the investigator's IRB approval for the sponsor.

## Types of IRBs

There are two types of IRBs, those that are affiliated with an institution and those that are not. The unaffiliated IRBs are called independent, central or national IRBs, and can be used by any researcher who is not constrained by institutional policy to the use of a particular institutional review board.

If an investigator is affiliated with an institution (hospital or university, etc.) that has an IRB, and if that investigator is conducting the trial or any part of the trial at the institution, then he or she must usually use the institution's IRB. If the trial is being conducted at the investigator's private practice and is not affiliated in any way with an institution, then he or she is not normally required to use the institution's IRB. However, a few institutions have policies that require any person affiliated with the institution to use the institution's IRB, even for research conducted outside the institution. If an investigator is doing a study at more than one institution (e.g., two hospitals) then IRB approval is required from each institution where the study will be conducted.

Independent IRBs, those not affiliated with a particular institution, are available to any investigator who is not affiliated with an institution, or who will not be conducting clinical trials at an institution, or whose institution does not have its own IRB. Independent IRBs are frequently used for multi-center studies in non-hospitalized patients. Study sponsors prefer to use independent IRBs when possible because, in general, the time they take to review a study (turnaround time) is faster. The IRBs at some teaching hospitals, for example, can take three to six months to review a protocol, while most independent IRBs will have a review time of less than one month.

Sometimes sponsors or investigators may express concerns about having research reviewed by an IRB that is not local and may not be as familiar with the investigative site, the investigator or the community. To counteract these concerns, the better independent IRBs visit investigative sites and have methods of determining community attitudes and other local issues in order to appropriately approve or disapprove research.

# IRB Responsibilities

Whether the IRB is affiliated with a particular institution or not, its primary responsibility is to protect the rights and welfare of human subjects participating in clinical research. To fulfill this responsibility, the IRB must answer two basic questions:

1.  Should the study be done at all? (Do the benefits outweigh the risks?) and if so,
2.  What constitutes adequate informed consent?

### Should the study be done at all?
### (The benefit vs. risk assessments)
In determining whether or not the study should be done, the IRB must consider several items. The IRB members must have assurance that the study is scientifically valid, in other words, that there is a properly designed protocol; however, it is not the responsibility of an IRB to judge the scientific merit or worth of the trial. For example, it is not the function of an IRB to decide whether we need another drug for hypertension, but rather to determine if the research methods being used to study that potential antihypertensive are valid.

Risks to the subjects must be minimized, so the IRB will look for a sound research design that does not expose human subjects to unnecessary risk. They will also ascertain if the protocol uses procedures that would be performed on these patients, both diagnostically and treatment-wise, even if they were not in the study, when appropriate.

The IRB must determine whether the anticipated benefit to subjects and the overall knowledge to be gained from the research compares favorably to the risks. In this evaluation, the IRB considers only those risks and benefits that may result directly from the research, excluding the risks and benefits that the subjects would have encountered even if they had not been involved in the research (just in the standard treatment for the condition). Remember that there are always risks involved in doing research.

The IRB will also want to know what the subject selection process is, in order to ensure that the selection is equitable, and that no groups of potential subjects are routinely excluded or included based on non-study related characteristics. Depending on the particular study, some of these characteristics might include sex, race, ethnic background, weight, smoking, educational background, etc. In making this assessment, the IRB will consider the particular setting in which the research will be conducted, as well as the purposes of the research.

## What constitutes adequate informed consent?

If the IRB determines that the answer to the first question (Do the benefits outweigh the risks?) is yes, then they will consider the consent form submitted by the investigator. It is a regulatory requirement that informed consent is sought from each subject, or the subject's legally authorized representative, before that person may be enrolled in the research project. By regulation,[2] informed consent must be documented, which is usually done by having the subject sign a written copy of the consent document. Consents are discussed in detail in the next chapter.

Along with the written consent, there must be provisions in the research plan for ongoing safety monitoring of the data, with the goal of ensuring the safety of the subjects during the research. It's not sufficient, for example, to have all the adverse event data reviewed only at the completion of a trial—data must be regularly reviewed throughout the study period, in case problems arise as more is learned about the drug, device or procedure under investigation.

The IRB will also determine whether or not there are adequate provisions in the research to protect the privacy of the research subjects, as well as to maintain the confidentiality of the data, where appropriate.

Payments to study patients and advertising are considered by the FDA and IRBs as part of the consent process, as they both might encourage a subject to enroll in a trial. If subjects are to be paid for their participation in the research, the IRB will review the planned compensation to ensure that it does not constitute an undue influence, or coercion, that could influence the subject's decision to participate. Ideally, subjects would not take the risks involved in study participation simply because of the compensation. The IRB's decision will be based not only on the amount subjects may receive for being in the study, but the setting in which the study will take place. An amount that may be coercive in one setting may not be so in another.

The IRB will also review any proposed advertising to ensure it does not make misleading or untruthful claims and does not constitute undue influence. Glowing claims of success for a new treatment, for example, can also influence subjects to participate in a trial that they would not want to be involved with otherwise. (See Chapter 12 for more on advertising.)

## Vulnerable subjects

Sometimes special, vulnerable populations are studied in research trials. Vulnerable subjects include children, pregnant women, prisoners, handicapped or mentally disabled people, people with acute or severe mental illness and people who are economically or educationally disadvantaged. If any of these categories of people are going to be included in the research, the IRB needs to determine whether or not there are sufficient additional safeguards to protect them from coercion or undue influence. There are a number of National Institutes of Health (NIH) regulations (45 CFR 46) regarding research in various vulnerable populations. IRB members, investigators and others involved in these types of research, including CRAs, should familiarize themselves with this information.

## State and local regulations

The IRB must determine that the research does not violate any existing state or local laws or regulations, or any applicable institutional policies or practices. Some states, for example, California and Massachusetts, have regulations that may exceed the federal regulations. People working in these states, and others, should be familiar with their state requirements for doing research. As an example, California requires that a patient bill of rights be provided to every study subject in a trial. For an example of a subject's bill of rights based on California's patient bill of rights, see Table 1.

---

**Table 1: Example of a California Patient's Bill of Rights for Study Subjects**

Any person who is requested to consent to participate as a subject in a research study involving a medical experiment, or who is requested to consent on behalf of another, has the right to:

- Be informed of the nature and purpose of the experiment.
- Be given an explanation of the procedures to be followed in the medical experiment, and any drug or device to be used.
- Be given a description of any attendant discomforts and risks reasonably to be expected from the experiment, if applicable.
- Be given an explanation of any benefits to the subject reasonably to be expected from the experiment, if applicable.
- Be given a disclosure of any appropriate alternative procedures, drugs, or devices that might be advantageous to the subject, and their relative risks and benefits.
- Be informed of the avenues of medical treatment, if any, available to the subject after the experiment or if complications should arise.
- Be given an opportunity to ask any questions concerning the experiment or other procedures involved.
- Be instructed that consent to participate in the medical experiment may be withdrawn at any time, and the subject may discontinue in the medical experiment without prejudice.
- Be given a copy of a signed and dated written informed consent form when one is required.
- Be given the opportunity to decide to consent or not to consent to a medical experiment without the intervention of any element of force, fraud, deceit, duress, coercion, or undue influence on the subject's decision.

---

# IRB Review of Proposed Research

An IRB considers each research project submitted for review separately. In order to determine if the research meets all the criteria discussed above, the IRB will review:

- Investigator qualifications
- Study protocol and supporting documents
- Proposed consent form
- Subject compensation, if applicable
- Advertising, if applicable

## Materials submitted to the IRB by an investigator

To ensure an adequate review, the investigator submits a number of materials to the IRB for review, including the following:

- A current curriculum vitae (CV) that includes his or her qualifications for conducting the research, including education, training and experience
- The study protocol, which includes or addresses the following items, as applicable:
    - Title of the study
    - Purpose of the study, including any expected benefits
    - Sponsor of the study
    - Results from previous related research
    - Subject inclusion/exclusion criteria
    - Study design, including a discussion of the appropriateness of the research methods
    - Description and schedule of the procedures to be performed
    - Provisions for managing adverse events
    - Payment to subjects for their participation
    - Compensation for injuries to research subjects
    - Provisions for protecting subject privacy
    - Extra costs to subjects for participation in the study, if applicable
    - Extra costs to third party payers because of a subject's participation, if applicable
- The investigator brochure or package insert, if applicable
- The proposed informed consent document, containing all appropriate elements
- All subject advertisements and recruitment procedures. In general, advertising includes anything that is directed toward potential research subjects and is designed for recruitment.
- Statement of Investigator (1572) form, if applicable. This form is required for all FDA-regulated studies conducted under an Investigational New Drug Application (IND). (Some IRBs do not require this, but many do.)

- Grant application for federally funded research, if applicable
- Any other specific forms or materials required by the IRB, such as an application form

### IRB deliberations

After documents are received from an investigator, an IRB will schedule the protocol for review. For the initial review of a protocol, the committee will meet to decide whether or not to approve the proposed research. In order to make this decision, the group will review all the submitted materials and discuss the proposed research, followed by a vote. The IRB may approve the project or request changes or additional information in order to approve it or disapprove it. Please note that an investigator can sit on an IRB, but he or she cannot participate in the discussion leading to the vote or voting for his or her own research, as this would constitute a conflict of interest.

The IRB must notify the investigator in writing that the study is approved. If a study is disapproved, the IRB will also notify the investigator in writing of its action and must allow the investigator to address the IRB concerning the decision either in writing or in person.

Any planned advertising must be approved before use, although this does not have to be approved before the study begins. Advertising is often started after study initiation, especially when subject recruitment has not been as rapid as anticipated.

Most importantly, IRB approval of the study and the consent form must be obtained prior to patient enrollment.

### Investigator reporting responsibilities

Throughout the study, the investigator must report any protocol changes or amendments to the IRB. Any change that would increase risk to subjects must be approved by the IRB prior to implementation. The only exception to this is when the change is necessary to eliminate an apparent immediate hazard to the safety and well-being of the subjects, in which case the change should be implemented immediately, followed by a timely notification and submission to the IRB. For example, if it is determined during a trial that taking a particular concomitant medication is unsafe, investigative sites would be notified by the sponsor to immediately stop giving that particular medication to study patients. Sites would start doing this immediately, then notify their IRBs. These exceptions are quite rare.

The investigator must also promptly report "immediately reportable" adverse events to the IRB. These usually include deaths and other serious adverse events that are unexpected during the study. Occasionally deaths may be the expected outcome in a study; in this case, the reporting rules may change, and deaths will not be reported as immediately reportable adverse events. This exception is also quite rare. (Adverse event reporting is discussed in detail in Chapter 11.)

The investigator must promptly report to the IRB any unanticipated problems that arise during the research that involve risk to the study subjects or others.

The investigator is required to submit periodic reports to the IRB, detailing the progress of the study. This will be submitted at least annually and may be required on a more frequent basis.

## Continuing review of a research study

The IRB will review each research project at least annually, although the IRB may require updates on a more frequent basis, such as quarterly, based on the degree of risk to which the subjects are exposed. At the continuing review, the IRB will ensure that the risk-to-benefit relationship remains acceptable, that the consent and study documents being used are still appropriate and that the selection of subjects has been equitable.

To help in making these determinations, most IRBs will require the investigator to submit an IRB-specific form asking about the progress of the study, including enrollment figures, withdrawals, adverse events and unanticipated problems, protocol violations, etc., at each review period. The IRB will also want to see a copy of the currently used consent form, advertising and any other appropriate documents. The IRB will ask for any protocol amendments during the time period, especially if they were not previously reviewed by the IRB. This information allows the IRB to determine whether or not the research can continue.

All research must be re-approved at least annually. The investigator will receive written notification of each formal re-approval. Re-review and re-approval continue throughout the entire research project, until such time as all subjects have completed their participation and the project is closed.

If an investigator is not submitting the required study updates to the IRB for review, the IRB has several options. The IRB may send the investigator a reminder that he/she is required to submit the update, with a deadline for receipt of the requested materials. If the reminder does not work, the IRB may put enrollment on hold until the updates are received and reviewed. In the worst case, the IRB may withdraw approval of the study. It is important to remember that each approval is good only for a specified time period. If re-approval is not received prior to the expiration date of the previous approval, the study is out of compliance with the regulations.

## Expedited review

Upon occasion, an IRB may utilize an expedited review process for minor changes in previously approved research; this may be done only during the time period for which the approval was authorized. Expedited review may be done by the IRB Chairperson, or by experienced members who are designated as expedited reviewers. Items may be approved by expedited review, but they can not be disapproved. If the expedited reviewer(s) thinks something should be disapproved, it must go to the full board. The Board must also be made aware of all expedited review decisions, which is usually done at the first regular meeting following the review.

Expedited review is never used in circumstances where the risk to human subjects increases. It cannot, in general, be used for the initial review of a research study. There are a few exceptions where initial review of a project can be done using expedited review, but these are not the kinds of studies in which CRAs would normally be involved; these exceptions are published in the Federal Register. If you are interested in reading more about this, there is a guidance document called Categories of Research That May Be Reviewed by the Institutional Review Board (IRB) through an Expedited Review Procedure.

## IRB Membership

An IRB must have at least five members. IRB membership should be selected to assure appropriate diversity, including representation by multiple professions, multiple ethnic backgrounds and both genders, and must include both scientific and non-scientific members. The members must possess appropriate professional competence to review the diverse types of protocols that are received. Most IRBs also have alternate members so that they will have a quorum if a regular member is unable to be present.

There must be at least one member who is not affiliated with the institution (and who has no immediate family member affiliated with the institution) other than his/her IRB membership. There must also be one member whose interests and background are non-scientific (layperson). It is acceptable for one IRB member to fulfill both of these criteria. In addition, an IRB that reviews FDA-regulated products (drugs, biologics and devices) will have at least one member who is a physician.

## IRB Operations

IRBs are required by regulation to follow written procedures. IRBs are audited by regulatory authorities, and they will be held responsible for having appropriate written procedures and for following them. They must also carefully document their decisions and retain this documentation appropriately.

# Conflict of Interest

No IRB member may participate in the initial or continuing review of any project where they have a conflicting interest in the research. A person whose research is being reviewed may be present at the IRB meeting to answer questions and give information about the project, but they should not be present for the discussion leading to the vote, and during the actual voting. The minutes of the meeting need to reflect that the person was not present, to alleviate any claim of conflict of interest.

# Key Takeaways

- IRBs are one of the primary safeguards for the protection of human subjects of research.
- CFR Part 56 contains the regulations that pertain to IRBs.
- An IRB must approve a study and the informed consent document before the study can start.
- There are two types of IRBs, those that are affiliated with an institution and those that are independent, i.e., not affiliated with an institution.
- The IRB must make a risk versus benefit assessment for each proposed project.
- There are special regulations concerning research in vulnerable subjects (children, pregnant women, prisoners, etc.).
- State and local research regulations must be followed.
- IRBs must approve advertising and subject compensation.
- An investigator must report adverse events and study progress to the IRB at least annually.
- Continuing review of a study must be done at least annually.
- Expedited review may not be used for the initial review of a project, except in particular instances published in the Federal Register.
- IRB members may not vote if they have a conflict of interest.

**References**
1. 21 CFR 56.102(g).
2. 21 CFR 50.27.

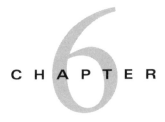

C H A P T E R

# Informed Consent

One of the main safeguards for the protection of human subjects in research is informed consent. In this chapter, we will discuss informed consents, including the regulations governing consent, the writing of consents, and the administration of consents.

The decision of whether or not to participate in a study is not an easy one. There is the hope of help and the desire to please the physician, as well as apprehension and fear of the unknown. To help a potential subject make a decision that is not based purely on emotions such as fear and hope, everything possible must be done to provide complete information in a format that is accessible and easy-to-read, along with sufficient time to make an informed decision.

Informed Consent is defined by the ICH Guidelines for Good Clinical Practice as:

> "A process by which a subject voluntarily confirms his or her willingness to participate in a particular trial, after having been informed of all aspects of the trial that are relevant to the subject's decision to participate. Informed consent is documented by means of a written, signed and dated informed consent form."[1]

The two key words in this definition are "voluntarily" and "informed." These words form the cornerstone of ethical conduct in clinical research and are in place to protect the rights and safety of the subjects who participate in research. Potential subjects of clinical research must understand what they are getting into and must be free to decline to participate.

The freedom to say "no" with a clear conscience and no fear of repercussion is an aspect of the consent process that must be considered. Many people have a certain reverence for their personal physicians; they want to please their physicians and will do as they direct. This carries over into the informed consent process and needs to be understood by physicians involved in research. CRAs should advise investigators to be conscious of this phenomenon. Investigators must make every effort to help potential study subjects understand that it is entirely acceptable if they choose not to participate.

# Monitoring Informed Consent

Informed consent should be one of the primary areas of concentration during a CRA's monitoring visits, both because it is so important ethically and because it is a frequent deficiency found during clinical investigator inspections conducted by the FDA. The problem is not that the consent process is not being done, but it is not being done correctly. Common problems are:

- The timing of the administration of consent may not be correct, meaning that the consent is not always obtained before any study-related procedures take place.
- Proper signatures are not always obtained.
- The consent form is poorly written.
- There are missing required elements.
- Amended informed consent is not signed.

The first step in monitoring informed consent is to be familiar with the requirements, both for the document itself and the process. There are three basic requirements that a consent form must meet:

- It must completely and accurately describe all of the activities required by the protocol and what the subject's participation will involve.
- It must be able to be read and understood by the study subjects.
- It must contain all the elements required by regulation (21 CFR Part 50, see Appendix G).

In other words, consents must inform, be comprehensible and comply with regulations. Let's look more closely at each of these requirements.

### Activities and participation

Potential study subjects need to be told about the study and their involvement in detail to be able to make an informed decision regarding their participation. Subjects need to know they will be participating in research, what is required of them and the potential benefits and risks they will face. The required elements of consent will be discussed later in this chapter. All the requirements (tests, procedures, activities, etc.) of the protocol must be described, including a description of how these various activities will have an impact on the subjects, both in terms of personal discomfort and any lifestyle changes. Subjects also need to know when each activity must be done and how long it will take for each activity and study visit.

### Readability and comprehension

It is difficult to adequately inform potential subjects about a study without overwhelming them. A consent form may contain a very detailed description of protocol activities and consequences, but if it is a long, multiple-page document, a subject may not have a good feel for what will happen because the document is just too long and simply presents too much information to comprehend. Writing a consent that properly informs without overwhelming is mostly the result of common sense and experience. It is important to keep this balance in mind if you are writing or reviewing a consent form.

Writing a comprehensible consent is as difficult as making it informative without being overwhelming. The consent form needs to be technically correct, yet intelligible for non-medical people. Consent forms should be written at approximately the sixth- to eighth-grade levels. This is a challenge in an industry filled with jargon, acronyms, medical terminology and highly educated people.

In general, the shorter the sentences and the fewer syllables per word that there are in the text, the easier it will be to understand. Make a conscious effort to use terminology such as "teaspoons" instead of "cubic centimeters" or "milliliters," or "high blood pressure" instead of "hypertension." There is no substitute for experience; after you have written a few consent forms, it becomes easier. There are formulas that will give you a good estimate of the grade level of your document; for example, Microsoft Word includes the Flesch-Kincaid Grade Level tester, which pops up after spelling and grammar checks have been done on a document.

### Elements

The last of the three requirements for a proper consent form is to make it compliant with federal regulations. 21 CFR part 50.25, which contains the elements of informed consent, is one of the more straightforward regulations. It clearly lists the elements that must be present in a consent form (basic elements) and those that are optional (additional elements).


# Basic Elements of Consent[2]

The basic elements of consent, taken from the federal regulations, must be present in all consent forms. They are:

- A statement that the study involves research, the purpose of the research, duration of the subject's participation, a description of procedures to be followed and identification of any procedures that are experimental.
- A description of any reasonably foreseeable risks or discomfort to the subjects.
- A description of any benefits to the subjects or others, which reasonably can be expected from the research.
- A disclosure of appropriate alternate procedures or courses of treatment, if any, that might be advantageous to the subject.
- A statement describing the extent, if any, to which confidentiality of records identifying the subject will be maintained and that notes the possibility that the FDA and study sponsor may inspect the records.
- For research involving more than minimal risk, an explanation as to whether any compensation and an explanation as to whether any medical treatments are available if injury occurs and, if so, what they consist of, or where further information may be obtained.
- An explanation of whom to contact for answers to pertinent questions about the research and research subject's rights and whom to contact in the event of a research-related injury to the subject.
- A statement that participation is voluntary and that refusal to participate will involve no penalty or loss of benefits to which the subject is otherwise entitled, and that the subject may discontinue participation at any time without penalty or loss of benefits to which the subject is otherwise entitled.

## Additional Elements of Consent

The additional elements of consent,[3] which should be included as appropriate, are:

- A statement that the particular treatment or procedure may involve risk to the subject (or to the embryo or fetus, if the subject is or may become pregnant) that is currently unforeseeable.
- Anticipated circumstances under which the subject's participation may be terminated by the investigator without regard to the subject's consent.
- Any additional costs to the subject that may result from participation in the research.
- The consequences of the subject's decision to withdraw from the research and procedures for orderly termination of participation of the subject.
- A statement that significant new findings developed during the course of the research that may relate to the subject's willingness to continue participation will be provided to the study subject.
- The approximate number of subjects involved in the study.

Since ICH guidelines mandate the inclusion of these additional elements, they usually appear in most informed consent forms, if appropriate.

One way of ensuring that all the elements are present in a consent form is to have an explicit heading for subsections that address each element. In any case, it must be clear that each of the elements is addressed in the form so that subjects are properly informed and so that the form will not be found deficient in a regulatory review.

Some states and institutions also have requirements that may have an impact on the content of the form. California, for example, requires that a Patient Bill of Rights be attached to all consent forms. (See Chapter 4)

In addition, the final Health Insurance Portability and Accountability Act (HIPAA) rule was published on August 14, 2002, which allows the authorization form for all uses and disclosures of a patient's protected health information to be combined with the informed consent form. This authorization form can also be signed separately. The choice is up to the individual investigative site. The compliance date for HIPAA is April 14, 2003, which means that a site that begins recruiting for a study before that date and continues to recruit for that same study after that date could potentially use two different informed consent forms for the same study. For more on HIPAA, see Chapter 10.

# Obtaining Informed Consent

Informed consent must be obtained from subjects at the proper time and in the proper manner. The first thing to remember is that no person may be involved as a research subject unless the person, or the person's legally acceptable representative (LAR), has given consent. According to "Guidance to Industry, E-6 GCPs" produced by HHS and FDA (See Appendix F), an LAR is an individual or juridical or other body authorized under applicable law to consent, on behalf of a prospective subject, to the subject's participation in the clinical trial. Secondly, a subject's consent must be obtained before the subject is involved in any study-related activity. A CRA should always check consents and when they were signed during the study enrollment period. The time of consent versus when the subject started the study is almost always checked during FDA inspections of investigative sites.

There are two types of consent forms, the short form and the long form. Both must be approved by an IRB before use.

### The Short Form Consent[4]
The short form consent may be used in circumstances when, in the best judgment of the investigator, it would be the most appropriate way for the subject to comprehend and give informed consent. This form supplements

and documents an oral presentation of the information provided to the study subject as part of the consent process. If this method is used:

- The form must state that all elements of consent required by regulation have been presented orally to the subject or subject's legally appointed representative.
- There must be a witness to the oral presentation.
- The IRB must approve a written summary of what is to be said to the subject or their representative.
- Only the short form itself is to be signed by the subject or their representative.
- The witness will sign both the short form and a copy of the written summary.
- The person obtaining the consent will sign a written copy of the summary.
- A copy of the short form and the summary will be given to the subject or their representative.

### The Long Form Consent

This is the standard consent form and process and is the consent method of choice whenever possible. The main difference between the two forms is that the long form spells out in writing everything that is presented orally when the short form is used. Consequently, no summary is needed. The subject signs and dates two copies, one to keep and one for the investigator.

## The Consent Process

As a CRA you will not be involved in the actual consent process. However, since it is a CRA's responsibility to ensure that investigative sites conduct their studies in accordance with GCPs, the CRA should be able to advise investigators and their staffs on consent activities. Here are some suggestions that can be discussed with investigators and study coordinators regarding the informed consent process; these may be particularly helpful for those at the site who are inexperienced with the consent process:

- Have someone read the consent form while the subject follows along. This usually improves comprehension and is helpful for subjects who may not read well.
- Have the presenter summarize what was read, emphasizing the important points of the consent and the procedures the subject will need to perform.
- Always ask the subject if there are any questions. Answer them completely and truthfully.
- Never try to convince a subject to participate.

- Ask the subject some questions about the consent material to determine how well the subject understood what was presented. This will often generate additional questions from the subject.

- A video presentation of the consent form can be an effective tool. If the investigative site has a person who is a particularly good presenter, this person could describe the study in the video. Camcorders are relatively inexpensive and can produce good quality recordings. In addition to ensuring that all subjects hear the same thing, the video documents what was said. Videos, however, should never be used in lieu of the involvement of the investigator, who should always be present to talk with subjects and to answer questions.

- The consent process should not be rushed. Subjects must be given ample time to assess, evaluate and discuss the information they have been given before having to make a decision. A subject may want to take the form home to discuss with family members before making a decision and should be encouraged to do so.

- The physician should have a written progress note detailing: the consent was given; no study-related procedures were done prior to signing informed consent; and a copy of the informed consent document was given to the subject, signed and dated.

## Exceptions from Consent

There are two situations in which exceptions to consent may be made for patients using investigational products. The first is for research involving the individual emergency use of a test article in a single individual, as provided for in 21 CFR 50.23. The second involves entire studies in which, because of the expected circumstances, it is not generally feasible to obtain consent before patients must be treated (21 CFR 50.24). Both of these situations are discussed below.

### Individual Exceptions[5]
Occasionally, a circumstance will arise where an investigator feels there is a subject who would benefit from the use of an investigational product, but who is not in a study or who would not qualify for the study. For example, there may be a patient who is near death from a severe infection, where all suitable marketed antibiotics have been tried, but the infective bacteria are resistant to all these drugs. The patient does not qualify for any ongoing study. Under this exemption this patient may be treated with one of the new, powerful antibiotics that might cure his infection. Although a physician may treat a patient with an investigational product in a case like this, he must follow the regulations discussed below.

According to the regulations, obtaining informed consent is feasible unless, before use of the investigational product, both the investigator and a physician who is not otherwise participating in the clinical investigation certify in writing all of the following:

- The human subject is confronted by a life-threatening situation necessitating the use of the test article.
- Informed consent cannot be obtained from the subject because of an inability to communicate with, or obtain legally effective consent from, the subject.
- Time is not sufficient to obtain consent from the subject's legal representative.
- There is available no alternative method of approved or generally recognized therapy that provides an equal or greater likelihood of saving the life of the subject.

The exception to this is if immediate use of the test article is, in the investigator's opinion, required to preserve the life of the subject, and time is not sufficient to obtain the independent determination in advance of using the test article. In this case, the determination of the clinical investigator shall be made and, within five working days after the use of the article, be reviewed and evaluated in writing by a physician who is not participating in the clinical investigation.

The documentation required must be submitted to the investigator's IRB within five working days after the use of the test article. If the investigator wants to be able to use the product for this type of patient more than just the one time, the necessary documentation must be submitted to the IRB and approved as for any study.

## Exception from Informed Consent Requirements for Emergency Research Studies[6]

In some types of studies, obtaining informed consent from study subjects prior to their participation may not be possible. Examples of these studies are those in which the subject is in a life-threatening, trauma situation, such as head injuries or heart attacks. Not only are the subjects in these studies not able to give consent prior to being treated, but there may not be time to identify and locate a subject's legally authorized representative before treatment must begin. Frequently, these studies have a relatively short window of opportunity for treatment; e.g., treatment must commence within two hours of the injury.

Exceptions or waivers from consent must be approved in advance of the study by the IRB. It is not the investigator or the sponsor who makes the determination of whether or not the exception is allowed. It must be approved by an IRB, with the concurrence of a licensed physician (who may or may not be a member of the IRB) who is not associated with the research project. In order for the IRB to make this determination, the following must be documented:

- The subject is in a life-threatening situation, available treatments are unproven or unsatisfactory, and the collection of valid scientific evidence is necessary to determine the safety and effectiveness of the particular intervention.
- Obtaining informed consent is not feasible because:
    - The subject will not be able to give consent because of their medical condition.
    - The intervention under investigation must be administered before consent can be obtained from the subject's legally authorized representative.
    - There is no way to identify prospectively the individuals likely to become eligible for participation in the study.
- Participation in the research may have direct benefit to the subject because:
    - The subject is in a life-threatening situation that necessitates intervention.
    - Previous research, both pre-clinical and/or clinical, provides supporting evidence of the potential for the intervention to provide a direct benefit to the subject.
    - Risks associated with the intervention are reasonable in relation to what is known about the medical condition of the potential class of subjects, the risks and benefits of standard therapy, and what is known, if anything, about the risks and benefits of the experimental treatment or intervention.
- The clinical investigation could not practically be carried out without the waiver.
- The protocol defines the length of the therapeutic window based on scientific evidence, and the investigator commits to attempting to contact the subject's legally authorized representative or family member within that window of opportunity and asking for consent, if feasible, rather than proceeding without consent. The investigator will summarize efforts to contact legal representatives and provide this information to the IRB and the time of continuing review.
- The IRB has approved the consent form and process to be used when informing the subject, when possible, or the subject's legally authorized representative or a family member.
- Additional protections of the rights and welfare of the subjects will be provided to include:
    - Consultation with the community in which the study will be conducted and the subjects selected.
    - Public disclosure (in the community in which the study is to be conducted) prior to initiation of the study of plans for the study and the risks and benefits associated with it.
    - Public disclosure following completion of the study of sufficient information to appraise researchers and the community of the study including demographics of the study population and its results.

– Establishment of an independent data monitoring committee to exercise oversight of the investigation.

The IRB also has a responsibility to see that the study subject is informed about the nature of the study and his or her involvement in it as soon as that can be done. If the subject remains incapacitated, then the legally authorized representative or, if not available, a family member, must be updated. The legally authorized representative (or family member) should also be told that they may request that the subject be removed from the study at any time without penalty or loss of benefit.

## Conclusion

A primary safeguard for the rights, safety and well-being of human subjects of research is informed consent. The informed consent process is a complex and important part of conducting clinical research. CRAs must have a working knowledge of consent forms and processes so that deficiencies can be recognized and corrected immediately. It is recommended that CRAs read the regulations governing informed consent (CFR 21 part 50). A checklist for reviewing informed consents is found in Appendix C.

## Key Takeaways

- Informed consent is a cornerstone of the ethical conduct of clinical research.
- Informed consent documents must be approved by the IRB before use.
- Informed consent must be obtained before a subject enters a study.
- Informed consent must be documented.
- Proper preparation of forms and conduct of the procedure is vital to ensure truly informed consent.
- Informed consent is usually required for all subjects involved in a research project.
- There are exceptions to the consent process under certain circumstances.

### References
1. ICH Guideline for Good Clinical Practice, as published in the Federal Register May 9, 1997. Part I. Glossary.
2. 21 CFR 50.25.
3. 21 CFR 50.25.
4. 21 CFR 50.27.
5. 21 CFR 50.23.
6. 21 CFR 50.24.

7

# Preparing for a Study

In this chapter we will discuss some of the primary activities that must be done before starting a study. These activities are: determining the study design, writing the protocol and developing case report forms. Since working with studies, protocols and case report forms are critical parts of a CRA's job, the CRA must have a good understanding of each of them even if he or she is not involved in determining study designs, writing protocols or developing case report forms. We will begin by discussing some aspects of design, followed by protocols and then case report forms, since this is the usual pattern of their development in a research program.

This chapter is designed to give you basic information. Much of the material that follows is in the form of an annotated outline that gives you the basic considerations for these documents.

## Study Design

CRAs should have a basic understanding of the critical aspects of study design. In this section, we will look at some of the terminology that CRAs should be familiar with, as well as a few of the more common study designs. In general, the statistician, in consultation with the medical monitor for a study, will determine which design is appropriate to use. We will also discuss sample size, the controls used in studies and methods for minimizing bias.

# Determining sample size

There are a number of factors that must be taken into account when determining how many subjects should be entered into a trial. The first of these is the sample size. The sample size for a trial is usually computed by the statistician and is based on three variables:

1. The magnitude of the effect expected between the treatments
2. The variability of the endpoints to be analyzed
3. The desired probability of observing the effect with a defined significance. (This is known as the power of the test, and is commonly set at at least 80%.)

The magnitude of the effect is the difference in what you expect to see with your drug and with the comparator (placebo or another drug). For example, if you expect your drug to work in 70% of the subjects, and the drug you are using as a comparator to work in only 50% of the subjects, the magnitude of the effect (the effect size) is 20%. It is always a bit of a guess to determine the effect size, especially in the phase II studies with a new compound. This is because you don't have much information about the effect size of your compound until a number of studies have been completed.

In advance of any studies, the effect size is determined by making educated guesses. The problem of approximating the effect size is like the chicken and the egg—you need to know something about the effect size to calculate a sample size, but you can't calculate the sample size without an effect size. What happens is that you make a guess in the early phase II studies, then information gathered from these studies will help determine the effect size; this information is then used to calculate sample sizes for subsequent studies. As the development program progresses and more is known about the investigational drug, the effect size estimates become more accurate, and sample sizes become easier to calculate. By the time phase III studies are done, the effect size estimates are reasonably accurate.

As the effect size increases, the necessary sample size goes down; that is, it takes fewer subjects to show a statistically significant difference between two treatments when the difference in the effect of the treatments is large.

As for effect size, the estimate of the variability is based primarily on educated guesses in phase I and early phase II studies, but becomes quite accurate by the time the phase III studies are done. Variability is also a statistical parameter and will be determined by the statistician, based in part on information from past work and from the clinician involved in the trial.

Given the effect size and the variability, the statistician can construct power curves that will show the sample size needed for various choices of power. These help ensure that enough subjects are entered into the study to show the treatment effect.

The sample size that results from these calculations tells how many subjects are needed at the end of the trial for valid analyses. However, it is rare that everyone who starts a trial completes it; subjects drop out along the way for many reasons (See Chapter 12). Consequently, you must start with more subjects than you need to compensate for those subjects who do not complete the study. If it is expected that 25% of the subjects will drop out along the way, then at least 25% more subjects than your sample size calculation must be entered. For example, if the sample size was calculated to be 300 subjects per treatment group, it would need to be increased by at least 75 (25%) for a total of 375 subjects per group.

Most of the time a larger sample size is better than a smaller sample size, but cost control and time both become harder to manage as the sample size increases.

### Placebo response versus placebo effect

It would be nice to be able to assume that the subjects receiving a placebo treatment during a trial would have no treatment effect at all, but this is far from true. People respond to treatment with placebo, sometimes quite dramatically. For example, in trials for depression or anxiety, it is commonplace to see placebo response rates of 25% to 40%.

Remember that in clinical trials, subjects get a great deal of care, including frequent visits, lots of medical tests and attention from both the investigator and the study coordinator—all this extra attention could be enough to make them feel better, even if they are only treated with a placebo. There have also been numerous studies showing that an actual disease state can respond measurably to placebo, including, among others, the lowering of blood pressure,[1] alleviation of postoperative pain[2] and relief of psychiatric conditions such as anxiety, depression, agoraphobia and schizophrenia.[3] Pundits have gone so far as to suggest that placebo might be the next wonder drug.

There has been much written about placebo response, but it is outside the scope of this book, so we will not discuss it further. However, you must be aware that it is a real phenomenon and has a significant impact on clinical trials.

Subjects do not have to receive a placebo to benefit from the "placebo effect" while in a trial. Remember that all subjects are receiving the same benefits from the trial—more tests, more visits and more attention. Therefore, subjects receiving the active treatment are as apt to experience a placebo effect as are those subjects being treated with the placebo. Ideally the placebo effect will balance out between groups so that the differences seen can be attributed to the actual drug effect.

### Statistical significance

Statistical significance relates to the probability that an event (such as the difference between two treatments) is due to chance alone. When a sponsor is doing a study to compare a drug to a placebo or to another active drug, it is hoped that there will be a statistically significant difference in favor of the sponsor's drug. The significance level is most commonly set at 5%, or $p = 0.05$, where p stands for probability.

If the drug appears to be better than placebo in a test at the 0.05 level, it does not prove that the drug is actually better, but it gives you a comfort level that there really is a difference in the effect of the two treatments.

Note that seeing a statistically significant difference does not say anything about the magnitude of the difference or the clinical significance of the difference. Inferences about the actual clinical value of the difference must be made based on the actual value of the variables being studied. For example, let's assume that the final average Hamilton Depression Rating Scale for Depression (HAM-D) total score was 10.6 in the investigational drug group and 13.2 in the placebo group, and that the difference (2.6) was statistically significant at p=0.05. This means, roughly, that the probability of this difference being due to chance alone is only 5%. Whether or not the difference of 2.6 points that separates the two groups is significant clinically would need to be decided by medical personnel.

## Control groups used in clinical trials

What is a control group? Subjects in comparative trials are divided into two (or more) groups: the treatment group and the control group. Subjects in the treatment group receive the investigational drug, while those in the control group receive placebo or an active drug that is already marketed for use. Control groups are used in clinical trials as a baseline against which to compare a new treatment to test that it is both safe and effective.

Three main types of control groups—placebo control, active comparator control and historical control—are discussed below.

### Placebo control

Use of a placebo control in a study means that one group is treated with the active drug and another group is treated with a placebo and the results are compared. Use of a placebo helps control for the psychological effect of being in a trial and helps to control for adverse events being attributed to the active drug when in fact they are simply the result of changes in the disease or other outside factors.

In the United States, placebo-controlled studies are common and are the most desirable to the FDA in all cases, except those for which the use of a placebo would be unethical (such as in an infectious disease known to respond to treatment). In many other countries, the routine use of placebo-controlled studies is less acceptable. However, if a placebo control is not used, it is difficult to tell whether the active medication was really effective, no matter what the size of the effect observed. This is because the result seen may have been due to the placebo effect rather than to the active treatment.

### Active comparator control

In cases where a placebo cannot be ethically used, the investigational drug may be compared to another active compound. The comparator will be an already marketed product; it is frequently an established, standard treatment used for the condition, although it may be the newest and most interesting treatment, or the market leader. It is usually the hope of a sponsor that its investigational drug will be shown to be statistically superior to the comparator drug. Remember, though, that the effect seen with one or both of the drugs may be due to the placebo effect, and there is no way to distinguish that in an active comparator trial.

Sometimes both a placebo and active comparator are used in a trial, making three treatment groups. This allows both drugs to be compared to the placebo as well as to each other, eliminating the potential placebo effect problem discussed above. In general, it allows for more subjects to receive an active drug rather than placebo. If one-third of the total number of subjects are randomized to each of the three study groups (investigational drug, placebo and active comparator), two-thirds of the subjects will receive an active drug treatment and only one-third will receive placebo treatment. Since most subjects would prefer to receive an active drug, this control scheme often makes a study more appealing.

### Historical control

Upon occasion a historical control will be used in a clinical trial. There are two types of historical controls. One type of historical control is the use of data obtained on the same subjects (on no treatment, the same treatment or a different treatment). Sometimes this is done by a crossover study, which will be discussed later in this chapter.

The other type of historical control is a comparison to data obtained in other patients, (again on no treatment, the same treatment or another treatment). This type of trial is seen rather often in the testing of new therapies for cancer, when no other treatment exists. The trial results will be compared to the remission rates or death rate seen in the general population of similar cancer patients when there is no treatment. For example, if the death rate in untreated people with a particular cancer is 35% over a particular period of time, and if the death rate in study subjects (getting the treatment) with this same cancer over the same period of time is 25%, this might show a significant difference with the use of the investigational drug.

## Minimizing bias

Bias, according to Webster's Dictionary, is "a systematic error introduced into sampling or testing by selection or encouraging one outcome or answer over others."[4] In clinical trials, these systematic errors distort the data, which may lead to an incorrect conclusion.

Bias may be introduced in a clinical trial from anyone who might be able to exert some influence over it, including the sponsor, the investigator, a monitor or study subjects. An investigator could introduce bias by placing subjects in study groups based on how the investigator felt each particular subject would react to one treatment over another. Bias may also be introduced in assessing a subject's response to a medication, based on how well the assessor (investigator, coordinator) thinks the given treatment will work.

It is difficult to give an impartial judgment if you have a particular point of view, in this case the expected result, of a treatment.

The two main techniques used in clinical trials to eliminate bias are blinding and randomization.

## Blinding

Blinding refers to a lack of knowledge of which treatment is being used with a subject in a clinical trial. The primary people who may be blinded in a trial are the subjects, the investigator (and staff), monitors and statisticians. Blinding is achieved by making the treatments look the same for each treatment group. If it is impossible to make the treatments look the same, blinding can be achieved by having someone who is not otherwise associated with the trial administer the treatment, while the investigator remains blinded while doing assessments of the subject. The most common blinding schemes are:

- Triple blind. The subject, the investigator, the sponsor's monitors and statisticians all do not know which treatment is being received by a particular subject.
- Double blind. Neither the subject nor the investigator knows which treatment is being received by a particular subject.
- Single blind. The subject does not know which treatment is being received, but the investigator does know.
- Open label. No blind is used. Both the investigator and the subject know which treatment the subject is receiving.

## Randomization

Randomization is the method by which study subjects are randomly assigned to treatment groups. It is usually done by means of a randomization code scheme, which is most often generated by a validated computer program. Randomization helps to reduce bias in a trial by ensuring there is no pattern in the way subjects are assigned to the treatment groups. It also allows the blind to be broken for one subject without breaking it for all other subjects at the same time.

If subjects were just assigned to treatment groups A and B one after the other as they came in, the investigator would not be blinded, as he or she would always know which treatment group would be assigned next, even if the drug itself is blinded. (See Table 1)

### Table 1: Assignment Scheme

| Subject | 1 | 2 | 3 | 4 | 5 | 6 | 7 | 8 | 9 | 10 | 11 | 12 |
|---------|---|---|---|---|---|---|---|---|---|----|----|----|
| Drug | A | B | A | B | A | B | A | B | A | B | A | B |

In a randomized assignment, the investigator will not be able to know the pattern, as it is random. When blinded study drugs are sent to an investigative site, they are labeled by subject number, Subject #101, Subject #102,…, etc. The investigator and site personnel will only know the subject numbers, not the underlying treatment, or the underlying randomization scheme. A random treatment pattern for the same two treatments, A and B, might look like:

**Table 2: Random Treatment Pattern**

| Subject | 1 | 2 | 3 | 4 | 5 | 6 | 7 | 8 | 9 | 10 | 11 | 12 |
|---------|---|---|---|---|---|---|---|---|---|----|----|----|
| Drug    | B | B | A | A | A | B | B | B | A | B  | A  | A  |

Note that there are twelve subjects in each randomization scheme, and that six subjects receive each treatment in each scheme. In the random scheme, however, it is not easy to predict the next treatment, as there is no particular order to the scheme. Sometimes randomization is done in blocks, where each block of subjects has the same number of people on each treatment. If you look closely at the randomization scheme above, you will notice that each block of six subjects has three people in each treatment group. This is called randomization in blocks. It is important that the subjects, the investigator and the CRA do not know this assignment pattern. If they did, it could effectively unblind them to the treatments, which might introduce bias and negate the benefits gained from randomizing and blinding.

Randomization and blinding are usually used together and constitute the best defense against bias in clinical trials.

## Common study designs

There are many different statistical study designs used for studies, but most of the clinical trials that CRAs work on employ only the two designs, or variations of them, that are briefly discussed below. If you are interested in reading more about study design, the Guide to Clinical Trials by Bert Spilker[5] has a good basic discussion on this topic.

### Parallel

This is the most common and most straightforward statistical design used in clinical trials. In this design, each subject is assigned to a treatment group, with all subjects following the same schedule and activities. The groups are followed in parallel. There may be two or more treatment groups. (See Table 3)

**Table 3: Parallel Study**

| Group 1 | Drug A | |
|---|---|---|
| Group 2 | Drug B | |
| | Start | Finish |

The analysis will compare the groups to each other.

## Crossover

A crossover design is somewhat more complicated, in that each group will receive both treatments. It starts off like a parallel design study, but halfway through, the groups switch to the other treatment. Frequently there is a washout period between the two treatments. A crossover study in its simplest form is shown in Table 4.

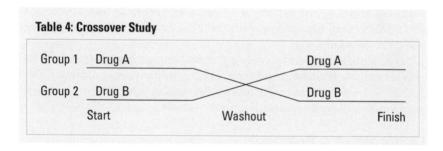

**Table 4: Crossover Study**

| Group 1 | Drug A | | Drug A | |
|---|---|---|---|---|
| Group 2 | Drug B | | Drug B | |
| | Start | Washout | Finish | |

In this design, each group can be compared to itself as well as to the other group. There is less variability in a crossover design as compared to a parallel design. However, many drugs have a carryover or residual effect after they are stopped, which is difficult to measure. This design is frequently seen in bioavailability trials, which allow a period between the treatments of usually ten or more half-lives of the drug to combat the carryover effect. There are many variations of crossover designs, but the general premise remains the same.

## Summary

Clinical trials are complex and have their own rules and terminology. CRAs should be familiar with at least the basics of trial design and with the terminology used. When the basic design elements have been determined for a trial, it is time to write the protocol. Protocol development is discussed in the following section.

# Developing a Protocol

In this section, we will look at how protocols are developed and what is included in a protocol. The protocol is the blueprint for a study and describes how the study will be conducted. If the protocol is well written and the study design is sound, the study will be able to generate valid data that are acceptable to the scientific community, including the FDA.

CRAs will almost never write a complete protocol, but in-house CRAs may be asked to prepare sections of protocols, or to draft a protocol plan, sections of which will be completed by others on the drug development team, such as the medical monitor and biostatistician. Even if CRAs are not involved in writing protocols, it is important for them to have an understanding of protocol basics. The protocol is the basic tool of clinical trials, and will be used in every study CRAs monitor. Knowing the basics of a protocol makes the CRA more effective and the job easier.

A CRA should be able to read a protocol and determine whether or not it contains all the elements important to a trial, as well as the critical medical information. A CRA should be able to determine if a protocol is realistically feasible to do, at least from a logistics standpoint. There is no other study document so important for a CRA to be knowledgeable about. (It is also a pet peeve of site personnel when the CRA does not thoroughly understand the protocol.)

Designing a study and writing a protocol require knowledge of the scientific method, regulations and the medical condition being addressed. Bert Spilker[6] has written a complete text on developing protocols for those who want a more in-depth dissertation on the subject.

## Contents of a Protocol

No two protocols are the same. Formats will vary from company to company and among different authors in the same company. The content will vary depending on the therapeutic area of investigation. Many sponsors have a pre-defined format for protocols that is dictated by their standard operating procedures (SOPs).

There are also differences in protocols because of the development phase of the compound. Phase I protocols are more flexible and less detailed than those for phases II and III because phase I studies are early in the development program and not much is known about how the investigational drug acts in humans. A phase I protocol is primarily an outline of the study and should include:[7]

■ A description of the number of subjects to be studied
■ A description of safety exclusions
■ The dosing plan, including duration, dose or method being used to determine dose
■ A detailed description of the safety procedures, such as vital signs, and laboratory evaluations.

Phase II and III protocols are very detailed and describe all aspects of the investigations. The FDA defines some minimal requirements for these protocols,[8] which must contain at least:

- A description of the objectives and purpose
- The name, address and qualifications of each investigator
- The names of all sub-investigators working under the direction of the investigator
- The institution where the research will be done
- The name and address of the IRB
- The inclusion and exclusion criteria for study subjects
- The number of subjects to be evaluated
- The design of the study, including the type of control group being used, if applicable
- The methods employed to minimize bias (usually randomization and blinding)
- The method used to determine dose(s) used, the maximum dose and the duration of administration
- A description of the observations and measurements being used
- A description of the measures (laboratory evaluations, procedures, etc.) being used to monitor the effects of the investigational drug and to minimize risks to subjects

These are minimum requirements; almost all protocols will contain additional elements as well. The common elements of a protocol, and the order in which they usually appear, are:

- Title page
- Protocol summary
- Abstract (optional)
- Table of contents
- Introduction
- Study objectives
- Study design
- Randomization and blinding
- Subject selection
- Subject enrollment
- Informed consent
- Screening procedures
- Replacement of subjects
- Treatment
- Concomitant medication
- Study activities and observations
- Adverse events
- Data recording instructions
- Data quality assurance

- Analysis plan
- Risks and benefits
- References
- Appendices

A brief description each of these elements in a typical protocol follows.

## Common Elements of a Protocol

1. **Title Page.** All protocols will have a title page. Essential information for the title page includes:

- Title: The title should be specific enough to distinguish the protocol from those for similar studies. It should be a concise description of the study providing the reader with the drug, disease, design and study phase.
  Example: A randomized, double-blind, phase III trial of (drug under study) in subjects with generalized anxiety disorder. A placebo-controlled, fixed-dose, parallel-group multi-center study of 12 weeks.
- Protocol Number: This should be a unique number that identifies the protocol. Most sponsors have a specific procedure for determining this number that identifies the drug, as well as the study.
  Example: 12AB345/0021, where 12AB345 is the drug identifier, and 0021 identifies the protocol within that drug development program.
- IND Number: The IND number of the drug, for studies done under an IND.
- Date: All protocols should be dated as part of their identifiers. This also allows various versions to be readily identified.
- Sponsor Medical Monitor: The name and contact information for the sponsor's medical monitor.
- Principal Investigator: The name and address of the investigator doing the study.
- Some protocol cover pages include the statistician, CRA, sub-investigators, study coordinator and laboratory contact information, but these are optional.

2. **Protocol Summary.** The protocol summary should give a good overview of the study and is highly recommended. CRAs can use the summary when they are interviewing potential investigators, even when the entire protocol is not yet complete. The summary will provide enough information for potential investigators to determine if they are interested in and have the capability to do the study.

The summary is usually one to two pages long and typically includes:
- Protocol Title: repeated from the title page.
- Study Objective: a statement of the main objectives and purpose of the study.

Example: The primary objective is to show that (study drug) is more effective than placebo in the short-term (12 weeks) treatment of generalized anxiety disorder. The secondary objective is to gain information on the short-term safety of (study drug).

- Study Population: a brief description of the type of subjects to be included.

  Example: Study subjects will be male or female, 18 years or older, with diagnosed generalized anxiety disorder and no clinically relevant co-morbid psychiatric conditions.

- Study Design: a brief description of design, e.g., single dose, multiple dose, pilot, safety, efficacy, randomized or not, single or double blind, open label, parallel, crossover, etc.

  Example: The study is a randomized, double-blind, fixed-dose, placebo-controlled, phase III, multicenter trial.

- Study Medication, including the:
  - Generic name and trade name (if known) of the compound.
    Example: alprazolam (Xanax®)
  - Dosage form. Example: 0.25 mg tablets
  - Route of administration. Example: oral
  - Dose and regimen. Example: 0.25 mg three times a day

- Duration of Treatment: the time period during which the study medication will be administered to the subjects. If the treatment is not continuous, it should be described.

  Example: Subjects will be treated for 10 weeks, followed by a two-week single-blind taper period.

- Methods and Materials: a general description of the procedures, tests, etc., required.

- Duration of Subject Participation: total duration of subject involvement in the study, including screen and any follow-up.

  Example: Subjects who complete the study will have 12 weeks of study involvement.

- Anticipated Maximum Number of Subjects: total number of subjects in all treatment groups.

  Example: There will be 440 subjects in each treatment group, for a total of 880 subjects.

  Number of Centers: if known.

**3. Abstract.** An abstract is optional. An abstract should be limited to one or two paragraphs describing the objective, design, population, sample size and major study activities.

**4. Table of Contents.** A detailed table of contents should be included in all protocols.

**5. Introduction.** The introduction should identify the reason for doing the study and place it in context with previous investigations and in the overall development plan. If the introduction is lengthy, subheadings should be used. Abbreviations and acronyms should be avoided when possible. Each abbreviation or acronym should be identified in full the first time it is used. Example: Hamilton Rating Scale for Anxiety (HAM-A). The introduction usually contains:

- A brief discussion of the study medication, including the medical need and rationale for use.
- A description of the design and major endpoints, including the rationale for use.
- A description of how this protocol differs from other similar protocols for the same treatment.
- An identification of the setting in which subjects will be studied (outpatient, hospital, etc.).
- The rationale for the dose and regimen, citing supporting data.
- A description of the study control (e.g., placebo) and/or comparator drug, plus the rationale for use.
- A general description of procedures and length of the study.

**6. Study Objectives.** These should clearly state the primary and secondary objectives and identify the endpoints that will be used to satisfy them. Primary endpoints are usually the key efficacy parameters to be studied. Secondary endpoints usually consist of efficacy variables that are of lower clinical significance and also the safety parameters of the trial. State whether the study is intended to show a difference or similarity between treatments (this could also be included under study design).

**7. Study Design.** This section should include a description of the study design, including:

- Type of study (methodology, pilot, tolerance, efficacy, pharmacokinetics)
- Controlled or uncontrolled
- Single or multiple dose (fixed or variable)
- Single site or multicenter
- Open label or blinded
- Randomization scheme
- Design (parallel, crossover, matched pair, block, sequential)

**8. Randomization and Blinding.** This section should describe the randomization and blinding procedure, including any stratification. It should also contain instructions for breaking the blind, if it becomes necessary.

**9. Subject Selection.** This section will include a description of the study population, indicating the number of subjects to be enrolled. If appropriate, it will differentiate between the maximum number of subjects to be enrolled and the minimum number of subjects required to meet protocol objectives. The subject selection criteria (inclusion and exclusion criteria) should include:

- A description of each requirement for subject eligibility. If there are any exceptions to a criterion, they should be stated.
- Specific disease-related criteria.
- Willingness to sign an informed consent form as an inclusion criterion.
- Allowed and disallowed concomitant medications.
- Criteria that will exclude subjects.
  - Subjects who are taking another investigational medication or who have recently taken an investigational medication within a specified time period (i.e., 30 days) are almost always excluded.

This section should also include a description of when the entry criteria must be met, e.g., before or following a screening period, after a washout period, etc.

In some trials, subjects who meet some basic study criteria are enrolled in a screening period. During this time, various tests are done (e.g., physical exam, laboratory tests) to determine if the subjects meet the criteria for entry into the entire trial. A washout period is a time when subjects are taken off their current (non-study) medications. When the carryover effect from these medications has had time to dissipate, subjects are entered into the main part of the trial.

**10. Subject Enrollment.** This section should identify the point at which a subject is considered enrolled. For randomized studies, this is usually at the time of randomization. Other possibilities might be after the informed consent form is signed or after successful completion of a screening period.

**11. Informed Consent.** The section about informed consent is sometimes located in the body of the protocol and sometimes in an appendix. It is always a good idea to provide the investigator with a draft consent form, instead of expecting each investigator to write one separately. Consent forms were discussed in detail in the previous chapter. The protocol section on informed consent should include:

- A complete description of informed consent requirements, emphasizing the requirement for obtaining consent prior to a subject's involvement in any study-related activity.
- The investigator's responsibility to obtain IRB approval of the consent.
- Specific instructions if vulnerable populations, such as minors, will be included in the study.

12. **Screening Procedures.** This section should contain the following:

- A description of all activities and tests related to the screening of subjects for study enrollment.
- Specify timing relative to tests, meals or the start of treatment.
- If results of any screening tests will be used as baseline for within-group comparisons, this should be stated.
- Describe discontinuation of any concomitant medications, if required.

13. **Replacement of Subjects.** This section should specify whether subjects who drop out will be replaced and any conditions associated with replacement. If replacement is allowed, the protocol should specify how replacement subjects would be assigned to treatment groups.

14. **Treatment.** This section should provide the following information about the investigational medication and any comparator medication, including a placebo.

- Generic, chemical and trade name (if known).
- Formulation of the placebo.
- Dosage forms and formulation, in general terms. If any medication contains excipients to which some subjects may be sensitive, such as lactose, this should be indicated.
- Packaging (e.g., bottles, blister packs).
- Special storage procedures and stability considerations. If the medication requires reconstitution, the stability in the reconstituted form should be specified.
- Route of administration; include any special instructions for reconstituting medication or preparing individual doses. If it is administered intravenously (IV), specify the infusion rate.
- The dosage regimen and time schedule for each dose. Clarify the duration of administration, including any medication-free periods or washout periods. As appropriate, specify the timing of dosing in relation to meals.
- Rationale for the dose and regimen.
- Procedures for dosage adjustments, if applicable.
- Compliance parameters, e.g., so many days allowable, etc.

15. **Concomitant Medication.** This section should include the policy on the use of concomitant medications, including over-the-counter (OTC) medications, herbals and vitamin supplements. Indicate that all concomitant medication must be recorded. If concomitant medications are allowed, there should be information about how they may be used and why the use will not confound the treatment effect. Interaction data should be cited as appropriate.

If the analysis will be stratified based on concomitant medication, this should be stated, with reference to the analysis plan.

If smoking, alcohol, caffeine or illicit drugs are prohibited or restricted, this should be mentioned in this section.

**Table 1: Example of a Protocol Activity Schedule**

| Study Activity | Baseline | Week 1 | Week 2 | Week 4 | Week 6 | Final (W8) |
|---|---|---|---|---|---|---|
| Informed consent | ■ | | | | | |
| Medical history | ■ | | | | | |
| Physical exam | ■ | | | ■ | | ■ |
| Labs | ■ | ■ | ■ | ■ | ■ | ■ |
| EKG | ■ | | | ■ | | ■ |
| Treadmill stress test | ■ | | | ■ | | ■ |
| Office visit—general assessments | ■ | ■ | ■ | ■ | ■ | ■ |
| Safety evaluations | ■ | ■ | ■ | ■ | ■ | ■ |
| Medication dispensing | ■ | ■ | ■ | ■ | ■ | |
| Final evaluation | | | | | | ■ |

**16. Study Activities and Observations.** This section will give all the activities that are to be done at each study visit. It should also include an overall activity schedule that shows at a glance each event, procedure, observation and evaluation that will be done for each visit. An example of a protocol activity schedule is shown in Table 1. Other considerations to keep in mind for this section are:

- Each time period should be clearly defined.
- Avoid the use of "Day 0", as it is confusing to most people.
- If "Time 0" is used, it must be carefully defined. This is usually the time of the initial dose of medication within a given evaluation period.
- List and describe all study activities, observations and evaluations to be made during each period.
- If any non-study medications are to be discontinued during a period (usually a screening period), describe the procedure.
- Specify the acceptable leeway or "treatment window" for each visit. This is the amount of time that is allowed before or after the scheduled visit date, such as the date plus and minus two days. Specify how the investigator should handle visits that occur outside the acceptable window.
- If there is a tapered discontinuation of the investigational medication, describe the exact procedures, including the specific dose adjustments and time schedule to be followed. Consider a tabular display of the taper schedule.

Clinical assessments also need to be described in this section. Things to keep in mind when discussing clinical assessments are:

- Describe and provide specific criteria (as appropriate) for the various observations and assessments at each study period. To avoid confusion, be sure to use the same terminology and categories that will be used in the case report forms (CRFs) (See "Case Report Forms" later in this chapter). Relate the various clinical assessments to the primary study observations they support.
- If a detailed description of a particular procedure or assessment tool is needed, consider describing it in general terms in this section, but in more detail in the appendix.
- Provide the rationale for the selection of specific endpoints or assessment tools unless discussed elsewhere.
- Discuss the accuracy, precision and relevance of any nonstandard assessment tool or procedures, citing references when appropriate.
- Specify any special conditions under which assessments are to be made or specific equipment that should be used. Quantify descriptions when feasible and appropriate (e.g., indicate that 15 minutes of rest should precede a "resting" blood pressure reading).
- As appropriate, identify who should make clinical assessments and indicate whether the same evaluator should be used for a given subject throughout the study or for all subjects. List any assessment forms that are to be completed by the subject.
- Specify the rules or criteria for changing the management of the subject if there is either marked improvement or worsening of the subject's condition.

**17.  Adverse Events.** There should be a very explicit section covering adverse events and adverse event reporting. Adverse events are discussed in detail in Chapter 11.

**18.  Data Recording Instructions.** This section should:

- Indicate how data will be collected. If detailed instructions have been prepared, specify their location (e.g., study manual, appendix, etc.).
- Discuss the use and management of source documents.
- Discuss the procedure for correcting errors.

**19.  Data Quality Assurance.** This section should:

- Describe procedures for assessing subject compliance.
- Describe any special training or other measures for site personnel to ensure valid data.
- Discuss source document review.
- Provide Good Clinical Practice (GCP) references.

**20. Analysis Plan.** Generally the analysis plan will be developed and provided by the biostatistician. Items that may be included are:

- Discussion of the general study design issues.
- A statement of the planned sample size, reason for choosing it, and power calculations.
- Classification of study variables (e.g., primary versus secondary).
- Identification of statistical model(s) to be used.
- Description of specific analyses, including any subgroup analyses.
- Information about the timing and purpose of any planned interim analyses.
- Handling of missing or non-evaluable data.

**21. Risks and Benefits.** This section should briefly summarize the risks and potential benefits associated with the use of the test compound or procedure. If there is any exposure to radiation, it should be discussed here. Note that this section should be consistent with the consent form.

**22. References.** Put all references for the protocol in this section.

**23. Appendices.** Appendices may be used to detail information that might be confusing if placed in the body of the protocol.

- Include an appendix describing investigator responsibilities, including the requirements for compliance with GCPs and sponsor SOPs. (Investigator responsibilities are discussed in the next chapter.)

## Summary

A good protocol forms the backbone of the research process and is essential for conducting a high quality study. CRAs must understand what makes a good protocol and the importance of protocols in research. For each study the CRA is monitoring, he or she must have a clear understanding of the protocol and what must be done to ensure adherence to it during the study.

After the protocol is written, case report forms can be developed. This is discussed in the following section.

# Case Report Forms (CRFs)

Case report forms (CRFs) are used during a clinical trial to record the protocol-required data for each study subject. CRFs standardize the collection of study data and help to assure that the medical, statistical, regulatory and data management needs of the study are met.

The mere mention of case report forms can evoke images of piles of paper and seemingly endless corrections. However, dealing with CRFs is a large part of a CRA's workload and they play a major part in the performance of a clinical trial. The CRA's involvement in monitoring CRFs is discussed in Chapter 10.

Many sponsor companies have designated people or departments that are responsible for developing the CRFs, or this work may be contracted out to a company that specializes in CRF development. Consequently, CRA involvement and input in developing CRFs vary considerably from company to company. However, the impact of CRF design on data quality is so significant that CRAs should have an understanding of the issues involved in CRF design and development. Being aware of the problems with poorly designed CRFs will also help the CRA when reviewing the forms at investigative sites.

## Case Report Form Design and Development

Unfortunately, sponsors often cause themselves significant problems because the design and development of CRFs are not given adequate attention. So much time and energy goes into protocol development that CRFs are sometimes almost an afterthought. However, taking the time to design good forms pays major dividends during the course of the study.

Past experience is extremely valuable, and time should be taken to utilize previous company CRF experiences. Try to use ideas that worked well for other studies. Get input from some of your more knowledgeable sites. Study coordinators know from experience what works well and what doesn't and will usually be willing to share their thoughts about good and bad CRFs.

Good case reports come from consistent improvement over time. Since CRAs are in an excellent position to monitor the quality of CRFs during monitoring visits, they should make notes of which forms or parts of forms seem to produce the most errors and those that are relatively error free; this information should be shared with those involved in forms design.

Some of the issues involved in producing high quality case report forms are discussed below.

### Standardization of CRFs

Everyone in this business is busy. One way to make better use of time is the judicious use of standardization. An approach to form design that has been used successfully by many companies is "modularization," which employs the benefits of standardization, while also capturing and utilizing corporate experience.

The modular process is simple. There are data that are always collected on study subjects regardless of the drug or disease being studied, such as header information, demographics, laboratory work and physical exams. There are also other procedures (ECGs, stress tests, etc.) where the information gathered is standard across different disease areas. When the group of fields to collect the information for one of these items is created for a study, it should be saved as a form module that can be used for other studies.

Over time, the catalog of form modules will become comprehensive. When new studies are planned, those involved in designing the CRFs can check the catalog to see which form modules will be appropriate for the study in question. Not only does this save design time, but the modules can also be pre-coded by data management, which saves additional time.

### Terminology used in CRFs
Always use standard terminology that is familiar to clinicians. Industry jargon will not be understood in a clinical setting.

### Selection of the media for CRFs
A decision must be made about whether paper or electronic forms will be used. If the answer is "electronic," the software that will be used for electronic data capture (EDC) will usually define the CRFs. With EDC, data may be entered into a laptop computer placed at the investigative site by a sponsor, or data may be entered into electronic forms that are transferred between the sponsor and the site via the Internet. In general, CRAs will have little or no input on the design or layout of electronic CRFs.

As we write this book, the majority of clinical trials still employ paper CRFs. Eighty-eight percent of data collection in the United States is still being done on paper forms.[9] Many of the concepts and principals discussed for paper forms are also applicable for electronic forms. This is important because more and more investigative sites will be using web-enabled systems for case report form capture and collection on the majority of their trials in the months and years to come.

### Determination of the data that need to be collected
One of the first things to be done is the determination of what information should be collected on the case report forms and how it will be coded, including acceptable ranges and any exceptions. The best way to do this is to go through the protocol and list all the data that are required, keeping in mind that the forms must collect these data in a way that allows for appropriate analyses. When this has been determined, the forms design process may start. For example, it is never a good idea to ask for the same data in more than one place in a case report form because, when this happens, the data do not always agree. Sometimes the case report forms ask for both date of birth and age, for example, and they frequently do not match when calculated; it is much better to ask only one question.

### Determination of CRF layout
If a module catalog is available, the next step is to determine which modules are appropriate for the study. If not, or if the modules do not cover all the necessary information, then the necessary fields to collect the remaining data must be laid out. Some things to consider during this process are:

**Header and footer information.** There should be standard header information on all forms. The sponsor name or ID, the medical monitor, the protocol number, the page title and a place to enter subject identification information should be preprinted on all forms. All forms should also be annotated as CONFIDENTIAL. Each form should also have a place for a signature and date; this usually appears at the bottom of the page in a footer.

**Number of fields per page.** It's tempting to crowd as much information on a page as possible to save costs. However, this approach usually turns out to be "penny wise and pound foolish" as crowding increases the chance for error. There is no easy way to quantify form density; it is a judgment call. The best way is to develop a feel for the amount of information on a page that is optimal and count the number of fields. Then try to stay within 10% of that number on all forms.

**Font size.** Use a font size and style that is easy to read.

**Spatial relationships.** The fields on a page, particularly the check boxes, should be lined up as much as possible. It is easier to enter data and to notice missing data when the alignment is straight.

**Location of fields on a page.** Something that is almost never considered during form design is where on the page to put specific fields. In one of our development programs, we paid close attention to data collection error rates and what contributed to them. We discovered that most errors on the CRFs occurred in fields that were on the bottom third of the forms. From that point on, we always put primary endpoints and other critical data on the top third of the forms. Although unsure why this phenomenon occurred, it was assumed to be eye fatigue as one worked through the form entering data.

Another consideration related to the position of fields on the form is the use of a logical layout. The material on the form should be organized in a manner that makes sense relative to medical practice. Group fields together for activities that are usually done together or in sequence in a clinic setting. For example, a module for collecting data on eye exams should not be put in the middle of a page that is collecting data from a physical exam and vital signs. In addition, vital signs—pulse, heart rate and respiration rate—should be grouped together rather than in different locations. Remember that the "customers" for your case report forms are the site personnel who must fill them out. Make your forms as user friendly for these people as possible to help reduce errors.

**Narrative fields.** As much of the data as possible should be collected using numeric fields or check boxes. Include a check box for "other" as appropriate, as exceptions do occur.

Written comments on case report forms are a problem because it is difficult to computerize and analyze comments. Everything on a case report form must be coded for computer entry and analysis; consequently, comments need to be interpreted and converted to code. The true nature of the comment is often lost or distorted during the translation. On the other hand, there may not be a better way to document an occurrence than by a comment. There should be places for comments on case report forms, but only when really necessary and valuable.

It is incumbent on the CRA to instruct site personnel on the use of comments on case report forms. Many CRF designers intentionally reduce margin space on case report forms to discourage comments. It is a difficult issue, but one that can be dealt with effectively if appropriate attention is given to it.

**Shading.** There are many opinions on the value of shading. Based on our experience, adding shading to forms can reduce error rates more than any other single design feature. If a form is shaded except for the places data are to be entered, it makes the fields stand out so clearly that errors of omission are almost eliminated. If an error does occur, finding it is much easier with shading than without. However, shading adds considerable expense to the cost of forms.

**Cross-visit forms.** The most difficult forms to design are those that collect data across visits, such as adverse event and concomitant medication report forms; consequently, a lot of care should be given to the design of these forms. Based on our experience, almost 75% of the errors occurred on about 15% of the case report forms, including the adverse events and concomitant medications cross-visit forms.

## Packaging CRFs

After the forms are designed, there is still a major decision to be made: how to "package" the forms. One decision is whether or not to use "no carbon required" (NCR) paper. If so, three seems to be a good number of copies per page, which allows one for the investigative site, one for the sponsor and one to use as a work sheet for corrections. Each copy should be a different color and clearly marked for the appropriate recipient and use.

Another consideration is whether or not the forms will be bound. There are several binding choices: stapled, stitched and glued, spiral bound, wire bound or in a three ring binder. Each has advantages and disadvantages. The number of pages per subject limits some choices. The primary binding options are:

- **Stapled.** This is easy and not expensive, but can be used only if the number of forms per booklet is relatively small. It can be done locally.
- **Stitched and Glued.** This needs special equipment and is limited to books of no more than one inch thick. Books can be difficult to use, because they don't open flat and the binding can break.

- **Spiral Bound.** These are easy to use (pages lay flat), but the booklet size should not exceed ½ inch or the spiral tends to break.
- **Wire Bound.** Same as for spiral, except the book size can be up to one inch. This is more expensive than spiral bound.
- **Three Ring Binder.** These are easy to use and can be up to 3 inches thick, although the larger binders are difficult to handle and store. Pages are easy to remove, which is nice for data entry, but they can also be lost or misplaced. They are bulky and expensive. If binders are used, the ones with pockets in the covers are handy for storing source documents and notes until the data can be transcribed. Three ring binders are the most common form of binding for CRFs.

Once the binding is determined, the next consideration is the arrangement of the pages. They can be arranged by visit or by form type, but most site personnel prefer to have them arranged by visit. It is good to include a tabbed cover page (printed on heavyweight paper) for each visit, followed by all the forms required for that visit. The cover page can include any special instructions and a list of all the forms required for that visit. The advantage of this method is that all the required data for a visit can be collected without having to refer to the protocol or go through the binder looking for the required forms. It is also valuable to have a foldout flap in the binder that can be placed between pages when entering data to prevent "bleed through" on other NCR pages.

Two other useful things to include in case report form booklets are an activity schedule from the protocol and a calendar, so that the person working with the study subject has an activity schedule handy and does not have to look for a calendar when scheduling the subject's next visit. The foldout flap mentioned above is a good place to print the activity schedule and/or calendar. Remember, making things as easy and convenient as possible for the people who record the data will reduce errors and sponsor workload.

## Ordering, Storage and Shipping of CRFs

When determining how many case report form books to order for a study, keep in mind that it is almost always cheaper to throw extra books away than to reorder more books partway through the study. Because of this, many companies order between 20 and 25 percent more than the number of subjects they plan to enroll.

If you have forms for screening subjects, it's appropriate to order about twice as many as the number of subjects that you plan to enter, in order to cover screen failures. It is good to place the screening forms in a separate binder; that way, in case of a screen failure, you have not spoiled an entire CRF book.

Because the enrollment rate at each site is not known in advance, and because many sites do not have much extra storage space, CRF books are often shipped in fairly small quantities at a time. Many of the larger printers will ship directly to the sites, which saves the sponsor time and storage space.

The CRA will need to instruct investigators and coordinators in how and when to order replacement forms, keeping in mind the amount of time it takes for the order to be processed and shipped. It helps if there is contact information for reordering inside the front cover of each CRF book as a reference for the site personnel.

### Miscellaneous Issues

Case report form design and production are complex and time-consuming tasks. Based on your company's capabilities and the specialized equipment required for the production of case report forms, it is often cost effective to contract this function with outside vendors. However, if you are employed by a smaller company or find yourself involved in forms design, some of the more popular software packages being used for this purpose are: Page Maker, Delrina Form Flow, Interleaf, Frame Maker and Claris Draw.

Many years ago in a course called "Managing Accelerated Performance," the instructor said something that is very applicable to case report form design. We were talking about things that could be done that would significantly improve performance and/or productivity (the "silver bullet"). He told us not to think that way because the silver bullet is seldom there. Instead, it is usually small improvements done consistently over time that have major impact. So, as a CRA, when you are monitoring your studies, notice what kinds of errors are occurring, and where. Think about what could be done in the design of the form to help prevent them. Take notes. Help your company to capitalize on good design features and eliminate the bad ones. These are the small steps that lead to continuous improvement.

### Summary

Determining study design parameters, writing good protocols and developing appropriate case report forms are the backbone of study preparation. Doing these activities well will help to ensure the success of the trial. Since CRAs work with these things at every investigative site they monitor, they should have a good understanding of the issues and processes involved.

# Key Takeaways

### Study Design
- Determining the sample size for a study is a statistical computation based on the expected effect size, variability and power.
- Both placebo response and placebo effect have an impact on clinical trials and must be considered when a trial is designed.
- Placebo controls and active controls are most often used in clinical trials. Historical controls are also used but much less frequently.
- Randomization and blinding are the two primary methods of reducing bias in clinical trials.

- In blinded trials, it is important that the subject and the investigator (and usually the CRA) do not know which treatment individual subjects are receiving.
- The most commonly used statistical design in clinical trials is the parallel group design. Crossover designs are also used, especially in bioavailability trials.
- CRAs should be familiar with the common designs and terminology used in clinical trials, as well as the reasons for the use of these various methodologies.

### Protocol

- The protocol is the blueprint for a study. It contains all the information necessary to do the study correctly and well.
- CRAs must have a thorough understanding of the protocol for each study they monitor.
- The writing of a protocol is usually a team effort, involving the medical monitor, the statistician and others.
- Protocols for phase I studies are relatively flexible, while those for phases II and III are more rigid and detailed.
- Certain information is required by regulation to be in protocols.

### Case Report Forms

- Case report forms have a significant impact on data quality.
- Standardize and use modules as much as possible.
- Shading, aligning and limiting the number of fields per page can materially reduce errors.
- Remember that the investigative site is the customer for your CRFs. Design them with the site in mind. Make them medically and clinically sensible.
- It's almost always cheaper to throw away unused forms than to reorder more; order 20 to 25 percent more than the number of subjects you plan to enroll.
- Continually improve your forms by noting good and bad design features.
- Investigative sites should be given clear procedures for ordering additional CRFs.

### References

1. Benson, H., & Epstein, M.D. (1975) The placebo effect. Journal of American Medical Association, 232, 1225-1227.
2. Lasagna, L., Mosteller, F., von Felsinger, J.M., & Beecher, H.K. (1954). A study of placebo response. American Journal of Medicine, 16, 770-779.
3. Klerman, G.L., & Cole, J.O. (1965). Clinical pharmacology of imipramine and related antidepressant compounds. Pharmacology Review, 17, 101-104.

4. Webster's Ninth New Collegiate Dictionary. Merriam-Webster. Springfield, MA. 1990.
5. Guide to Clinical Trials. Bert Spilker, Lippincott-Raven. 1996
6. Guide to Clinical Studies and Developing Protocols, Bert Spilker, Raven Press, 1984.
7. 21CFR 312.23 (6).
8. 21CFR 312.23 (6).
9. Pharmaceutical R&D Statistical Sourcebook 2000 (Parexel, Rose Tree Corporate Center, 1400 N. Providence Rd., Ste, 2000, Media, PA.

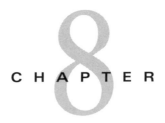

C H A P T E R

# Clinical Investigators

Investigators are responsible for the conduct of studies at investigative sites. In the first part of this chapter we will discuss investigators and their responsibilities. In the second part, we will discuss the evaluation and selection of investigators and investigative sites. During subsequent chapters, we will discuss the things a CRA can do to help investigators meet their responsibilities during clinical trials.

## Investigators and Their Responsibilities

### What Is an "Investigator"?

According to the regulations (21 CFR 312.3), "investigator means an individual who actually conducts a clinical investigation (i.e., under whose immediate direction the investigational drug is administered or dispensed to a subject). In the event an investigation is conducted by a team of individuals, the investigator is the responsible leader of the team." Sometimes the investigator is called the principal, or primary, investigator (PI). Other members of the team may be referred to as sub-investigators, especially in the case of other physicians who are involved with the study. On occasion, there will be co-investigators for a trial. In this case, both individuals are equally responsible for the trial.

Usually, but not always, the investigator is a physician. Sometimes, a person with a Pharm. D. or a Ph.D. degree may serve as an investigator; in that case, there should be (at least for FDA-controlled studies) a physician as a sub-investigator.

## The Statement of Investigator Form (FDA Form 1572)

The Statement of Investigator Form (FDA Form 1572) must be completed and signed by the investigator before he or she may begin a study. The investigator then sends it to the sponsor, and the sponsor submits it to the FDA. A copy of this form is in Appendix G. The 1572 form contains:

- Name and address of the investigator
- Title (and number, if any) of the protocol, including the IND number
- Name and address of the facility where the research will be conducted
- Name and address of any clinical laboratories that will be used
- Name and address of the IRB used to approve the study
- Names of any sub-investigators who will be associated with the study
- Investigator commitment section (discussed below)

There is also a section of the 1572 that lists responsibilities of investigators. These include a commitment by the investigator that he or she will:

- Conduct the study according to the protocol.
- Comply with the regulations.
- Personally conduct or supervise the trial.
- Obtain informed consent from subjects.
- Report adverse events properly.
- Read and understand the material in the Investigator Brochure before starting the trial.
- Assure that other people assisting in the trial are aware of their obligations.

When the investigator signs the 1572 form, a legally binding commitment has been made to conduct a study according to the regulations and constraints of the 1572. CRAs should be very familiar with the 1572 form, and should be prepared to discuss the commitments in depth with potential investigators. CRAs will also need to assure that these forms are properly completed and signed and dated by the investigator before a study commences.

## Investigator Responsibilities

The investigator has ultimate responsibility for the safety of participants in a clinical trial. Research participants are under the immediate care of the investigator and subject to the judgment and professional abilities of the investigator. This is why investigators must be qualified through training and experience before beginning to study a drug or device.

The general responsibilities of an investigator during a trial include ensuring that the trial is conducted according to the signed investigator statement (FDA Form 1572), following the protocol and the regulations, and protecting the rights, safety and welfare of subjects in the trial. In the next sections, we will discuss some of the other specific responsibilities that an investigator has during a trial.

### Control of the Investigational Drug

One of the important responsibilities of an investigator is maintaining control of the investigational drug at all times. The drug may not be used by anyone other than trial subjects, who are under the supervision of the investigator or sub-investigators. Remember that the investigator has responsibility for any sub-investigators assisting in the trial.

If the investigational drug is a controlled substance,* then the drug must be stored in a locked area with limited access. This is a good idea for the storage of all investigational drugs, when possible, as it eliminates potential problems. When not controlled properly, you run the risk of study drugs being used for patients who are not in the trial, or being used by other physicians for non-trial purposes. Losing track of the study drug supply can be a major problem and have a negative effect on the trial.

The CRA will want to ensure that the study drug is properly stored at an investigational site and that provisions have been made to properly administer and account for the drug. This will be covered in more detail in Chapter 10.

### Investigator Recordkeeping and Retention

An investigator must maintain case histories of all subjects and data collected during a trial. These case histories include the case report forms and all supporting documents such as patient charts and progress notes, signed and dated consent forms, laboratory reports, EKGs and any other relevant patient-related documents. The histories must show that the consent form for each subject was signed and dated prior to participation in the study.

The investigator must also maintain complete records of the dispensing and disposition of the study drug, including dates, quantities, use by study subjects and amounts returned.

All study documents must also be maintained and retained, including copies of the signed 1572, the protocol and consent forms, the IRB approval letters, CVs for the investigator and sub-investigators, laboratory normal ranges and correspondence with the IRB and the sponsor. A complete listing of this documentation is found in Appendix C.

All these records must be maintained for a period of two years after the approval of the drug for marketing, or two years after the investigation is closed and the FDA is notified that the company is not pursuing further inves-

---

* Under the definitions found in the Controlled Substances Act.

tigation of the drug. In reality, most sponsors expect the investigator to maintain the records for a much longer period, if not indefinitely. Most contracts between the sponsor and investigators require the investigator to retain all study documents until the sponsor has informed the investigator in writing that they may be destroyed. Although we will discuss this in more detail in Chapter 10, the CRA should make it very clear to the investigator that the records must be kept until written notification that they may be disposed of is received from the sponsor.

**Investigator Reports**

There are reports that the investigator must provide to the sponsor throughout the duration of the trial. They include regular progress reports, which usually consist of the completed case report forms, plus periodic updates on enrollment and study status. Safety reports must also be furnished to the sponsor, including reports on any adverse events that may reasonably be regarded as having been caused by the study medication. Serious adverse events, those that are immediately life threatening or deaths, must be reported to sponsors immediately. A final report must be provided to the sponsor shortly after completion of the study. These reports are necessary in order to allow the sponsor to meet the regulatory requirements for reporting study progress to the FDA.

**IRB Review**

The investigator is responsible for assuring that the IRB he or she is using for the study meets the requirements for IRBs that are found in 21 CFR 56. The investigator must submit and wait for approval of a protocol and informed consent form before beginning a study, as well as promptly reporting to the IRB any changes in the protocol or any unanticipated problems involving risk to study subjects or others. The responsibilities of the investigator with respect to the IRB were delineated in detail in Chapter 5.

## Disqualification of Investigators

Investigators who do not comply with the regulations governing clinical research, or who falsify data in the investigation or reports to the sponsor and/or the FDA, may be disqualified from receiving investigational drugs and doing studies in the future. The FDA maintains a list of restricted and disqualified investigators, known in the business as the "black list." This list is available on the FDA web site (www.fda.gov). Once an investigator is put on the list, the name stays there forever, even if all conditions for reinstatement are met and the investigator is allowed to do research again. Most sponsor companies will not use an investigator who is on this list, even if the person has been reinstated to do research. More information on this topic is included in Chapter 14. CRAs should always check the "black list" before contacting a potential investigator.

In summary, investigators have enormous responsibility when they agree to participate in clinical research. A good investigator will enable the research to proceed smoothly, while a study conducted by a poor investigator will most likely be fraught with problems. Consequently, the selection of investigators is a crucial element of the research process.

# Evaluating and Selecting Investigators

One of the most important tasks that CRAs undertake is the evaluation and selection of investigators. The success of a study depends in large part on the investigator—his or her experience, expertise, commitment, staff, resources and facilities. In this section we will discuss the qualities of a good investigator/investigative site and how a CRA can locate and evaluate sites for successful studies.

### Types of Investigative Sites
There are many types of investigative sites conducting studies. It is useful for a CRA to have an understanding of these different organizations when looking for and assessing potential sites for study placement. Some of the more common investigator site organizational types are listed below.

### Part-Time Sites
Investigators at part-time sites participate in research studies, but also maintain their regular practice. Sometimes these investigators do only one or two studies at a time, while others may participate in research to a greater degree, depending on their interest and the resources they have for doing studies. Most sponsors like this kind of site because there is greater potential for study subjects readily available and because the physician, if used, will become familiar with the drug, so by the time it is marketed will be more likely to prescribe it to his or her patients.

As a CRA, this type of site has both advantages and disadvantages. Because the site may not be as experienced, the CRA can train the site to do things in the way the sponsor would like them to be done, without having to "un-train" or change the way the site is used to doing things. On the other hand, since these sites may have less experience, they may need more training and "hand-holding" throughout the study.

### Dedicated Sites
These sites are dedicated just to conducting studies; no other medical practice is carried out at these sites. They are generally very experienced and need less help from the CRA in learning how to do studies, although they still need instruction in how to do each particular study, with its unique characteristics. These sites are usually very productive and have the advantage of being consistent in their practices. They tend also to be very aware of which studies they can do successfully and are less apt to accept studies for which they do not think they can enroll sufficient subjects within the given time period.

Concerns are sometimes expressed about these sites being "study mills" and having "professional study subjects," but, as long as they are not in violation of the protocol, this does not seem to be a problem.

For the CRA, these sites are usually easy to manage. Since they rely on studies for their business, they are usually accommodating as well as compliant.

## Academic Sites

Academic sites are those located in universities and teaching hospitals. They tend to do original research on their own and government-sponsored clinical trials, as well as industry-sponsored clinical trials. Often these organizations are headed by "thought leaders," the top specialists in their fields. Clinical trials may or may not be the academic site's primary interest, although in the past few years, sponsors have been using academic sites more frequently. It is sometimes the industry trials that provide added funding to allow these sites to carry on other research.

It is desirable for a sponsor to use some academic sites in their development programs. This allows thought leaders to become familiar with the new compounds and, hopefully, to become spokespersons in favor of the compound when it is marketed.

Unfortunately, these sites can present some difficulties for a CRA. It can be difficult for the CRA to meet with the very busy investigator; these investigators have been labeled "phantom investigators" because they never seem to be around during the trial. It can also be difficult if industry-sponsored research is not the primary interest of the site, in which case enrollment may wane and study activities may not receive proper attention. It is important for CRAs to be aware that sometimes investigators at academic sites are more likely to want to deviate from the protocol due to their curiosity about where the research will lead them. Also, because publishing is a key issue at academic sites, sponsor policies regarding publication of the trial results should be clearly delineated prior to the initiation of the study. That being said, there are many excellent academic sites with dedicated researchers who add an extra dimension to clinical development programs.

## Site Management Organizations (SMOs)

SMOs bring together a group of sites and organize them centrally to do studies. They standardize procedures across sites and often provide standardized materials (SOPs, study file procedures, etc.) to each site in the organization. Many SMOs also provide training for their sites and assist the site in compiling and submitting the required regulatory documents. They usually provide centralized services for marketing the sites (attracting studies) and for subject recruitment. There are several types of SMOs, from those that own the sites in the group to those with other partnership agreements.

The main difference for a CRA when using an SMO is that control over study processes may not reside at the site, but may be handled centrally. If the CRA is working with only one site in the SMO, this can cause a bit of difficulty, although it may be advantageous if working with multiple sites in the SMO because of the consistency on study practices.

A variation of an SMO is the Coordinator Organization. This is usually a group of experienced study coordinators who have formed a business. They recruit investigators to do trials and then place an experienced coordinator in the investigator's office to manage and help conduct the trial. These coordinators usually act as the interface with the sponsor/CRO and manage the operational aspects of the trial; the physician is utilized for his or her medical expertise and patient base. The only difference for the CRA is that the coordinator is the main contact for all business aspects of the trial, including grant payments. [Note that the investigator is usually paid a fee by the coordinator organization.]

Regardless of how the physician's research practice is organized, the CRA must still monitor and manage the trial for the safety of the subjects and the integrity of the data.

## Locating Potential Investigators

There are a number of ways to locate potential investigators. One of the best ways is to ask other people in your company for suggestions. In large sponsor companies, people working in one medical group may not be aware of good potential investigators who are being, or have been, used by another medical group. Some companies keep a database of their investigators; if your company has such a database, that is the best place to start identifying potential investigators for your trial. An investigator database is especially valuable if statistics are kept on enrollment rates and numbers, timeliness of data submission and error rates on case report forms. If your company does not have an investigator database, ask for suggestions from other therapeutic groups.

Another excellent way to find good investigators is to ask investigators you know and/or are currently working with. "Dr. Smith, you've been doing a terrific job on this rheumatology study. I have some cardiovascular studies coming along soon. Do you know any physicians who might do as good a job on those studies as you are doing on this one?" If your investigator has some suggestions for you, he or she may be willing to call the other physician as an introduction for you. Some CRAs have had great success using this technique.

There are web sites that list investigators and their areas of specialty. These sites will give you names and contact information by region and specialty and make it fairly easy to start a list of people to contact. There are references to some of these web sites in Appendix A.

Another successful method is networking with colleagues from other companies. Ask colleagues if they have worked with anyone in the therapeutic area you are interested in who did a good job for them in the past.

This is often a very useful method, but be sure to reciprocate when you can. Other potential methods for locating investigators are:

- Look in medical journals for articles dealing with the therapeutic area you are interested in and contact authors of relevant articles.
- Look at regulatory submissions from other companies working in the same therapeutic area and contact the investigators they used.
- Contact professional organizations that may have listings of physicians.
- Contact patient advocacy groups that may keep lists of investigators.

Once you have collected a list of potential investigators for your program, you will want to contact them.

## Initial Contact

If you have no previous company experience with a potential investigator, a telephone call is probably the best initial contact. Try to call the physician directly, rather than leaving messages with staff people. When you call, if you say only that you are from a pharmaceutical company, the person answering the phone may think you are a salesperson, and you are apt to have a difficult time reaching the physician. You might say that you are from the "research division of the XXX company," and that you are interested in talking with Dr. Smith "about becoming involved in research studies." If you are still encountering some difficulty, you may want to tell the person that you are not in sales. If you have too much trouble trying to get through, call the next person on your list and forget this one—if they are that hard to reach, you'll probably always have trouble trying to contact them directly.

Once you reach the physician, introduce yourself and say why you are calling. If the physician appears to be interested, give a brief overview of the program and the study to be done. Find out if the physician has research experience and, if so, the types of projects he or she has done in the past or is doing currently. Ask questions about the patient population, the staff and the facilities.

If interest is high on the part of the potential investigator, and if you feel there is good potential for placing a study at the site, arrange a time to visit the site in person. This will enable you to better evaluate the investigator's capability to do your project. Depending on your company policies, you may be able to send the potential investigator some materials about your drug and/or program, such as a protocol or a protocol summary, before you visit. If your company requires a signed confidentiality agreement before sharing these materials, arrange to fax or mail it to the site and have it completed and returned before sending any other materials. One clue to the interest of the investigator is the speed with which the signed confidentiality agreement is returned to you. It is a good idea to send a letter to the investigator confirming the date and time of your visit to the site.

## Site Evaluation Visits

When the CRA makes an evaluation visit to a potential investigative site, the CRA will be evaluating the investigator's experience, expertise and interest in the trial, as well as the staff, facility and potential patient population available. The sponsor company may have a specific checklist that will guide the CRA in making an assessment. The advantage of using a checklist is that the CRA won't inadvertently forget to assess some important items. A sample site evaluation checklist is found in Appendix C.

### Investigator Experience, Expertise and Interest

The investigator's curriculum vitae (CV) will help you make a general assessment of the investigator's experience and expertise. Conversing with the investigator in person, however, will allow you to determine in depth his or her research activity, especially in the therapeutic area of interest. This is a good time to determine if the investigator has conducted trials similar to the one being proposed, or has worked with similar compounds.

While listening to answers to your questions, you should also be aware of the non-verbal clues to the investigator's interest in your project. Is the investigator actively listening to you? Asking pertinent questions? Being attentive to the conversation and materials? If an investigator professes great interest in doing a study, but is also getting and replying to his email during the meeting—obviously his interest level isn't very high. One of the most critical factors for the success of a study is the interest of the investigator. If the investigator isn't truly interested, the study won't be foremost in his or her mind and it will probably suffer because of it.

The CRA will also want to assess the investigator's reactions to the protocol. Is there anything in the protocol that the physician objects to doing? Is the investigator willing to follow the protocol as it is written? Is the physician comfortable with the study design, and the use of a placebo, if applicable? Does the protocol match his or her generally accepted clinical practice, except for study-specific parameters? Making assumptions that everything is acceptable without checking is a risky path to follow—it's better to find out about potential problems and conflicts before the study is offered to him or her.

This is also a good time to review the following differences between clinical practice and clinical research with the investigator. This is particularly important if he or she is new or relatively inexperienced. Failure to understand these differences can lead to protocol violations, which could have a serious impact on the quality of the study, or lead to its termination. Some of these differences are:

- During a clinical trial, the definitions used for adverse events are regulatory definitions, and are not necessarily based on usual clinical observation (See Chapter 11 on adverse event reporting).

- Concomitant medications that would normally be prescribed for the subject may not be allowed by the protocol, or, if allowed, the dose and regimen may differ from standard practice.
- The protocol treatment period for the disease being studied may differ from normal medical practice. It could be longer or shorter, and is very apt to involve more frequent visits.
- If the study is placebo controlled, the investigator must be comfortable using placebo in subjects with the condition being studied.

## Staff and Facility

It is not enough for an investigator to want to do a study; sufficient staff and an appropriate facility are also necessary for success.

It is not a good idea to place a study at an investigative site that does not have a research coordinator (also called a study coordinator). The research coordinator is essential for the administration of the study; he or she coordinates patient enrollment and visits, manages the study documentation, completes the case report forms and is the primary contact for the CRA throughout the study. The CRA will want to meet and spend some time interviewing the research coordinator during the evaluation visit. If the trial calls for other specialized site personnel (a dietician, for example) then the CRA should ask about these people during the evaluation visit. Is the staff experienced in doing clinical trials? Ask about turnover among the staff.

Not only must there be appropriate people available for a study, but they must have sufficient time to do the necessary work. Upon occasion, an investigator may assure the CRA that there are plenty of people to do the work, but when the CRA talks with the research coordinator, it is apparent that there is already too much work and that adding an additional study would severely compromise the abilities of the coordinator. Are the people in the office pleasant and friendly? If you were a study subject, how would you feel about interacting with them?

Most investigators will want to show the CRA their facilities during an evaluation visit. The CRA should always accept this invitation and look closely during the tour. Is there space to store the study drug and other supplies? Is there a secure area for the study drug? Is the necessary equipment for your study present? For example, if your study calls for treadmill testing, you should see a treadmill somewhere. Is there room for a CRA to work during monitoring visits? It's hard to work while balancing the case report forms and source documents on your knees or while bending over an exam table. Is the facility clean and well maintained? Are there any clinic or hospital policies that would limit the CRA's ability to review source documents, such as patient charts?

**Patient/Subject Population**

One of the primary problems facing the smooth execution of clinical trials is enrolling appropriate patients within the allotted enrollment time. Consequently, when interviewing possible investigators, the CRA will want to thoroughly assess the enrollment potential of the site. The CRA will want to ascertain if the subjects will come from the investigator's current patient population or if they will be drawn from elsewhere. Will the investigator be able to draw patients from other physicians in the same hospital or clinic? Will the site need to advertise for patients? (Advertising will be discussed in Chapter 12.)

It is usually easier to assess enrollment potential for chronic disease studies than it is for acute disease studies. For chronic diseases such as arthritis or diabetes, the investigator should already have appropriate patients among his or her current patient base. It does not necessarily follow that these patients will qualify for or want to participate in the research study, but it gives a base from which to start. For acute studies, one must rely on past statistics. For example, if a pneumonia study is being discussed, the CRA will want to know how many patients with pneumonia the investigator saw over the past year. In either case, the more thorough the records are concerning the patient population, the better the enrollment estimates will be.

Unfortunately, estimates of subject enrollment are almost always too high. Some CRAs use the "halving" technique to arrive at a final estimate: for each major exclusion criteria in the protocol, cut the original number of patients in half. The final number will be much closer to the enrollment you can actually expect to achieve.

---

**The "Halving" Technique**

The investigator says, "I have 500 patients with the disease of interest in my practice." Your protocol has five major exclusion criteria. Cut the 500 in half for each one.

$$500 \rightarrow 250 \rightarrow 125 \rightarrow 63 \rightarrow 32 \rightarrow 15\text{–}16$$

This is probably about the number of subjects you can plan to have enrolled.

---

## Miscellaneous Factors

There are several other items a CRA will want to discuss during an evaluation visit. One is whether or not the site is doing, or is planning to do within the same time period, any competing studies. A competing study is usually one in which similar subjects are to be enrolled. In order to meet the enrollment targets, it's important that your study does not have to compete for subjects with another sponsor's study. In assessing competing studies, it is not enough to assess only those studies being done at the investigator's site, but those being done in the same community. Those studies will also be in competition for subjects, and can have a great impact on the ability to meet enrollment targets.

Another factor is the timing for the study. If the site has too many active studies at the same time, your study may not get the attention it needs to be done well.

The CRA will want to check on the laboratory and/or pharmacy, if either will be used for the study. Are their accreditations current? Are the facilities adequate to perform the necessary study activities? If a pharmacy will be involved in drug dispensing, it is valuable to discuss the study with the pharmacist.

The CRA should be certain that the investigator is familiar with the IRB process and should determine which IRB will be used for the study. How often does the IRB meet and how long does it usually take for the IRB to review and approve a study? The time it takes to review and approve a study or documents related to a study is called "turnaround time."

Some preliminary budget discussions can take place at an evaluation visit. The CRA can discuss with the investigator how the sponsor prefers to work with respect to the budget and payments for trials. The CRA may also want to find out how the investigator normally puts together a budget. If the site looks promising, it might be appropriate to talk about the grant range that the company is willing to pay to ensure that both parties are at least in the same ballpark. Details can be left until the CRA is sure that the site is desirable to use for the study.

The CRA should be sure that a thorough evaluation of the site has been made before leaving and that notes have been made for future reference. It is appropriate to send a thank you letter to the site within a few days of the visit. If the investigator is selected to do the study, a telephone call can be made to finalize the site's willingness to participate, followed by a confirmation letter.

## Pre-Study Visit

If a study starts soon after an evaluation visit for a selected investigator, the evaluation information is current. Sometimes, however, several months can pass between the evaluation visit and the actual start date for a study. In this case, it can be valuable to do a pre-study visit to re-evaluate the site's capability to do the trial. This visit does not vary much in content from the evaluation visit, except that the investigator is already committed to do the trial. The purpose of the visit is to assure the sponsor that the site is still appropriate for the work.

At this meeting, the CRA should take time to go over the protocol in detail with the investigator. Does the investigator have a good understanding of what needs to be done, when it needs to be done, subjects that are suitable, etc.? Has the investigator changed his or her mind about any aspects of the medicine or clinical aspects involved? Are there any problems with using a placebo control or with using the comparator medicine? Sometimes if there has been quite a long time between when the protocol was written and the study is due to start, other new medications have become standard treatment for a condition and physicians may not want to use an older drug as a comparator in a trial.

Pay close attention to the investigator's attitude, interest and reactions during your discussions. The investigator may be saying one thing, but communicating something much different. Interpreting the non-verbal clues takes experience and good human relations skills; over time, a CRA can become very adept at "reading" people.

It is much better for an investigator to back out of a program before it starts than to fail at it later. An experienced CRA will let investigators know that saying a project is not right for his or her site is not a negative; saying it can be done and not doing it means a sponsor will rarely come back.

Reassess the staff and their ability to do the study at this visit. Are the same people at the site? Has there been any major staff turnover? Ask the investigator and the staff if there are plans for anyone to be away for an extended period of time during the study—you might be surprised at what you hear.

Check again for competing studies. Since several months may have passed since the last evaluation visit, the site may have started other studies in the interim. It is important to ascertain if these studies will be competing with your study for patients, coordinator time or other resources.

Be sure that the facilities are still acceptable, including storage areas for the study medication and supplies. Ensure that the pharmacy and laboratory are aware of and ready to handle their study responsibilities. If a pharmacy is to be used, find out how much storage area they have for the study drug. It may be necessary to make multiple drug shipments over time instead of sending it all at once if space is limited. (Space in pharmacies is almost always at a premium.) Be sure that the storage requirements for the study drug are clearly understood and that appropriate storage conditions are available. If, for example, your drug requires refrigeration, there should be enough capacity to store an adequate supply of the drug.

The CRA should discuss with the investigator the subject population for the study. This is a good time to review the inclusion and exclusion criteria of the protocol in detail. There may have been changes in the physician's practice since the last evaluation that could adversely affect the site's ability to enroll subjects in the trial.

Hopefully you will have all the documents necessary to start the study in-house by this time, but if not, try to collect the rest of them at this visit. (These documents are listed in Appendix C.) If the IRB has approved the study, the investigator should have a copy of the approval letter. Make a copy for your company while you are at the site if you do not have it already. If the study has not yet been approved by the IRB, find out when the IRB is meeting and when approval can be expected. If there have been any changes in the study team personnel, be sure that the correct people are listed on the 1572 form. If they are not, have the site revise the 1572 and give you a copy while you are there.

Usually the grant for the study has been agreed upon prior to this visit, but if not, now is the time. You don't want any last minute delays in a study initiation because of stalled grant negotiations. Large organizations (hospitals, university medical centers) may have a separate office that handles grants and contracts. If so, the savvy CRA will get to know this office staff, which may smooth the way for speedier negotiations.

The bottom line is whether or not you still feel comfortable about using this site to do your study. If you are having doubts, pay attention to them. Chances are that if something doesn't feel quite right, it isn't. You will always come out ahead dealing with problems before the study starts rather than later.

If the evaluation and/or pre-study visits have gone well, if you thoroughly and accurately assessed the site's ability to do your study, and if you feel comfortable about doing a study at the site, you have done the best you can to ensure a successful study start. In Chapter 10, you will learn how to help ensure the continuation of a successful study at your site.

## Key Takeaways

- The investigator is the individual who actually conducts and is responsible for a clinical investigation.
- The Statement of Investigator Form (FDA form 1572) contains pertinent investigator and site information, as well as a listing of investigator responsibilities.
- Investigators have the ultimate responsibility for the safety of subjects in a clinical trial.
- Investigators must be qualified by training and experience to study a drug/device.
- Investigators may be disqualified if they do not comply with the regulations concerning clinical research, or if they falsify data or reports of the trial.
- Some of the best ways to locate potential investigators are asking:
  - within your own company
  - for suggestions from current investigators
  - colleagues from other companies.
- A site evaluation visit is the best way to assess a site's capability to conduct a clinical trial.
- A prestudy visit should be done to reassess a site if there has been a lengthy period of time between the evaluation visit and the start date for a study.

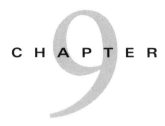
# Study Initiation

In this chapter we will discuss a number of activities that must be completed before a study site can start enrolling subjects. Topics included are: study initiation documents, financial disclosure, investigator meetings, study initiation meetings, investigator study files, and grants and contracts. CRAs are very involved in these activities and need to have a thorough understanding of them.

## Study Initiation Documents

Before a trial can begin, a number of documents must be collected for each site. Most of these are required by FDA regulations, although some sponsors may require their own additional documents. Both the sponsor and the investigator must have copies of each of these documents; usually, the originals are kept at the investigator's site, while copies are sent to the sponsor. It is recommended that the CRA also keep copies of most of them, in case one is misplaced or disappears and needs replacing during the study.

The documents listed below are the ones that a sponsor company must have before the trial may start. Note that most sponsors will not ship the study drug before receiving all of the documents.

- Signed, IRB-approved protocol and any amendments
- IRB-approved informed consent, preferably containing an IRB-approved stamp
- IRB approval letter, verifying approval of both the protocol and consent document
- IRB approval of advertising and subject recruitment materials, including subject compensation, if applicable
- Signed, completed FDA 1572 form (Statement of Investigator)
- Financial disclosure forms for the investigator and any other study personnel listed on the 1572 form
- Appropriate CVs of everyone listed on the 1572 form
- Current laboratory certification and laboratory normal ranges
- Signed contract or letter of agreement (not required by regulation, but required by most sponsors)

Some sponsor companies have specific people whose primary responsibility is to collect and maintain these documents, while in other companies the CRAs gather the documents for their sites. Since the CRA is the person who visits the site, he or she will probably be involved in the collection and maintenance of documents even if another internal group has the primary responsibility.

The one document that generally takes the longest time to get is the IRB approval letter. This is the only document not under the direct control of the investigator. The IRB may have approved the study, but until the investigator receives written notification, it is not official. The CRA may need to encourage the investigator to keep contacting the IRB, as some are slow to issue approval letters.

Most sponsors will not ship the study drug until all the documents have been received. Note that some companies do ship the case report forms and other non-drug supplies before receiving all the documents in an effort to speed the process, while others wait and ship everything only after documentation is complete.


## Financial Disclosure

On February 2, 1998, the FDA published the final rule for financial disclosure.[1] The requirement became effective a year later, and applies to any study of a drug, biologic or device that is used to support a marketing application. The regulation requires that sponsors certify the absence of certain financial interests of clinical investigators, disclose these financial interests, or certify that the information was impossible to obtain. If a sponsor does not do this, the FDA may refuse to file the application. A full description of the requirements is found in 21 CFR 54, which is included in Appendix G.

Disclosable financial arrangements, as taken from the FDA's "Guidance for Industry: Financial Disclosure for Investigators," are:

*(a) Compensation affected by the outcome of clinical studies means compensation that could be higher for a favorable outcome than for an unfavorable outcome, such as compensation that is explicitly greater for a favorable result or compensation to the investigator in the form of an equity interest in the sponsor of a covered study or in the form of compensation tied to sales of the product, such as a royalty interest.*

*(b) Significant equity interest in the sponsor of a covered study means any ownership interest, stock options, or other financial interest whose value cannot be readily determined through reference to public prices (generally, interests in a nonpublicly traded corporation), or any equity interest in a publicly traded corporation that exceeds $50,000 during the time the clinical investigator is carrying out the study and for 1 year following completion of the study.*

*(c) Proprietary interest in the tested product means property or other financial interest in the product including, but not limited to, a patent, trademark, copyright or licensing agreement.*

*(f) Significant payments of other sorts means payments made by the sponsor of a covered study to the investigator or the institution to support activities of the investigator that have a monetary value of more than $25,000, exclusive of the costs of conducting the clinical study or other clinical studies, (e.g., a grant to fund ongoing research, compensation in the form of equipment or retainers for ongoing consultation or honoraria) during the time the clinical investigator is carrying out the study and for 1 year following the completion of the study.*[2]

Financial disclosure became an issue with small biotech companies in their start-up phases, as sometimes investigators and companies had closely tied financial interests, leading to conflict of interest in the testing of potential new products.

Having a financial interest in a company or product does not mean that an investigator cannot be involved in a trial; it simply means that all parties must be aware of the potential for conflict of interest. The sponsor will want to evaluate the potential for bias based on an investigator's financial interest before deciding whether or not to use that investigator. The FDA will do the same when reviewing an NDA.

Financial disclosure applies to all the people listed on the FDA form 1572 for a study, plus their spouses and dependent children. This is one good reason for not listing unnecessary people on the 1572 form.

Financial disclosure information must be collected at study start.[4] Any changes that result in exceeding the threshold(s) must be reported during the course of the study and for one year following its completion. There is no required form for the collection of this information from the investigator. Consequently, sponsors develop their own forms and ways of collecting and maintaining this information.

Financial disclosure information must be reported to the FDA on FDA forms 3454 (certification of absence of financial interest) or 3455 (disclosure of financial interest). These forms are submitted as a part of the NDA.

Although not popular with investigators or sponsors, financial disclosure information is required to be collected, and usually CRAs are involved in the collecting of that information. Because of their involvement, it is recommended that CRAs read the FDA's "Guidance for Industry, Financial Disclosure by Clinical Investigators," which is available on the FDA's web site (www.fda.gov).

# The Investigator Meeting

For a clinical trial with six or more sites, most sponsors hold an investigator meeting. Although not required by regulation, this meeting, which includes all investigators, their coordinators and appropriate sponsor representatives, is one of the most important activities pertaining to the conduct of a good trial. This meeting is often the first time the investigators and study coordinators meet the sponsor personnel; it creates an initial impression and sets the tone for the rest of the study.

Investigator meetings may be held when there are fewer than six sites, depending on the complexity of the study. Six sites is merely a rule of thumb. Some investigator meetings include two or three hundred people, if the trial is very large. Frequently, if the meeting would be very large (e.g., over 150 attendees), two or three smaller meetings will be held instead. Smaller meetings allow more opportunity for questions and interaction among the participants. These smaller meetings may be held regionally to lessen travel. The division may also be based on which sites are ready to start the study and which sites still have documents outstanding.

Investigator meetings are scheduled and conducted by the sponsor (sometimes with the help of a contract company). The purpose of these meetings is to allow the participants to get to know each other, which facilitates communication throughout the study, and to review the entire study and its conduct. The major advantages of holding these meetings are that everyone hears the same thing at the same time, and people become acquainted. If done properly, the investigator meeting can also be a powerful motivational and training tool.

Since this meeting is so important to the success of a trial, and since CRAs are frequently very involved in these meetings, both in meeting planning and as attendees, the investigator meeting will be discussed in detail.

There are a number of things that require serious thought and planning when it comes to investigator meetings. These include when to hold the meeting, the location, who should attend, social activities and the agenda.

## Timing and location of investigator meetings

The first decision that needs to be made is when to have the investigator meeting. Since these meetings are expensive, CRAs must make every effort to ensure that all their sites are ready to start the study before the meeting. Sites that start the study more than a month or two after the investigator meeting might as well not have attended, as they will have forgotten much of the information by the time they actually start. Ideally, the study drug is shipped while the meeting is going on and the motivated investigators and their coordinators return home to immediately enroll the first patients. Unfortunately, this rarely, if ever, happens.

Getting numerous sites for a multi-center trial ready to start all at the same time is nearly impossible. Given this scenario, the sponsor should try to hold the investigator meeting when as many sites as possible are ready to start, and within a month of when the last site will be ready. The problem of determining when to hold the meeting is compounded by the fact that the meeting has to be planned so far in advance that good estimates of site readiness will not be available.

The meeting location requires a balance between business and pleasure. Everyone wants to go to a nice place for a meeting, preferably warm, with lots of things to do or see. However, from a pure business sense, the ideal place is probably at the sponsor company or at least in the same town.

If the meeting is held at the sponsor's primary location, there will be few budget restrictions on company representatives attending. Consequently, all the clerical personnel needed to make things run smoothly will be available. It will also be possible to have the professional support needed from groups such as Quality Assurance and Regulatory who attend infrequently when travel is involved. CRAs not involved with the study and other clinical or support people can attend as a learning or training experience. In addition, the investigators and coordinators can see the company and meet more employees than they would if the meeting were held elsewhere.

We tried this at our company, but the concept was not very popular because our own people wanted to "go somewhere nice" for our investigator meetings, rather than staying home. The one legitimate complaint was that it required the investigators to make a commuter air trip and many people object to that. Also, because of our location in the Midwest snow belt, local meetings between December and April were problematic.

Wherever the meeting is held, it should be in a place that is pleasant (without being too distracting) and relatively easy to get to. If possible, it should be centrally located relative to the geographic locations of the participating sites. Another important factor to keep in mind when determining a location is the budget; some locations are less expensive, both to get to, and for meeting accommodations, while others are always more costly, usually due to popularity. Expensive places cost considerably less during the off-season, but Scottsdale, Arizona, is really hot in the summertime.

## Planning and Logistics

Once the date and location have been determined, it's time to start making arrangements. Many sponsors have meeting planners who put these meetings together, so CRAs are not usually involved in this aspect of the meeting. If you do have input, remember that the meeting should be informative, yet pleasant for those attending.

An agenda and general information regarding transportation, hotel information (swimming, tennis, golf, etc.) and reimbursement procedures should be sent to all investigators at least a month prior to the meeting. If the sponsor is providing the airline tickets, they should be sent well in advance of the meeting date. Additional information and handout material should be available for participants when they check in at the hotel, if it would be useful to have prior to the meeting.

One important decision is how much time will be required for the meeting. Normally, one day is sufficient unless it is a large complicated trial. Physicians are busy people and being away from the office more than a day usually causes problems. If one day is sufficient, the meeting can be held all in the same day or during the afternoon of one day and the morning of the next. Both have their advantages and disadvantages. Many prefer the split day format as it allows attendees to arrive in the morning, and because it is split into two shorter sessions. If the agenda is planned properly, often the investigators can leave after the afternoon session if they wish. The primary disadvantage is there is little time to relax or rest prior to the start of the meeting and it may make leaving that same night difficult. Airline departures and connections for investigators must be considered.

It is appropriate to plan a social event, such as a dinner or reception, so the site and sponsor people can get to know each other in a less formal environment.

Table 1 summarizes major activities required in planning. Note that the meeting planning starts about four months in advance of the actual meeting date. The bigger the meeting, the more time it will take to plan and execute the preliminary activities.


## Preparation for meeting presentations

Frequently, the presentations for investigator meetings get the least attention, which can spell disaster. First it must be determined who from the sponsor will be attending and who will be presenting material. In cases where key personnel are simply poor speakers, or have a fear of speaking in public, someone else should do it for them. The key person should still be present and introduced as the expert in that area. That way, no one loses face.

Remember, Chapter 1 stressed that good CRAs must have good communication skills. Investigator meetings are one activity where that is very important. CRAs frequently present some topics during the meeting. If you are asked to do this, you should be prepared and should follow basic presentation procedures, e.g., speak clearly, engage the audience and use visual materials effectively.

We have all have seen copies of typed pages put on a screen and read to the audience by a presenter facing the screen. The speaker often begins by saying, "I know you probably can't read this . . ." The reaction of most attendees is, "Then why, for goodness sake, are you showing it?" Do not use visual materials that are unreadable by the audience.

**Table 1**

| Activities | Month 4 | Month 3 | Month 2 | Month 1 |
|---|---|---|---|---|
| Budget | ■ | | | |
| Select location | ■ | | | |
| Contact hotels | ■ | | | |
| Prepare reference/ instruction manuals | | ■ | | |
| Letters of invitation | | ■ | | |
| Rooming lists/requirements | | | ■ | |
| Final agenda | | | | ■ |
| Follow up letter with agenda | | | | ■ |
| Rehearsal | | | | ■ |
| Meal selections/reception | | | | ■ |
| Ship materials to hotel | | | | ■ |
| Final transportation reservations | | | | ■ |

Another key part of preparation is rehearsal, a full run-through. Unfortunately, very few companies take the time to do this. At a minimum, everyone who will be attending the meeting should be present for the rehearsal so that everyone gets a chance to hear what the others have to say before the meeting.

One of the most embarrassing things we have seen occur at an investigator meeting was when the speaker was interrupted by one of his colleagues who said, "That's not right, we don't want it done that way." Not only was it very embarrassing for the presenter, but the sponsor representatives, as a group, immediately lost credibility.

Rehearsals can prevent things like that from happening. Everyone attending from the sponsor should be instructed that if a speaker does say something that is incorrect, wait until the break, discuss it and if it needs restatement, the speaker can come back and say, "I think I misspoke when I said ..."

Another benefit from a rehearsal is that it allows the presenters to run through their material in front of an audience and also helps for checking the timing, both for individual presentations and overall. This allows for editing and overall planning.

The rehearsal should be open to people other than the attendees, as it is a good learning opportunity for less experienced people and will help prepare them for the time they become involved as a presenter. Everyone, including CRAs, should try to attend a rehearsal, or an actual meeting before having to organize and/or participate in one. It is also valuable to have some experienced people from other units or divisions attend to act as advisors. Their experience and ability to look at presentations with a fresh view are very useful.

It is recommended that a moderator be used for an investigator meeting. Companies that use moderators seem to have better meetings. The moderator should be a good speaker and a "people person." He or she usually opens the meeting, makes introductory remarks about the company, gives an overview of the meeting, makes administrative announcements, introduces company speakers and injects humor as appropriate. The moderator is a huge asset for keeping the meeting running smoothly and on time; this allows the medical monitor and other presenters to concentrate on their presentations and meeting the investigators and coordinators without having to worry about logistical matters.

## The Agenda

There is no one agenda that fits all investigator meetings. However, they will almost always contain the items shown in Table 2. An example of an expanded agenda is shown in Table 3. These can be used as starting points for planning a meeting, with other items added and deleted as appropriate.

---

**Table 2: Investigator Meeting Agenda—Basic**

- Introduction of attendees
- Introductory remarks about the company in general
- Background of the project
- Discussion of the protocol
- Administrative responsibilities of investigator and sponsor (and/or CRO) personnel involved in the study
- Sponsor procedures and expectations
    - Monitoring
    - Data collection
    - Adverse event reporting
    - Other sponsor specific issues
- Financial matters
- Miscellaneous

---

## Table 3: Investigator Meeting Agenda—Expanded

- Welcome
  - Introductions
    - The company (very brief promotion)
    - Individuals and their roles
    - Investigators and their staff members
- Overview of the drug development program (include significant timelines, dates)
- Discussion of the Protocol (avoid a page by page review)
  - Objectives
  - Study overview
  - Main protocol areas
  - Design
    - Primary efficacy endpoints
    - Entry criteria
    - Drug (formulation, dosing and regimen)
    - Risk/benefit
    - Medical events
    - Methods and materials
    - Any special procedures required
- Administration
  - Responsibilities and obligations of the investigator
  - Informed consent
  - The IRB
  - Forms requiring signatures
  - Study documents
    - Protocol, IRB approvals, etc., and filing requirements.
  - Financial matters
- Study Materials
  - Clinical supplies
    - Packaging, ordering and receipt (have sample packages if there is anything unique or unusual)
    - Drug accountability
    - Drug dispensing procedure, forms
    - Reorder procedure
    - Storage
    - Inventory and return
- Laboratory
  - Exhibit forms, supplies, mailers, etc.
  - Demonstrate any unusual procedures
- Special Procedures and Forms
  - Diaries (if used)
  - Demonstrate special medical procedures if appropriate (treadmill, Holter monitor, etc.)
  - Training, rater certification

### Table 3: Investigator Meeting Agenda—Expanded (continued)

- − Procedures for randomization and breaking the blind
- ■ Case Report Forms
  - − Design
  - − How /when to complete
  - − Source document management
  - − Correction procedures
- ■ Closing remarks and questions

## Attendees

Who should attend investigator meetings? Key people from both the sponsor and the sites should be there; other attendees may be determined by the budget. Table 4 shows the usual cast of mandatory and optional attendees from both the sponsor and investigator sites.

### Table 4: Investigator Meeting Attendees

| Investigator site attendees | Sponsor attendees |
|---|---|
| Mandatory attendees: | Mandatory attendees: |
| ■ Investigator | ■ Investigator |
| ■ Clinical research coordinator | ■ CRA(s) |
| | ■ Biostatistician |
| Optional attendees: | ■ Project manager |
| ■ Co-investigator | ■ Data manager |
| ■ Research Manager | ■ Laboratory person (usually from a |
| ■ Pharmacists | central lab) |
| ■ Dietician | ■ Moderator, if one is used |
| ■ Others as appropriate | ■ Designated presenters |
| | ■ Meeting facilitator, if needed |
| | |
| | Optional attendees: |
| | ■ Management (Medical director, etc.) |
| | ■ Other monitors, CRAs |
| | ■ Regulatory representative |
| | ■ QA person |
| | ■ Secretary |
| | ■ Consultants, if appropriate |

Remember that one main purpose of the meeting is for sponsor personnel and site personnel to become acquainted. Sometimes the CRAs are the only ones who know people in both groups before the meeting. The CRA should take responsibility for the people attending from his or her sites. The CRA should ensure that the investigators and coordinators are introduced to the appropriate sponsor representatives they may come in contact with during the study, that they are taken care of and have all the meeting materials, and that they have a good and informative meeting. If site personnel have any unanswered questions at the end of the meeting, the CRA should get the information to them within a few days.

As a CRA, you should act as the host for your sites. Let the physicians and the coordinators know that they are critical to the success of your study. Ask your site people questions and listen to the answers. Spend time with them. This meeting is an excellent opportunity to establish good relationships with your site personnel, which can make the study go smoothly for you as it gets under way.

### Evaluation and Critique

It is important to evaluate how the investigator meeting went and was perceived. To help with this, it is useful to have evaluation forms that attendees will complete. They do not need to be complicated. Sample evaluation forms are shown in Tables 5a and 5b.

---

**Table 5a: Investigator Meeting Evaluation Form**

Protocol_____     Date:_____

Please complete this form before you leave to assist us in evaluating and improving our meetings. (Include instructions for where to leave the form.) If you forget, please mail it to us at: (insert address)

| Please rate the level of satisfaction with the facility: | High | | | | Low |
|---|---|---|---|---|---|
| ■  Accommodations | 5 | 4 | 3 | 2 | 1 |
| ■  Food | 5 | 4 | 3 | 2 | 1 |
| ■  Meeting room | 5 | 4 | 3 | 2 | 1 |
| ■  Location | 5 | 4 | 3 | 2 | 1 |

| Meeting planning: | High | | | | Low |
|---|---|---|---|---|---|
| ■  Pre-meeting communication | 5 | 4 | 3 | 2 | 1 |
| ■  Organization of meeting | 5 | 4 | 3 | 2 | 1 |
| ■  Agenda | 5 | 4 | 3 | 2 | 1 |

[ ]   Too long
[ ]   Too short
[ ]   Too little (much) time on some items (specify)

Sessions of least value _____

Sessions of most value_____

Suggestions for improvement _____

---

After each investigator meeting, the sponsor should have a critique of the meeting, including a discussion of the evaluations. This should help in determining what was done well and should be repeated at future meetings, as well as what should be changed or eliminated. Critiquing past meetings is an excellent tool for improving future meetings; each meeting should be better than the last one.

**Table 5b: Session Evaluations**

| Session: _____ | Presented by: _____ | | | | |
|---|---|---|---|---|---|
| Please rate the presenter of this session in the following areas: | High | | | Low | |
| ■ Speaking quality | 5 | 4 | 3 | 2 | 1 |
| ■ Adequately established objectives at the beginning of the session | 5 | 4 | 3 | 2 | 1 |
| ■ Presented material in a clear understandable manner | 5 | 4 | 3 | 2 | 1 |
| ■ Material was in a logical sequence | 5 | 4 | 3 | 2 | 1 |
| ■ Provided useful information | 5 | 4 | 3 | 2 | 1 |
| ■ Effective use of audio visual aids | 5 | 4 | 3 | 2 | 1 |
| ■ Adequately summarized material | 5 | 4 | 3 | 2 | 1 |
| ■ Provided adequate opportunity for participation/questions | 5 | 4 | 3 | 2 | 1 |
| ■ Responded satisfactorily to questions and comments | 5 | 4 | 3 | 2 | 1 |
| Comments: _____ | | | | | |

# Study Initiation Meetings

The study initiation visit (sometimes known as the startup visit) is held at the investigator's site just before the study begins. The CRA (and sometimes additional sponsor personnel) will meet with the investigator and the supporting staff. The purpose of the meeting is to review the study protocol, processes and procedures to ensure that all site personnel understand what is necessary to perform the study.

The study initiation should be held at the point when all regulatory paperwork is complete for the site and the study drug and other supplies have been shipped, but before any subjects have been enrolled. Many sponsors will not allow the site to begin enrollment until after this meeting is held.

The CRA must be flexible when it comes to scheduling the meeting; to maximize attendance, it may need to be held early in the morning, in the evening, or even on a weekend. A good, thorough, informative initiation meeting may take half a day, or even longer for a very complicated study.

The CRA is almost always in charge of the initiation meeting, although the sponsor medical monitor and/or an in-house associate monitor may also be present. It is important that all site personnel who will be involved in the study attend the meeting, including ancillary personnel such as the sub-investigators, other coordinators, the pharmacist, dietician, lab person, etc.

If the investigator and coordinator attended an investigator meeting, the initiation visit will serve as a review and amplification of the topics covered during that meeting. If there was no investigator meeting, or if it was held a month or more prior to initiating the study, then the entire protocol, processes and procedure should be discussed in detail. Since the investigator and study coordinator are usually the only site people who attend the investigator meeting, other site personnel will not be as familiar with the study. The initiation meeting provides an opportunity for everyone at the site to become familiar with the study and to understand everyone's study role.

## Preparing for the Initiation Visit

Proper preparation for an initiation visit is important. The CRA should think about how to conduct the meeting and what should be addressed. On occasion, the sponsor's medical monitor will want to attend the meeting, particularly if it is the first time the investigator has done work for the sponsor. In this case, the CRA will need to determine what role the medical monitor would like to play and plan accordingly. However, the CRA should be in charge of the meeting.

The CRA must prepare an agenda. Much of the same material will be covered at the initiation meeting that was covered at the investigator meeting, if one was held. The agenda and the amount of detail to be covered at the initiation visit will depend on: if there was an investigator meeting and who attended; how long it has been since the investigator meeting was held; the involvement of other personnel at the site (pharmacist, etc.); the complexity of the program; and how much time you are allowed for the meeting.

**The items to be covered at an initiation meeting are:**

- Detailed discussion of the protocol, including:
  - Inclusion and exclusion criteria
  - Study procedures
  - Administration of the study drug
    - Randomization and blinding
  - Primary outcome measures
  - Other pertinent details
- Drug accountability
- Adverse event reporting
- Case report forms (going over each unique form in detail)
  - How to avoid errors (See more about this in Chapter 10—Monitoring)
- Monitoring visits—how often, what should be ready, what will be covered
- Regulatory requirements

- Investigator responsibilities
- IRB interactions
■ Any other study-specific or sponsor-specific items of importance
  - Periodic reports of enrollment

It is recommended that the CRA rehearse before the meeting—even if it's in front of the mirror—to check for timing, to be sure the material is clear and understood and even for word pronunciation. It is embarrassing to find out that you don't understand, or can't pronounce, something at the time you are presenting it. There is nothing harder than explaining a process to someone else when you don't understand it yourself.

If the CRA is not comfortable with any of the study procedures, he or she should ask for help and/or clarification before the meeting. For example, if the CRA is not comfortable with the data management and correction process, it should be reviewed with the data management people supporting the study.

If a study instruction manual has been developed, the CRA should be familiar with what is in it and how the site is expected to use it; if the site does not have one yet, plan to take it with you to the meeting. [Note: The study instruction manual is simply a guide for sites that explains study procedures in detail. It is a quick reference, and will usually include practical hints and tips that would not be found in a protocol.]

## During the initiation visit

This meeting involves several people. Since the CRA is in charge, he or she should always be on time or a little early. If you have a morning meeting and it's out of town, plan to arrive the day before. Be sure you know where you are going and how long it will take to get there, allowing for problems like morning rush hour traffic, and plan accordingly. Depending on the time of day, it is a nice gesture to arrange for coffee and rolls, or other refreshments.

Start the meeting by saying how pleased you are to be there and how much you are looking forward to working with them on the study. If people don't know each other, let everyone introduce themselves. Then start on the agenda.

It is important that people know they can ask questions as you go along. The main purpose of the meeting is for everyone to have a clear understanding of what is involved in doing the study. It is far better to answer questions now than to have things done incorrectly later. Take your time. Solicit questions periodically. Look around and see if people look perplexed or look comfortable. This is one of those times when a CRA's interpersonal skills are critical.

If certain attendees are not able to stay for the entire meeting (investigator, pharmacist), be sure to cover the items critical to their participation while they are there. Other items, such as completing case report forms, can be covered with the coordinators (and others who may be involved) in a smaller group.

When the formal presentation part of the meeting is complete, there are some additional activities the CRA should do before leaving. One is to check the study drug and other study supplies to be certain they arrived in good condition, and are appropriate and in the proper quantities. If computer equipment was provided, be sure it is in order, set up properly and working. Check with the pharmacy to be sure that they understand the drug dispensing, if appropriate. Check the investigator's study file to be sure that all the necessary documents are present and correct. If the file has not yet been set up, the CRA can help with this. (See next section, "Investigator Study Files.")

When everything has been covered, the CRA should be sure to thank everyone involved before leaving. One of the important intangibles at this meeting is the opportunity it gives the CRA to establish good working relationships with all the site personnel. Do everything possible to make the people at the site feel good about you, the study and the sponsor. This will pay huge dividends as the study progresses.

After the meeting, the CRA must complete a visit report detailing what was discussed and completed during the visit. Many companies have a special visit report for this meeting. ICH guidelines call for a trial initiation monitoring report that documents that trial procedures were covered with the investigator and his or her staff; this report is to be kept in both the sponsor and investigator study files.[3] The same purpose can be accomplished by sending the investigator a letter listing what was covered during the meeting.

If questions arose during the meeting that need further follow up, the CRA must be sure to find out the information and relay it to the site. A written thank you letter is a nice gesture on the part of the CRA.

Doing this meeting well will go a long way in helping the site do a successful study. It deserves the full attention of the CRA.


## Investigator Study Files

Either before or during the initiation meeting, the CRA should discuss with the investigator and coordinator how to establish and maintain an investigator study file. This file will have significant impact on the quality assurance for a study and, subsequently, the validity and usability of the data.

If the site is experienced, this will be a routine activity. If the site is new or relatively new, the CRA should be prepared to recommend how the files should be organized and to instruct the site regarding the documents that must be maintained in the file.

By regulation (21CFR 312.62), the investigator must keep records relating to disposition of the study drug, including dates, quantity and use by study subjects, and case histories, including case report forms and all supporting documentation. Supporting documentation includes the signed and dated consent form, medical records, progress notes, hospital charts, nursing notes and any other source documents. It should also be documented that informed consent was obtained prior to the subject's participation.

This is the minimum by regulation. In reality, study files contain much more information. One recommendation is to have three major categories for study files: Regulatory, Administrative and Clinical. Investigator files organized under this system would look like this:

### In the regulatory files, the following will be kept:

- Completed FDA form 1572 (Statement of Investigator)
- Copies of the CV for the investigator and sub-investigators
- IRB approved consent form
- Written IRB approval of the protocol (study) and consent form, and advertising and subject compensation, if applicable
- Signed copy of the protocol and any amendments
- Copies of the laboratory certification and normal ranges
- Investigator brochure

### In the administrative section of the file, the following will be kept:

- Correspondence and telephone logs, including contacts with the sponsor, CRO (if involved), IRB and the institution (if applicable)
- Instructional material
  - CRF completion/correction
  - Guidelines for handling adverse events
  - Procedures for handling and storing laboratory specimens
  - Study drug information, including instructions for storing, dispensing and accounting
- Drug shipment, dispensing and return records
- Sponsor/CRO contact information
- Log of study subjects (Master Study Subject Roster)
- Records of meetings and contact with the sponsor and/or CRO
- Monitoring log (a record of CRA monitoring visits)
- Miscellaneous

### The investigator will also have a clinical file for each study subject, which will include:

- CRFs and supporting documents for each subject
- Signed consent form

Files will vary depending on the site, the sponsor and the nature of the studies.

There are two items not mentioned in the list above: the grant and any reports from sponsor QA audits. This information is not routinely made available to FDA auditors and should not be kept in study files.

File retention is discussed in Chapter 13, Study Closeout. However, investigators must be aware from the start of the study that all study documents must be retained long after the study is over.

The CRA can be a valuable help to the site in assisting it with setting up and maintaining its files throughout the study. The CRA must also check the files regularly throughout the study and again at study closure. Being sure that the files are in order periodically during the study will ensure that they are in order in the event of an audit of the site by the sponsor, the IRB or the FDA. Some companies provide clearly marked containers for study files to help minimize loss after the study is completed.

# Grants and Contracts

Involvement of the CRA in grant negotiation and investigator contracts varies considerably among sponsors. In general, the larger the company, the less the CRA is involved; this is because large companies tend to have a separate department that handles the financial aspects of trials. However, CRAs need to have an understanding of the grant and contract process in order to work well with study sites.

## Grants

The average grant per patient received by sites in 2002 was $6,716, and this figure has been growing steadily, but slowly, at less than 5% annually over the past ten years.[4] When this figure is adjusted for inflation, it has stayed essentially flat, although protocols have become more difficult and call for significantly more procedures, on average, during the same time period. This means that sites must be careful about whether or not they can actually afford to do a study, without losing money, and that they will most likely be much more selective about the projects they decide to take on.

A good CRA will have an understanding of how grants are determined, both by the sponsor and by the investigator. Frequently the CRA can help negotiations along to everyone's benefit.

Most sponsors operate on a fee-for-service basis. This means that they will pay for actual work performed, i.e., subjects enrolled and subject visits. Most grants are formulated on a per-subject amount and prorated for the number of visits a subject actually completes. The amount per visit will often vary, as some visits are more labor- and time-intensive than others. Sponsors feel that they are buying a service from the investigator and do not expect to pay if the work (subjects and data) is not delivered.

There are a few different ways in which grant figures are determined. Many of the larger companies subscribe to a service from DataEdge called PICAS. PICAS is a computer program that is used to calculate grant figures. Briefly, all the subscribers put their grant information into the system (blinded, of course) by the type of study, the procedures involved, site loca-

## Table 6: Budget Worksheet—Protocol XXX

| Study Activity | Number of visits | Cost | Expanded cost |
|---|---|---|---|
| Phone pre-screen | 1 | 50 | 50 |
| Medical history | 1 | 50 | 50 |
| Physical exam | 3 | 150 | 450 |
| Labs | 8 | 150 | 1200 |
| EKG | 3 | 200 | 600 |
| Treadmill stress test | 3 | 250 | 750 |
| Office visit—general assessments | 8 | 75 | 600 |
| Phone assessments | 2 | 50 | 100 |
| **Sub-total for procedures** | | | **$3800** |
| Coordinator time | 8 | 50 | 400 |
| Pharmacy charge | 8 | 35 | 280 |
| **Subtotal** | | | **$680** |
| **Total** | | | **$4480** |
| Overhead—15% | | | 672 |
| **Grand total per completed subject** | | | **$5152** |

tions and amounts. The data from all the companies form a huge informational database. When starting a new protocol, the subscriber can enter all the protocol procedures into PICAS and get back subject costs, including ranges, averages and deciles, overall and regionally. This gives the sponsor a very realistic grant range to work from when determining how much they wish to pay for per patient grants. PICAS is probably the best method available for determining realistic grants based on actual data.

Some sponsors will determine a range or a single per-subject grant figure that they will pay and will not budge from this figure. Investigators either accept it or will not be able to do the study. Other sponsors will allow more flexibility, depending on experience with an investigator or geographic location. Costs do differ in different parts of the country, so it makes sense to allow some flexibility.

Some companies expect their CRAs to negotiate grants with their investigators. Ideally, there will be a range or a starting figure given for the negotiations. A CRA must understand enough about calculating reasonable grants to help a site, especially if the site is inexperienced and has not done this before.

A good way to come up with a grant figure is to look at each study activity, have the investigator attach a cost to it, add an additional amount for overhead and other required activities and total it up. An example of a grant worksheet for a hypothetical study is shown in Table 6.

For this hypothetical study, there are eight visits. One common way to determine a prorating schedule is to look at the visits and the amount of work to be done at each visit. If some visits demand considerably more work than others, count them as two visits; generally speaking, the baseline visit and the final visit are the most demanding.

In the example shown in Table 7, there are three visits that are more labor-intensive, (Visits 1, 5 and 8) the three that involve physical exams and stress testing. To determine the prorating dollar amount, each of these visits should count as two and the other five visits should each count as one, for a total of eleven. If the cumulative amount of $5,152 is divided by 11, the cost per visit is $468.36. Based on this, the three more intensive visits should be prorated at $937, and the other five at $468 (with the extra dollar added to the cost of the last visit). Note in Table 7 that if a subject drops out after visit 3, the investigator would be paid $1,837. For a subject dropping at Week 7, the payment would be $4,214, and so forth.

### Table 7: Grant Amounts for One Subject

|  | Visit 1 | Visit 2 | Visit 3 | Visit 4 | Visit 5 | Visit 6 | Visit 7 | Visit 8 |
|---|---|---|---|---|---|---|---|---|
| Amount per visit | $937 | $468 | $468 | $468 | $937 | $468 | $468 | $938 |
| Cumulative amount | $937 | $1405 | $1837 | $2341 | $3278 | $3746 | $4214 | $5152 |

This is a simple way of calculating grants and prorating visit costs, but it is quite effective if the initial amounts for each procedure and activity are realistic. It is easy to explain and should help the CRA in negotiating a grant amount that is fair to both the sponsor and the investigator.

When a grant has been agreed upon and the study is under way, the CRA's responsibilities for grant activities are again variable. Some companies utilize the CRA in determining when grant monies should be paid, while others handle all grant payments in-house without the CRA's involvement. These companies usually pay either on a timed schedule, such as quarterly, or on the basis of case report forms received in-house. Whatever the scheme, the CRA should understand what it is, and be able to discuss it with the investigator.

Note that many companies will pay a small amount of the grant up front (maybe two subjects' worth), but will then apply this amount to the work being done. This allows the investigator to set up study procedures, pay for initial labs and other tests, etc., without having to use site funds.

If grant payments are based on input from the CRA, the CRA will need to keep track of the work done and payments made. It is advisable not to pay in advance, with the exception of a possible up-front payment, just in case the site does not enroll any subjects at all. If an investigator is paid in advance and doesn't earn that amount, there is always the sticky business of trying to get the funds back. This is unpleasant for both the sponsor and the investigator, and even more so for the CRA, who is often caught in the middle.

Although some CRAs find it difficult to be involved in negotiating and paying grants, it does add stature in the eye of the investigator, and does give the CRA more clout at the site. No matter how involved the CRA is, he or she should have a good understanding of both the process and the specifics for a site, in order to be able to discuss the grant with the investigator and answer any site questions.

## Contracts

A contract between the sponsor and the investigator will be signed before the trial starts at a site. This document usually contains the responsibilities of the investigator, including the number of subjects the site is expecting to enroll, timelines for enrollment, grant amounts and the regulatory requirements for the investigator. It also contains the responsibilities of the sponsor, including when and how grants will be paid, monitoring of the study and sponsor regulatory requirements. It will be signed by the appropriate company representative, and by the investigator. [Note that in large institutions contracts may be signed by someone in the contract office rather than by the investigator.]

Contracts are rarely written, negotiated or signed by the CRA. The CRA may, however, be asked to take the contract to the investigator and/or collect the signed contract. The CRA will want to have a copy of the contract, if possible, to know what was agreed to for enrollment, timelines and payment schedules.

# Key Takeaways

### Study Documents

- There are a number of documents that are required before a study can begin at a site.
- Most sponsors will not ship the study drug until all required documents are collected.
- Copies of all documents must be kept in both the site's and the sponsor's study files.
- The CRA should keep track of the IRB approval process and letter, so the study is not unduly delayed.

### Financial Disclosure

- The purpose of financial disclosure is to identify any potential conflict of interest that could bias a clinical trial.
- Financial disclosure information must be gathered for all people listed on the 1572, and their immediate family members.
- These data are collected for the time period of the study and one year following.
- Financial disclosure information is reported to the FDA when the NDA is filed.

### Investigator Meetings

- All investigators and coordinators, as well as relevant sponsor personnel, should attend the meeting.
- The meeting should be held at the time when most sites are ready to enroll.
- The purpose of an investigator meeting is to ensure that all sites have the same understanding of all protocol and administrative procedures.
- Sponsors should always have a full rehearsal before the meeting.
- CRAs should act as the host for their respective sites and ensure that site personnel meet the sponsor representatives.

### Study Initiation Visit

- The purpose of an initiation meeting is to ensure that everyone at the site has a clear and accurate understanding of how the study is to be done.
- This meeting should be held after a site has all the study supplies, including the study drug, but before study personnel enroll any subjects.
- All relevant site personnel should be present for the meeting.
- The CRA is in charge of the meeting.
- The meeting should be documented in both the investigator's and sponsor's study files.

### Investigator's Study Files

- Investigators are required to keep study records and documents both during the trial and after the trial is closed.
- CRAs can help the investigator set up and organize these files and must check them regularly throughout the study.
- Maintaining files appropriately will ensure that they are in order for an audit.
- It is often simple to catch and correct problems with the files on an ongoing basis throughout the study. It may be impossible to correct the files when the study is over.

### Grants and Contracts

- A CRA should be knowledgeable about grants and how they are calculated.
- If involved in payments, the CRA must track the study progress to keep abreast of money owed.
- Most grants are prorated by visit for each subject.
- Contracts between the sponsor and the investigator are signed before the study starts at the site.

### References

1. Guidance, Financial Disclosure by Clinical Investigators www.fda.gov/oc/guidance/financialdis.html.
2. 21CFR312.53 and 21CFR812.43 (devices).

3. ICH Guidelines for Good Clinical Practice 8.2.20.
4. DataEdge, CenterWatch analysis.

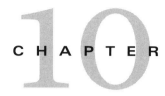

# Study Monitoring

This chapter will discuss the CRA's main activity: study monitoring. In previous chapters, we discussed the importance of a good protocol, case report forms, investigator selection, investigator meetings and startup and initiation meetings in producing high quality clinical trials. Without good study monitoring, however, the best preparation will not produce a high quality study. Poor study monitoring is probably the largest single contributor to inferior study quality.

A good CRA can produce good studies under a variety of circumstances, with investigators and protocols of varying quality. On the other hand, a poor CRA will almost always generate a substandard study, regardless of the quality of the protocol and experience of the investigator. Good CRA site monitoring and management are essential for good studies.

## The Game Plan for Monitoring

The game plan used in athletics is a strategy that the coach and players develop before each game and includes what needs to be done to maximize the chance of winning. It changes for each game because the conditions, circumstances and opposition are different each time. So it is with monitoring. No two study sites are the same, even if they are following the same protocol. A CRA should spend some time putting together a monitoring plan, including both general and specific information for each site. The primary components addressed in this plan are: how the study will be monitored, how often and specific activities to be performed.

## How to Monitor

How to monitor a study in the field (meaning you must travel from your company to the study site) requires considerable thought. Almost all field monitoring requires regular visits to the site by the CRA throughout the period of the study. On very rare occasions, an extremely simple, low risk study might be monitored almost exclusively by telephone except for the startup and closeout visits.

A CRA must determine how to integrate telephone, email, fax and regular mail communications into a monitoring strategy. This will differ for different programs and sites. It will depend on the technologies available, sponsor and site SOPs and personal preference, both at the site and at the sponsor company. In monitoring, like any business, many problems can be traced back to a lack of communication, inappropriate communication and/or unclear communication. A good communication strategy should have a high priority in your monitoring plan.

The intensity of monitoring will vary across studies and among sites. Must or should the CRA be present while the site is seeing study subjects? Will the CRA have any interaction with study subjects? In early phase I studies, the CRA may be required to be present during all or part of a subject's treatment. Therefore, the CRA must determine how long he or she will need to be there and make appropriate arrangements.

Sometimes a CRA is the sole monitor for a site, while at other times the CRA will team monitor with other CRAs. Establishing who will monitor requires consideration of the sponsor's SOPs for field monitoring, the complexity of the protocol, the condition being studied, the experience of the investigator and his or her staff and the training and experience of the CRA.

The CRA's overall monitoring plan should remain fairly consistent, but the strategy for individual sites may change considerably during the course of the study, depending on study conditions and site performance.

## Frequency of Monitoring Visits

Another key determination in a monitoring plan is the frequency with which the CRA will visit each site. There are a number of factors that must be considered in making this decision:

- Complexity of the protocol
- Disease being evaluated
- Experience of the investigator/staff
- Number of study subjects enrolled at the site
- Rate of enrollment

- Site performance
- Sponsor monitoring SOPs
- CRA experience and effectiveness

The protocol dictates the conduct of the study by establishing the procedures that subjects must undergo and their frequency. The more activities that are required during a study visit, the more monitoring will be required. The disease being studied also dictates the frequency of visits. If, for example, the CRA is monitoring an infectious disease study, the course of therapy will probably be complete for each subject in about ten days. This requires a different frequency of visits than a cholesterol-lowering study with a treatment period of one or two years.

All sites should be visited soon after the first subject or two are enrolled just to be sure the site understands and is correctly following protocol procedures. Catching and solving problems early will save a lot of extra work as the study progresses.

The rate of enrollment will also affect monitoring frequency. Generally speaking, the more subjects a site has, the more frequently the CRA will have to visit. The faster a site enrolls and the more data generated, the more frequently the site will need monitoring.

The CRA should visit a site regularly even though enrollment may be slow or non-existent. Slow subject enrollment may indicate a lack of enthusiasm on the part of site personnel regarding the study. In that case, a bit of CRA encouragement may help, which will probably involve visits. Site personnel often view frequent visits by the CRA as an indication of the importance of their study to the sponsor. Not only that, but seeing the CRA walk through the door reminds the site of their commitment to enroll subjects and complete the study on time. Call it encouragement or call it guilt—it generally works. Sometimes a few extra visits are all that is necessary to get a study back on track or to re-establish priorities at the site.

The frequency and duration of monitoring visits will also vary from site to site depending on the experience of the investigator and their staff. A less experienced site may require more or longer monitoring visits, especially at the beginning of the study. Once the site has demonstrated the ability to do the study well, the CRA may be able to space the monitoring visits further apart.

In some instances, sponsor SOPs dictate the frequency of monitoring visits. If so, the SOP normally establishes a minimum schedule, e.g., "all sites must be visited every six weeks or less." In this case, the CRA must adjust the visit schedule to ensure compliance with the SOP.

The frequency of monitoring visits may change as the study progresses. Some sites will do a better job complying with GCPs than others and may need less frequent monitoring. Subject enrollment may complete or level off after a period of time, allowing for more time between monitoring visits. Subject visits may spread out over the course of long-term studies and require less review; for example, weekly visits may be required initially, followed by monthly, and perhaps even quarterly, visits as the study progresses. In short, a CRA must visit each site often enough to stay on top of the activities that are required for good monitoring. The more experience the CRA has, the easier making this determination will be.

Another factor that has an impact on CRA visit frequency is the number and location of sites for which he or she has monitoring responsibility. There is always the chance that the CRA simply cannot physically visit the sites as often as he or she would like to or need to because of travel time and the actual number and location of sites. Here again, the CRA will have to spend some time integrating travel requirements with site experience and study complexity.

The CRA should schedule four hours at the very least for a site visit. With the complexity of protocols, regulatory requirements and good monitoring practice, the CRA will need to spend a day or more at most sites. Creative scheduling of your travel itinerary is a must. It helps to use the "loop method" for travel, where the sites closest together are linked in your itinerary for a single trip. (See Appendix B for additional tips on traveling.)

As a general rule, a good CRA should be able to effectively monitor twelve to eighteen sites. The number will change depending on the complexity of the study, site and CRA experience and locations. If the CRA is in a situation where it is simply impossible to be able to visit sites with the degree of frequency necessary for good monitoring, this should be discussed with his or her supervisor.

## Monitoring Activity

The CRA should have a general plan for what will be monitored at each site visit. Most sponsors have a site visit report or monitoring report that the CRA completes during and after a site visit. This report is a standard document that a CRA will use for all field monitoring visits. It serves as both a checklist for the CRA and as documentation of the visit. However, the CRA must not view this as the only list of activities that must be done.

To be successful as a CRA, it is important to develop a sense for what you should monitor at each site and how much attention should be given to each activity. It helps to be aware of where problems are most likely to arise during the conduct of a study. A good indication of potential problems is the list of activities that receive the most deficiencies during FDA audits. This list is published annually by the Center for Drug Evaluation and Research (CDER) and has remained essentially unchanged for over a decade. The most recent top five deficiency categories for site inspections, as reported in 2001 Report to the Nation,[1] are:

- Failure to follow the protocol
- Failure to keep adequate and accurate records
- Problems with the informed consent form
- Failure to report adverse events
- Failure to account for the disposition of study drugs

These areas, in addition to the things the sponsor wants emphasized, should receive specific attention during monitoring visits. Sponsor expectations for studies are important. Independent CRAs and those employed by CROs need to spend enough time with sponsors' representatives to clearly understand those expectations.

Many successful CRAs rely heavily on checklists that they have developed and refined over time. Basic checklists cover those things that should always be reviewed, regardless of the program, sponsor or site. This list can be modified as needed to fit each monitoring assignment. Sample checklists are in Appendix C. If a CRA thinks experience is a substitute for checklists, remember that all airline pilots use checklists every time they fly, regardless of how many hours of flying time they have. Which plane would you prefer to fly on? One whose pilot uses a checklist or one whose pilot figures personal experience is enough to ensure the safety of the flight?

---

**Checklists**

*"I have trained new CRAs and CRA Managers, and I always impress upon these folks the importance of using a checklist, no matter how brief it is. Toward the end of my career as a CRA, I was training a new CRA in Pittsburgh. We were going to do site/investigator evaluations that day, and I had told him to have a checklist for the various meetings. The first interview went fairly well, but he left out a few things. After the visit, we discussed the fact that he had not used a checklist. The second interview went the same as the first, and the ensuing discussion was the same. It was the third interview that really gave me pause to wonder if the person would make it as a CRA. Once again, no checklist was utilized. The person seemed to have asked all the right questions, except for one: "How many patients do you have, doctor, who might qualify for this study?" I had to ask it for him. On our way back to the car, the young man looked at me and said, "I guess I should have used a checklist."*

*—A CRA Friend*

---

## Preparing for a Monitoring Visit

Once the CRA has a good idea of how to monitor, what to monitor and how frequently to monitor, it is time to prepare for the visit. There is a military saying: "Proper Preparation Prevents Poor Performance." Remembering the "5 Ps" will serve you well. A CRA should spend a considerable amount of time preparing for each site visit.

In addition to a working knowledge of good clinical practice (GCP) and any state and/or local requirements, the CRA must know everything possible about the activity at the site, the protocol and the sponsor's monitoring SOPs before arriving at the site. A CRA's preparation will be evident to the investigator and his or her staff; a lack of preparation can cause a loss of credibility. Once a CRA has lost credibility, control of the site and the ability to generate a good study diminishes significantly. It takes an enormous amount of extra work to re-establish lost credibility, if it can be done at all. Remember that "you only get one chance to create a good first impression." Establishing and maintaining a high level of credibility should be among a CRA's primary goals. The easiest way to achieve credibility is to be prepared.

One of the things a CRA should do is set up travel files for each site he or she monitors. These files should contain the items shown in Table 1. It is also useful to have a small travel kit containing mailing envelopes and labels, paper clips, pens, pencils, Post-It® notes, note pad, and your calendar/planner/PDA. Your files should also contain any other items you think would be of value when you are at the site. These files should be kept current. When preparing to leave for a monitoring trip, the CRA can simply pull the files for the sites to be visited. It also helps to have a generic travel file that includes checklists and a copy of the regulations (there are copies of some of the pertinent regulations in Appendix G). When leaving for a monitoring visit, the CRA can easily pack the generic file, the site-specific files, and any other necessary supplies, and he or she is ready to go.

---

**Table 1: Travel File Content**

- Personal notes
- Copies of the last site visit report
- Study progress or enrollment logs
- Key site documents
  - Protocol
  - 1572
  - Latest drug shipment form(s)
- Pertinent correspondence

---

Prior to a site visit, the CRA should check with colleagues who are involved in the development program for the investigational drug, particularly the sponsor's medical monitor. This is especially important for CRAs who are based regionally and may not be aware of correspondence or other communications that have occurred between the site and the sponsor since the last visit. The CRA should also check for any authorized protocol deviations or other changes in the conduct of the study at the site, as well as changes in enrollment or other study-related activity.

Some sponsors have in-house CRAs who oversee study activity, particularly error correction and data management, by monitoring incoming case report forms. Some of these in-house monitors have frequent contact with study site personnel. If a CRA is field-based, he or she should check with the in-house CRA to see what has transpired at a site since the last monitoring visit. The in-house CRA may also maintain some site performance or status logs; the CRA should review current copies of these documents prior to a site visit.

Before leaving for a monitoring visit, the CRA should contact the site by phone to confirm the visit. This serves a number of purposes. First, it reminds the site of the visit. Second, it confirms that the necessary site personnel will be there and available; if key people will not be available during the visit, it should probably be rescheduled. This call also allows the CRA to remind site personnel of expectations for the visit, any prior preparation that is needed and approximately how long the visit will last. Finally, it can help to avoid a wasted trip if the site is not prepared for the visit, or if there has been a scheduling change or misunderstanding about the date.

Lastly, know where you are going. This may sound funny, but there are stories of CRAs who have become hopelessly lost on their first visit because they did not take the time to get directions or study a map. (There is more on travel in Appendix B.) As a hint, place the directions for finding each site in its travel file—including how to find the office in the hospital, etc. It's easy to forget when monitoring several sites and visiting only every six weeks or so.

If the CRA has prepared properly for a visit, the site will be expecting his or her arrival and will also have prepared for the visit.

# Site Monitoring Visits

### Professionalism

Before getting into the details of monitoring a site, it is important to have a short discussion of conduct and appearance. Even in today's casual environment, it's important to look and act professional. CRAs can get off to a bad start because of the way they work and dress. The CRA should wear appropriate business attire and should always arrive at the site on time or a little early. The CRA must remember that he or she is an official representative of the sponsor and should always behave in an appropriate business-like manner.

Monitoring requires a lot of unsupervised time "on the road;" consequently, CRAs must have excellent self-discipline. There are many temptations when traveling that can distract a CRA from work—shopping, museums, television or the latest bestseller. Although there may be some down-time when in the field, the CRA can use this time to catch up on writing reports, reading protocols and catching up on other tasks. An employer deserves an honest day's work, whether the CRA is in the office or on the road.

### Meeting with the Investigator

If possible, the CRA should spend a few minutes with the investigator at the start of the visit, so he or she knows you are there and what your activities will be while at the site. This is a good time to update the investigator on the overall progress of the study, including enrollment, timelines and any changes or other news from the sponsor.

Exit visits with the investigator should be routine. Since the investigator has ultimate responsibility for the study, the CRA should keep the investigator apprised of findings during the visit and how the study is going in general. The exit meeting is a good time to discuss how the study is progressing at the site, any corrective actions that need to be taken, grant or budget matters, and any other items that need to be discussed with the investigator.

Investigators tend to be very busy and occasionally, after the study gets under way, they become less accessible. A CRA must make certain from the beginning that the investigator knows that a short meeting is expected each time the site is visited. Good communication with the investigator is essential for a good study. If a CRA is having problems trying to meet with an investigator, discuss this with the sponsor medical monitor. Often the monitor can help, perhaps by calling the investigator personally—doctor-to-doctor contact sometimes will work wonders.

Another aid for dealing with difficult investigators is to occasionally review with them the responsibilities that appear on the 1572 (Statement of Investigator) forms that they signed. That can be a reminder that they agreed, in writing, to good study conduct, which includes good communication with the CRA. Sometimes nothing will work and an investigator will simply not meet with a CRA. In this case, the CRA must to do the best he or she can to keep the study on track. CRAs should always discuss these situations with their supervisor so that everyone is aware of the problems. Problems like this should also be documented in a visit report so that informed decisions can be made regarding future use or possible termination of the site.

## Working with the Study Coordinator

For actual study conduct, the study coordinator or clinical research coordinator (CRC) is the most important person at the site. A CRA must establish a good working relationship with the coordinator. The coordinator can make monitoring relatively easy and enjoyable or a nightmare, and the choice is usually dependent upon the CRA.

A CRA needs to spend time developing a rapport with the coordinator and developing a monitoring routine that works well for both. Each should understand how the other works. The CRA should determine the best times and methods for routine communication with each coordinator and let the coordinator know what your expectations are as the field monitor.

Some CRAs have such a good relationship with their coordinators that all the materials to be reviewed at a visit are laid out and ready when the CRA arrives at the site. With others, the relationships are not as good, so study materials are not ready for review, and monitoring becomes a challenge. A good relationship is worth nurturing; a bad one is costly.

Some CRAs simply have better interpersonal relationship skills than others do. It's amazing what a smile and good manners will do. Taking the coordinator to lunch occasionally is a nice gesture. Remember, however, to always maintain a professional relationship. It's easy to develop a friendship over the course of a long study. However, the CRA must still be able to enforce compliance if the study gets out of line. It is not easy to maintain your position of authority if the relationship becomes too friendly.

## Site Management

There are a number of general things the CRA will want to be aware of when monitoring a site, including interpersonal relationships, the stability of the staff, organization, how site personnel manage their time, and an overall impression and feeling about the site. The reason for this is that the atmosphere at a site affects the study. The better it is, and the smoother things run, the better the study will go.

Be observant when monitoring a site. Do people get along well with each other? Do they work together? Are there obvious antagonisms, one-upmanship, etc.? If one person is very busy, do others help out? If there are problems, the CRA may need to work around them in order to achieve the monitoring objectives. At the same time, however, the CRA will need to be careful not to add to any bad situations; the CRA should always treat everyone well, be pleasant and smile. Stay out of site politics.

How is the organization of the office? Are things running smoothly or are they always scattered? The study will often run the same way unless the CRA puts in additional time to help organize the study and study materials for smoother operation. Do site people have enough time to do their usual jobs plus the study? Are things always late or hurried? Were they ready for the monitoring visit? Again, a CRA may need to put extra effort into helping site personnel manage the study efficiently. Otherwise, the study may never be run as planned.

Another CRA responsibility is problem solving. Things rarely go exactly as planned, and clinical trials are no exception. The CRA must be prepared for a variety of potential problems such as enrollment difficulties, personnel turnover, waning interest in the study by site personnel, poor conduct of the study and protocol violations. Experience, knowledge and good common sense are your best tools for problem solving.

A CRA needs to think about how to approach a site that does sloppy work. Some CRAs try to crack the whip right from the very start, while others adopt a more moderate approach. In general, a moderate approach is the best, using the minimum amount of pressure required to get the necessary results. It is important for a CRA to learn how to take care of site problems without alienating the investigator and site personnel. If the site people are unhappy with the CRA, the study will languish and everyone loses.

If a problem arises that a CRA feels uncomfortable dealing with, or does not know how to solve, the CRA should speak with his or her supervisor or the sponsor's medical monitor. Don't ignore problems; they seldom go away by themselves. If there are problems with site management, the CRA may have to monitor more often to ensure that the study is run properly and that things get done in a timely manner.

## Monitoring Strategy

A CRA will need to develop an overall "hands on" monitoring strategy for site visits. In general, it is best to start with the most important activities, or at least the ones that must be done at each visit. This will ensure that if time runs short and everything cannot be completed, at least the most important things will have been reviewed.

One monitoring plan consists of the following activities, done in the order listed:

- Serious adverse event review
- Informed consent review
- Checking protocol adherence
- Case report form review and source document review
- Queries and error correction
- Investigational product review and accountability
- Review of laboratory samples
- Study document file review

### Serious Adverse Event Review

One of the first things a CRA should do at each monitoring visit is ask the investigator and coordinator if there have been any serious adverse events since the last visit, and if there have been, if they were reported to the sponsor. (The CRA should know about them if there were any reports to the sponsor, but sometimes there is a communication gap.) Whether or not the serious events were reported to the sponsor, the CRA should examine the information available about the events, including a review of the patient chart and any supporting documentation. If additional information is available that has not gone to the sponsor, the CRA can gather it and ensure that it is submitted to the appropriate person at the sponsor in a timely manner. The CRA can also discuss with the site personnel the need for any additional information that is necessary for complete reporting. Serious adverse event reporting is discussed in detail in Chapter 11.

### Informed Consent Review

At each visit, the CRA should check the informed consents for each new subject enrolled since the last visit. Informed consent forms should be signed and dated by the subject or the subject's legally authorized representative. Check the dates (and times, if available) against the date/time that the subject started the study; both should precede study entry. If other signatures are required on the consent form, such as the investigator's or a witness', those people should have signed also. The person signing the consent should also date it. Site personnel must never date the subject's signature on a consent form.

If the site is doing more than one study, the CRA should check to be sure the correct consent is being used.

---

### The Wrong Consent Form

*I was monitoring with a CRA and decided to check all the consents while he was doing the case report form and source document review. The site was a busy one, and doing a number of studies. As I looked through the consents, I noticed one that was different—in fact, it was not for our study at all. It was for a very similar study, but one being done for a different sponsor. It was interesting reading, but not the right consent.*

*The study coordinator was chagrined, as was the CRA. The subject was, in fact, in our study, the correct CRF was being used, and the correct activities being done. The coordinator had just inadvertently grabbed the wrong consent for him to sign.*

*To remedy this situation, the investigator contacted the subject, explained the problem, and had him sign a new, correct consent form. The situation was documented in the site's study file, including the changes they made to their procedures to ensure that it would not happen again. From that time on, the consents for each study were placed in a separate folder, clearly marked and stored in separate locations, rather than together in one file.*

*—Karen*

---

If the consent form for a study has changed, (e.g., protocol amendment) the CRA must be sure that all newly enrolled subjects are signing the appropriate consent. Except for a file copy, any copies of the old, inappropriate consent, should be destroyed so that they are not inadvertently used. If there are subjects who signed the old consent but are still on study, they should sign the new consent before continuing. The CRA should also check to be sure that this was done.

Periodically it is a good idea to go back and check all signed consents at the same time. One reason for doing this is to ensure that they are all still there and available. It is also a good idea to flip through and look at all the signatures at once; they should vary, and it should be obvious that they were signed by different people.

### Checking Protocol Adherence

Checking protocol adherence is something the CRA should check when monitoring each subject's data. It is easy to become so involved in checking the case report forms and source documents that the overall protocol adherence can be missed—it's the "not seeing the forest for the trees" syndrome. To ensure adherence, the CRA will want to check the following items:

- Subject eligibility. Did the subject meet all the inclusion and exclusion criteria?
- Randomization. Was the subject randomized to the correct subject number and did he or she receive the appropriate packages of investigational drug?
- Protocol activities. Were the correct activities done for or by the subject at each visit?
- Visit schedule and windows. The visit window is the number of days around the actual projected visit date when the subject can be seen. The window is usually the date plus and minus a number of days. For example, if the subject is due to be seen on May 6th and the window is plus or minus two days, the subject can be seen between May 4th and May 8th. Did the patient come in for each visit during the appropriate time period?
- Drug dispensing. Was the subject given the appropriate drug and the appropriate amount at each visit? Did the subject return any unused study drug? Was enough study drug taken so that the subject met the rules for drug compliance?

## Case Report Form (CRF) Review and Source Document Review (SDR)

Case report form review and source document review take most of the CRA's monitoring time. A suggested approach to this activity is to do the following:

- Start with new subjects, those enrolled since the last monitoring visit.
- Next, review the other currently enrolled subjects.
- Check all the CRFs for a subject before doing source document review.
- Then do SDR before checking the next subject's CRF.
- Finish one subject at a time.

The reason for starting with new subjects is that the CRA will want to be sure that they qualify for the study. If the subject does not qualify, or if other mistakes are being made, it is best to catch them soon after the subject is enrolled, rather than later.

CRF review and SDR require a different focus. It is easier to review the CRFs before looking at the source documents. We will look at each of these activities in more detail. Finishing one subject at a time is simply a good organizational tool. When the CRA has finished with the activities for a subject, put those items away. It is too easy to get things mixed up when trying to review multiple subjects at the same time.

## Case report form review

When reviewing the case report forms for a subject, the first thing to do is check each single page. The CRA should check for completeness, ensuring that each item has been completed and each blank is filled in. Are the forms legible? If the CRA has trouble interpreting what has been written, the data entry person will probably also not know what has been written. Are the answers within range? Is the header complete and correct? (The header is the top part of each form that lists the subject and study identifiers.) Is the form signed, if appropriate, and by the correct person?

Next, check all the pages for a single visit. Check for completeness, and correct dates. Is the visit within the window allowed? Check to be sure the timing of procedures was appropriate. If, for example, there was to be a blood draw, followed by another activity, then the blood draw should have been done first, and the times should reflect this. Any time there is a specific order to be followed for activities, that order must be followed. Check for consistency across forms. If the subject is getting better according to various ratings, then the overall rating should reflect an improvement. If a form says there was a concomitant medication administered for an adverse event, then the medication should be listed on the concomitant medication form and the adverse event entered on the adverse event CRF. In addition, the CRA should think about what appears in the forms, and whether or not it makes sense, given the subject condition and the study activities. If something does not make sense, the CRA should discuss it with the study coordinator and/or investigator.

The CRA should also check across visits. Are the data consistent from visit to visit? Is the timing of procedures appropriate? Do the data match where necessary? Are the visit windows correct over time? Usually each visit window is calculated by going back to the starting or baseline date, not from the previous visit. The reason for this is if a subject is always two days late, and if the window is always calculated from the last visit, you are adding two days and two more days and two more days...and so forth. After a while, there is not enough study drug for the subject to finish all the visits specified by the protocol.

Lastly, be sure it is the same subject at each visit, with the same initials, number and other identifier. It is always better to straighten out any problems while reviewing CRFs at the site, as compared with sending the forms in and having to make corrections later.

After completing the case report form review, it is time to do the source document review. Error correction will be discussed following the source document review section.

## Source document review

Source document review, sometimes called source document verification, involves checking the data recorded in the case report forms against data found in available source documents, including the patient chart, laboratory reports and other supporting documents. A source document is any document where the data are first recorded.

The purpose of source documentation is twofold: first, to verify that the subjects exist and, second, to verify that data in the CRF are consistent with the information found in the source documents, which verifies the integrity of the data.

One would expect to see basic demographic information in an office chart for a patient, including name, address, phone number, insurance information and a social security number. The CRA is not interested in the particulars of this information, but only that it exists. The usual office chart will also contain lab reports or reports of other tests. The name and identifying information should match the other information in the chart. This information is indicative that the person entered in the trial actually exists.

When the data in the case report forms are in agreement with data contained in source documents, it is an indicator of the quality and veracity of the information being gathered for the study. It is not necessary for every entry in a CRF to have a matching entry in a source document, but where the data do appear in both, they should agree. Neither ICH GCPs nor FDA regulations require that source documents be kept for all entries on case report forms. Under 21 CFR 312.62(b), "An investigator is required to prepare and maintain adequate and accurate case histories that record all observations and other data pertinent to the investigation...Case histories include the case report forms and supporting data including, for example, signed and dated consent forms, progress notes of the physician,...hospital chart(s) and nurse's notes."[2]

ICH GCPs say only that the study monitor shall verify that "the data required by the protocol are reported accurately on the CRFs and are consistent with the source data/documents."[3] Despite the lack of any regulatory requirement, many companies are currently insisting on a matching source document for every case report form entry. Whether or not this is the case, the CRA should be verifying that where matching data do exist in source records, they are consistent with the CRFs.

Upon occasion, the original collection of data may be done directly on the case report form; in effect, the case report form becomes a source document in this case. This is frequently seen in rating scales, such as the Hamilton Depression Rating Scale, because it is easier to collect the information directly on the CRF as opposed to transcribing it later. It is not wrong to do this, but a note should be made to the investigator's study file saying that this is being done. The sponsor may request/require this to be done.

What happens if there is a discrepancy between the case report form and the source document? Usually the source document takes precedence, but the CRA should always ask the investigator or coordinator to determine which one is correct, and to make the appropriate corrections. If the source document is corrected, the site person making the change should sign and date the document, including an explanation, as appropriate. CRAs should not make changes on either the source documents or the case report forms; this is the responsibility of site personnel. The CRA must remember, however, that even one change on a CRF can have an impact on other data. Be sure to check this, both within the visit and across visits.

There are significant differences among sponsors with respect to the amount of source document review that a CRA must do, and there are no guidelines in the regulations. Some companies require "100% source document review," but the definitions of 100% source document review also vary, from the expectation of a source document for every data point for every subject to 100% verification of the data insofar as it exists in source documents. Other sponsors have a sampling scheme, and these also vary considerably. Whatever the scheme, however, all subjects' case report forms are normally reviewed for critical information, such as the inclusion and exclusion criteria, a signed consent, adverse events and critical study-specific parameters. Some source document review sampling scheme examples are:

- 10% of the subjects are done.
- The first subject and then every other subject thereafter are done.
- The first two subjects are done. If there are no problems, every fourth subject thereafter is done. If problems are found, do two more subjects …iterate as needed.
- All subjects, but only certain variables are done.

No matter how much source document review/verification is done, it will never replace common sense. A CRA must think about what is being seen on the CRFs and in the source documents, and determine if it makes sense in terms of both the study and good medical practice.

### Errors, queries, and corrections

Perhaps the most important errors a CRA might find are those that result in protocol violations. These include such things as a subject not meeting the inclusion/exclusion criteria, a wrong diagnosis, a subject taking disallowed medications, problems with visit windows and others. Often these are found during source document review. Other errors are also found during source document review and run the gamut from incorrectly transcribed data to things that are just plain wrong. Then there are the case report form errors discussed earlier, such as missing data or out of range values.

Fixing errors is easier if the CRA has an effective procedure for dealing with them. It is helpful to have an Error Query/Correction form that is simple and easy to work with. A sample of this form is in Appendix C. Some CRAs rely heavily on Post-It® notes. Although they are good reminders, and mark CRFs nicely, they can fall off and get lost, and they do not generate an audit trail. A written correction form/log is more effective overall.

When potential errors are found, the CRA should note them in the corrections/questions log and discuss them with the study coordinator. When they are resolved, the coordinator should make the necessary corrections to the case report forms; CRAs do not make the corrections. Corrections are made by drawing a line through the incorrect entry, making the correct entry, and dating and initialing it. If the reason for the change is not clear, a reason should also be added to the form. It is never acceptable to use white-out or to erase a wrong entry before correcting it; anyone reviewing the forms must be able to see what was changed, when and why. Write-overs are also unacceptable. See the example below for a correctly done change.

Date 01/16/~~08~~ 09  JAK 2/5/09

It is in the CRA's best interest to find and have the coordinator correct errors at the site before sending the case report forms to the sponsor. Despite everyone's best efforts, additional errors are usually found when the CRFs go to data entry. Computer-generated errors will be sent back to the site and/or to the CRA. These are usually called queries. Different sponsors have different methods of doing queries, but usually there is a query form that is sent to the site; it lists what the errors are, where the errors are located on the CRF and asks for a correction or explanation to be made and sent in. Sometimes the CRA is involved in the correction process; sometimes it is solely between the site and data management.

Whether errors are found by the CRA or come in the form of queries, they should be used as training tools by a CRA. The CRA should explain to the site personnel why each one is an error and how it can be avoided in the future. It is important to review and enter the forms for the first few subjects as early as possible, in order to give timely feedback to the site, with the goal of eliminating similar errors in the future. This is especially important in the case of consistent errors, which are usually due to misunderstanding. Most study coordinators want to do the job correctly and will be pleased to have feedback if it is friendly and constructive.

Error rates should decrease as the study progresses, due to feedback and training by the CRA and data management, as well as to experience on the part of site personnel. If a site continues to have a high error rate due to carelessness, the CRA will need to discuss this with the investigator and coordinator.

Errors are very costly, both in terms of money and people hours to correct. Although most of the cost is borne by the sponsor, about one-third of the cost is borne by the site. From some informal work done looking at errors, each field that needs to be changed costs approximately $50 to correct (based on salary and benefits costs) and takes about 45 minutes. If a CRA is having difficulty with error rates at a site, these figures extrapolated over the number of errors being seen might make an impression on the investigator and coordinator. See Chapter 15 for additional discussion of errors.

### Electronic Data Capture (EDC)

After many years of piloting various electronic data submission methods, electronic data capture is beginning to be used for many studies. We will not discuss specifics in this book because of the number of different programs that are being used. However, according to the article entitled "Drivers of Change and Response," published in *CenterWatch* in January 2002, "EDC is gaining widespread acceptance as a necessary component of the drug development process. Research professionals throughout industry expect EDC to become routine practice within the next several years."[4] The same article goes on to say, "The roles of study monitors and investigative site personnel involved in capturing clinical trial data will be redefined."[5] CRAs should remain vigilant to changes in the industry, and be prepared to adapt as new technologies come along.

### Good, high quality data

We talk a lot in this business about "good, high quality data," but this term isn't usually defined. By asking a number of people how they would define good, high quality data, the following list of characteristics was generated.

**The general characteristics for good data are:**
- They can be evaluated and analyzed.
- They allow valid conclusions to be drawn.
- They are complete and accurate.
- They do not need to be queried.
- They are consistent across subjects and sites.

**More specific characteristics are:**
- Subjects meet the entry criteria.
- All fields are complete.
- Entries are legible and understandable.
- Values are within range.
- Entries make logical sense.
- The units (for measurements) are correct.
- There are no extraneous comments.

If these characteristics are met, the data should lead to valid conclusions and results that are reproducible. This is the goal for clinical studies.

There are a number of things that sponsors can do to help eliminate errors and generate good, usable data. First of all, the sponsor should develop good case report forms that are readable, easy for sites to use and have clear directions. Second, don't ask for the same information more than once in the CRFs; when this happens, the data frequently do not match. See the section on case report form development in Chapter 7.

Clear, detailed instructions and good training are also instrumental in minimizing errors. Most errors are due to misunderstandings, and these misunderstandings can be eliminated with training. CRA monitoring soon after the first few subjects are enrolled is a big help in clearing up misunderstandings. Fast turn-around on edits and queries will eliminate repeat errors, as well as cross-form edits of which the site was not aware. All of these items will help the site achieve lower error rates, with big cost savings in terms of both time and money for both the site and the sponsor.

## Investigational Product (Drug, Biologic, Device)

The CRA will want to check on the investigational drug or other product at each visit. The CRA will want to ensure that the drug is being used properly and distributed properly to study subjects. The CRA must check that the subjects are being dispensed the proper drug, according to the protocol and the randomization scheme, and should also ensure that the drug is being stored properly (in a secure manner and that any special conditions, such as refrigeration, are being met).

If sufficient study drug has not been sent to complete the entire study, and additional shipments are required, find out where the shipments are received, who receives them and when the receiving area is staffed. Avoid having drug shipments sitting on a receiving dock over a weekend or holiday. Not only is loss a concern, but it is also not a good idea for a product to be exposed to heat or freezing temperatures for very long. Know how long it takes a drug shipment to arrive at the site after an order is placed, and be sure that whoever is responsible for requesting shipments is aware of when new shipments to a site will be necessary. Whatever method of shipment is being used for investigational supplies, it should require a signature upon receipt. This significantly reduces lost or improperly handled study drug and provides an audit trail for the receipt of the product.

It is important to verify that the study coordinator is accounting for the study drug (product) on a regular basis as the study progresses. It does not work to wait until the end of the study and then try to reconcile how much study drug is left with how much study drug is supposed to be left; it is much more successful to do this on a continuing basis. The concept of drug accountability is pretty simple: the amount of study drug shipped to the site minus the amount of study drug used by the subjects should equal what is left at the end of the study. The problem is, it never seems to work out like this. It depends on how well the site manages the study drug. It is often better if the drug is stored and dispensed by a pharmacy; they tend do a better job of accounting for it and maintaining records, since that is their primary responsibility. A sample drug accountability form is in Appendix C.

Most sponsors require that unused study drug be returned to the sponsor company. In general, this is a CRA responsibility. On a periodic basis, the CRA will inventory and return to the sponsor the amount of study drug that was unused and returned by subjects, or not used at all because of early discontinuations. After it has been inventoried and packed by the CRA, the site can contact a shipper to pick it up for return. Again, it is usually better to do this periodically throughout the study rather than once at the end. It is easier to keep records straight, and it gets the unnecessary containers out of the way at the site/pharmacy.

## Sample collection

If blood or other samples are to be collected during the study, the CRA should ensure that this is being done, and is being done properly. The timing should be checked to verify that the collection is being done in accordance with protocol requirements. If the samples are stored and batched for shipping, the CRA should verify that storage conditions are appropriate.

The shipping must be done properly and according to all applicable laws and regulations. There are significant fines for not following appropriate packing and shipping procedures.[6] Proper shipment of dangerous material protects the shipper from exposure to these risks. To verify potential exposure, refer to 49 CFR 107.301 through 107.339 (hazardous material transportation regulations).

Reports generated on the samples should be reported and kept according to instructions.

## Study document review

Another monitoring task is checking the investigator's study document file. It is recommended that the CRA check this file at the first monitoring visit after the study starts, to ensure that copies of all pertinent documents are available and filed. If something is missing, it should be relatively easy to get a copy of it early in the study. The CRA may have a copy in his or her file, or the sponsor will. Having everything present and accounted for is a good way to start the study.

The CRA will not need to check the investigator's document file at every visit, unless the sponsor requires it. It should be checked periodically, however, especially if the CRA is aware of changes or when new documents have been added. It is also critical to check it at the end of the study, before it is filed for long-term storage.

Here are some hints for a CRA when checking study documents. Use a checklist for this activity, as it is easy to miss something without a list; a sample checklist can be found in Appendix C. Be sure that the current versions of documents, primarily the protocol and consent, are being used. Earlier versions should be retained in the file for reference only.

Copies of the 1572, IRB approvals and drug shipment invoices (the most common missing documents) should be in your travel file. This way, missing documents can be replaced with your copies. If you don't have a particular document, make a note to bring it with you the next time you come. Any time you replace a document, make another copy for your own file. These tips can save you time and hassles over the course of the study.

**Great Study, Wrong Protocol**

*"Once, while doing an antihypertension study in a physician's office in North Carolina, we discovered an unusual amount of errors in the case report forms (CRFs). We reviewed the study requirements, and then corrected the errors properly; yet, something did not seem quite right. Our in-house folks checked their records, and I, as the field CRA, checked his. We discovered that the physician had inadvertently been sent a different protocol than he had signed up for. But ... he had done the wrong protocol correctly! He had used the CRFs from the study he had signed up for, but performed an entirely different protocol! We never truly discovered how it happened, and we submitted appropriate documents to fix the problem. A CRA truth learned the hard way: Never assume the investigator has the correct protocol. Check the files and make sure the proper and current protocol is the one being done. Make sure the CRFs are for the protocol."*

*—Senior CRA*

# Confidentiality

During all monitoring activities, the CRA must be attentive to confidentiality. No study record, other than the consent form should identify the subject. The CRA has an obligation to help protect the confidentiality of all study subjects. The study documents are also confidential. During site visits, sometimes CRAs have seen competitor's protocols lying around unprotected. All one needs to see is the protocol cover page to know the name of the drug and phase of development. The CRA should periodically remind the investigator and coordinator of the confidentiality of these documents, and ensure that they are kept in a secure location.

### The Health Insurance Portability and Accountability Act (HIPAA)

The purpose of the Health Insurance Portability and Accountability Act (HIPAA) is to improve the efficiency and effectiveness of the healthcare system by encouraging the development of healthcare information systems using electronic data interchange for health-related administrative and financial transactions. In addition, HIPAA seeks to establish the required use of national transaction standards while maintaining patient privacy when business and patient information is transmitted electronically between organizations.

All vendors of electronic medical record (EMR) systems must conform to the standards in the Administrative Simplification component of HIPAA. This component encompasses four standards:

1. Electronic transactions and code sets
2. Privacy of individually identifiable health information
3. Security to preserve patient confidentiality
4. Creation of unique health identifiers for patients, health plans, providers and employers

The fourth standard is one part of HIPAA that will directly affect clinical research. It addresses standards by which unique patient-identifying information can be transmitted electronically, possibly over the Internet.

The final HIPAA rule was released on August 14, 2002, and has a compliance date of April 14, 2003. Specific areas of the final regulation that will affect researchers are: de-identification of patient health information, as mentioned above; single authorization from the patient required for all uses and disclosures of patient health information; the combining of patient authorization forms with the informed consent document; and the elimination of an expiration date or event for research authorization. The final regulation also now has one set of transition provisions for all forms of research regardless of whether they involve treatment or not. The full text of the final HIPAA rule and an explanation of modifications can be found at www.hhs.gov/ocr/hipaa.

# The End of the Visit

Before concluding a monitoring visit, there are some miscellaneous items to attend to. It is important to check the last site visit report for any noted problems or unresolved issues. These items should be followed up on until they are resolved, and the site visit reports must show what was done to follow-up. This is something that an auditor will look for if the site is inspected later, plus it is good monitoring practice.

The CRA will also want to see if more study supplies need to be ordered, including drug/product, case report forms, lab kits and anything else that may be necessary for the study. If so, the ordering should be done before the CRA leaves the site.

If the CRA is involved in grant requests, this should be discussed with the investigator and, if appropriate, a grant request should be submitted.

Before leaving, plan ahead for the next monitoring visit. Explain what materials should be ready for review. If there are scheduled enrollment updates planned, remind the coordinator about them. The CRA should always schedule the next visit before leaving the site, while both the CRA and the coordinator have their calendars available.

If possible, it is good to write the CRA visit report before leaving the site. If not, write it as soon as possible after leaving, while the details are still fresh. Before leaving, be sure you have everything you need to take with you and that it is organized. If you have collected case report forms, they should be inventoried, in order, and ready to mail. The investigator and CRA should have been debriefed about monitoring findings and the status of the study. Before leaving, the CRA should thank everyone for his or her time and efforts during the visit.

If the CRA has told site personnel that he or she will find out any particular information for them, be sure this is done and reported back. It is also nice to follow the visit with a letter recapping any pertinent information, thanking the site personnel for the work they have done, and verifying the date of the next monitoring visit.


# Monitoring Visit Reports

Most sponsors have a standard monitoring visit report form that is used to document visits to investigative sites. If a sponsor does not have one, the CRA will want to devise a form to use for this purpose; there is an example of a monitoring report in Appendix C.

The purpose of the monitoring visit report is to document the findings from the monitoring visit. The CRA should use this form to summarize what was done at the investigative site, including CRFs gathered for shipment to the sponsor. This is also where problems must be documented, including what was done to solve them, or to make recommendations of action items for the next visit.

It is important to remember that the visit report is a business document, and can be accessed by the FDA in case of a sponsor inspection. The language used should be business-like and factual; this is not the place to vent frustrations with a site. If the monitoring visit was not as successful as the CRA had hoped, these frustrations can find their way into the report; this is not appropriate. Here are some examples of unacceptable and acceptable language for a visit report:

**Unacceptable:** "Coordinator doing sloppy work!!! She is the worst coordinator I have ever seen."
**Acceptable:** "CRFs incomplete and needed many corrections. Coordinator was instructed in the proper way to fill in the forms."

**Unacceptable:** "Investigator shows no interest in the study. He is never available to meet with me and probably doesn't even know what is going on in the study."
**Acceptable:** "Investigator not available during this visit. Time with him was scheduled for my next visit, and a letter will be sent verifying the appointment time."

**Unacceptable:** "This study is so screwed up nobody can tell what's going on. We should close it and never let them do studies again. This is a really terrible site. The coordinator is a dunce, and the investigator thinks he walks on water."

**Acceptable:** "There are many aspects of this study that need clarification and correction. It is recommended that someone from our compliance department visit the site with me within the next two weeks so that we can determine what needs to be done to ensure that the study is brought into compliance with good clinical practices. After this visit, we will recommend any further actions that appear necessary."

Remember that monitoring visit reports are the official record of CRA visits and will stay in the sponsor trial file for many years. They should reflect what was done at the visit, what was transmitted to the sponsor and problems that were found, plus potential solutions. The ICH Guidelines for Good Clinical Practice summarize monitoring reports very well:[7]

- The monitor should submit a written report after each monitoring visit.
- Reports should include the date, investigative site, name of the monitor, name of the investigator and any other individual(s) contacted.
- Reports should contain a summary of what was reviewed and statements concerning significant findings/facts, deviations and deficiencies, conclusions, actions taken or to be taken and/or actions recommended to secure compliance.

## Conclusion

Successful monitoring is the result of experience, knowledge of the protocol, CRFs, the study drug, therapeutic area, regulations and SOPs, people skills and management ability. It is not easy, but can be fun and rewarding when done well.

To close this chapter, here is a story from a CRA friend that's a great example of the strange things a CRA experiences.

---

**The Most Fruitless Trip for No Real Reason**

*"Our company was doing a very large phase IV study to support changing a prescription drug to an over-the-counter drug. Subjects were recruited through pharmacies and they received a telephone call quarterly to check on their status. If subjects reported that they had been hospitalized, we physically went to their location to investigate the case.*

*I received notification to investigate a case of a person who had been hospitalized with "AH Blood Poisoning." This was a very unusual report,*

---

because no one had ever heard of such a thing. Besides being an unusual case, the person and his physician lived in Star Lake, New York.

It was January, and Star Lake is located in Upstate New York between Watertown and Lake Placid. The snow was about two feet deep, and I arrived late. The hotel was elderly, with one telephone, and a bar, whose keeper, elderly as well, was also the hotel room clerk. If one asked politely, he would make you a burger for dinner. The next morning breakfast was at the local grocery store, because there were no restaurants.

The hospital was very small, and the physician's office was just next door in a small building. The physician was pleasant and most helpful, but he, too, had no clue what "AH Blood Poisoning" was. He told me, that the man had an infection in his arm because his pet cockatoo had bitten him, and this resulted in cellulitis. The man recovered after a course of antibiotics.

I reported the cellulitis to our in-house study coordinator, and apologized for not being able to ascertain exactly what "AH Blood Poisoning" was. A few days later, he called me back and said, "I think I know what happened." He said, "The telephone operators who interview subjects take down whatever they say verbatim. I checked with the interview service and confirmed that the man had answered the question about whether anything untoward had happened with, 'I had, ah, (AH) blood poisoning.'" And that was the end of the great "AH Blood Poisoning" mystery.

—A CRA Friend

## Key Takeaways

- A CRA should develop a plan for monitoring each investigative site.
- The frequency and timing of monitoring visits depend on the complexity of the study, the rate of enrollment and site experience and performance.
- Investigative sites should be visited soon after the first subject or two are enrolled.
- CRAs should use checklists for various monitoring activities.
- CRAs should maintain a file for each investigative site.
- CRAs should confirm each scheduled site visit before leaving on a trip.
- CRAs should spend some time with the investigator and the coordinator at each monitoring visit.
- Serious adverse events should be checked at each visit.
- Informed consents must be checked for all study subjects.
- The bulk of CRA monitoring time is spent on case report form review and source document review.

- The purpose of source document review is to verify that the subjects exist and the integrity of the data.
- Quick feedback and explanation of errors and queries will help reduce the number of corrections needed in the future.
- CRAs must never correct or modify source documents or case report forms themselves. Corrections can only be done by site personnel.
- Drug accountability should be done throughout the study.
- Study documents need to be checked at the beginning and end of the study, and periodically throughout the study.
- The monitoring visit report should summarize the activities that took place during the visit, including what was reviewed, what was sent to the sponsor and any problems that were found, along with solutions.

### References

1. www.fda.gov/cder/reports/rtn/2001/rtn2001-2.htm.
2. 21 CFR 312.62 (b).
3. ICH Guideline for Good Clinical Practice 5.18.4(m).
4. "Drivers of Change and Response," CenterWatch, January 2002, vol. 9, Issue 1, CenterWatch Editorial, p. 6.
5. Ibid.
6. 49 CFR Part 173 (http://hazmat.dot.gov/rules.htm).
7. ICH Guidelines 5.18.6.

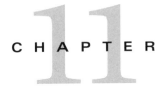

CHAPTER

# Adverse Events and Safety Monitoring

In this chapter, we will discuss adverse events and safety monitoring. It is critical that adverse events are monitored during clinical trials, for the protection of the subjects enrolled in the trial as well as for protection of the patients and proper use of the drug once it is marketed.

Monitoring safety during a clinical trial is one of the most important tasks a CRA performs. At the same time, safety reporting is one of the most difficult things for a study site to do correctly. There are often misunderstandings about what is necessary for reporting on safety issues in trials, stemming at least in part because of the differences in clinical studies as compared to clinical practice. Also, although the regulations charge the investigator with protecting the rights, safety and well-being of subjects in trials, they don't give much information about actual safety reporting. We will look at the regulations in detail.

## Regulations

21 CFR 312.64 (Investigator reports) requires investigators to report adverse events during clinical trials. It states:

> *Safety reports. An investigator shall promptly report to the sponsor any adverse effect that may be reasonably regarded as caused by, or probably*

149

caused by, the drug. If the adverse effect is alarming, the investigator shall report the adverse effect immediately.

By signing the 1572, the investigator also commits to reporting adverse events to the sponsor that occur during the course of a trial, in accordance with 21 CFR 312.64.

The ICH Guidelines for Good Clinical Practice have somewhat more information. In the glossary both adverse events and adverse drug reactions are defined as follows:

### Adverse Event (AE)

*An AE is any untoward medical occurrence in a patient or clinical investigation subject administered a pharmaceutical product. It does not necessarily have a causal relationship with this treatment. An AE can therefore be any unfavorable and unintended sign (including an abnormal laboratory finding), symptom, or disease temporally associated with the use of a medicinal (investigational) product.*

### Adverse Drug Reaction (ADR)

*In the preapproval clinical experience with a new medicinal product or its new usages, particularly as the therapeutic dose(s) may not be established, all noxious and unintended responses to a medicinal product related to any dose should be considered adverse drug reactions. The phrase "responses to a medicinal product" means that a causal relationship between a medicinal product and an adverse event is at least a reasonable possibility, i.e., the relationship cannot be ruled out.*

*Regarding marketed medicinal products: A response to a drug that is noxious and unintended and that occurs at doses normally used in man for prophylaxis, diagnosis, or therapy of diseases or for modification of physiological function.*[1]

The ICH GCPs also contain a section (4.11) on safety reporting. In this section, it states that:

*All serious adverse events (SAEs) should be reported immediately to the sponsor except for those that are designated in the protocol or investigator brochure as not needing to be reported immediately. The initial report should be followed by a detailed written report.*

*The investigator should comply with regulatory requirements for reporting unexpected SAEs to regulatory authorities and the IRB.*[2]

In clinical studies, sponsors are required to report serious, unexpected, related events that are fatal or life threatening to the U.S. Food and Drug Administration (FDA) by telephone and/or facsimile within seven calendar days of the date the sponsor first becomes aware of the event. The reporting clock starts when the first person in the sponsor company hears of the event.

If the sponsor company is using a CRO, the CRO becomes, in effect, the sponsor company; in this case, the reporting clock starts even if a person in the CRO is the first to become aware of the event. Note that the first person may be a secretary or any other person who happens to answer the telephone or receives the fax—it doesn't have to be someone involved in managing the study.

A written report detailing all the information the sponsor has about the event is sent to the FDA within a fifteen-day time period. This is a total of fifteen calendar days from the initial report of the AE, not fifteen days after the seven-day telephone or facsimile report. The sponsor must also send out IND Safety Reports, which will be covered later in this chapter.

Adverse events that are serious, unexpected and related to the investigational drug but not fatal or life threatening, must be reported to the FDA by the sponsor in writing within fifteen calendar days of the date that anyone in the employ of the sponsor first becomes aware of the event. Anyone in the employ of the sponsor is defined exactly as described above for seven-day reporting.

## Definitions

There are a number of definitions related to adverse event reporting that are important to know and understand. These are regulatory definitions, not clinical definitions, which is an important distinction to understand when working with investigative sites. These definitions are:

- **Adverse event.** An adverse event is any untoward medical occurrence in a subject administered a drug (biologic, device). It does not necessarily have a causal relationship with the treatment/usage.

- **Serious adverse event.** Serious adverse events are those that result in death, are life threatening (immediately as it occurred, not had it become worse at some time in the future), require hospitalization (or a prolongation of hospitalization in already hospitalized patients), result in a persistent or significant disability or incapacity, are congenital anomalies or birth defects. For clinical studies, these serious adverse events also include any other event that the investigator or the sponsor company judges to be serious, or is defined as serious by the regulatory agency in the country where the event occurred.

   It is important to distinguish between the terms "serious" and "severe." The term "serious" is used with the definition above and categorizes events (i.e., they either meet the definition for serious or they don't). The term "severe" refers to the intensity of the event and can be used with any event, without regard to whether or not it meets the criteria for being classified as "serious." For example, a subject can have a severe headache, but it is not a serious event.

- **Related to or associated with the drug.** This is defined to mean that there is a reasonable possibility that the event could have been caused by the investigational product (drug, biologic, device).

- **Expected/unexpected.** An expected event is one where the specificity and severity of the event are consistent with the information in the investigator brochure or labeling for the product. Unexpected events are all the others.

- **Life-threatening.** A life-threatening event is one where the patient is in immediate danger of death unless intervention is done. It does not mean that the patient may die at some time in the future from the event or may have died if the event had been more serious or specific.

- **Significant disability.** A significant disability is one that causes substantial disruption to the person's normal life and activity.

Later in this chapter, we will discuss ways that a CRA can work with sites to help investigators and their staff understand these definitions and how to apply them.

## Adverse Events (AEs) on Marketed Products

Companies must collect safety information on each of their products throughout the entire life cycle of the product—from the first time it is used in people during clinical trials to the time the last dose of marketed drug is sold and used.

Events collected after a product is marketed are called spontaneous adverse events. They are called spontaneous adverse events because they are reported spontaneously/voluntarily to the sponsor by medical professionals, patients or others, as opposed to being collected systematically during clinical trials. CRAs are not usually involved in the gathering or reporting of adverse events on marketed products. Since these events are reported voluntarily, they are all classified as "related" to the drug for reporting purposes. The reasoning behind this classification is that if someone feels there is enough of a relationship to report the event, it makes sense to assume it is related in some way. Remember, however, that an adverse event must meet all three criteria to need expedited reporting to the FDA; it must be serious, related and unexpected.

The bulk of spontaneous adverse event reports come to a pharmaceutical company from health professionals. Health professionals often call a pharmaceutical company to report unusual things they have seen in patients who are taking the drug; frequently these are calls asking for further information about the compound. Reports may also come in from patients, other consumers, or from the FDA or other regulatory agencies.

The requirement for reporting adverse events on marketed products stems from the fact that clinical trials are never sufficient to provide a full adverse event profile for a drug. Some of the differences between clinical trials and marketed use of a drug are shown in Table 1.

All these differences can have an impact on the adverse event profile of the drug. As an example, assume there is an adverse reaction to a drug that occurs only about once in every 50,000 people who take it. Chances are that this adverse reaction will never be seen during the clinical trial program, which usually consists only of several thousand patients. Even if the clinical program enrolled 20,000 subjects, an event occurring only once in 50,000 probably will not show up more than once, if at all. When the drug is marketed, however, and is available for use by millions of people, these events will become apparent. The purpose of the FDA's safety surveillance program is to ensure that there is a mechanism to report, and learn about, these events.

**Table 1: Differences Between Clinical Trials and Marketed Use of a Product**

| Clinical Trials | Marketed Use |
|---|---|
| ■ Relatively small number of patients | ■ Millions of patients |
| ■ Tight control | ■ No control |
| ■ Extra care | ■ Standard care |
| ■ Highly trained physicians | ■ Any physicians |
| ■ Narrow patient population | ■ Anyone prescribed the drug |

# Adverse Events (AEs) in Clinical Trials

The adverse events that CRAs will be most involved with are those that are collected during clinical trials of drugs that are usually not yet marketed, but are still in the development process. All adverse events that occur during studies are collected. They are further classified by the definitions for serious, related and unexpected, as given above.

Most of the adverse events seen during clinical trials will not be serious, as defined in the regulations. In general, these non-serious adverse events will be recorded regularly on case report forms and will be reviewed and collected by the CRA during regular monitoring visits. Remember that non-serious events can be severe in intensity but still not meet the definition of serious.

Most sponsors want all serious adverse events that occur during a trial to be reported to them by the investigator as soon as he or she becomes aware of them. This is for two reasons: first, to ensure the continued safety of subjects in the trial; and second, to meet the reporting requirements for the FDA. The FDA reporting rules for serious adverse events occurring during clinical trials are similar to those for spontaneous adverse events, although there are some differences.

Sponsors must still report (in writing) all AEs that are serious, related and unexpected to the FDA within fifteen calendar days, and those that are also serious and alarming (death, immediately life-threatening) must be reported by fax or phone within seven days, with a written report within fifteen days.

## Safety Reporting Sections in Protocols

Every protocol for a clinical trial should contain a detailed plan for the collection and reporting of all adverse events, both serious and non-serious. There are several key items that should be included.

**Definitions.** The protocol should include the regulatory definitions for an adverse event and a serious adverse event, as well as the definitions for related/associated and for expected/unexpected events.

**Sources of AEs.** In general, the standard sources of all adverse events will be the investigator reporting of:

- All directly observed events. [I see you have a rash on your arm...]
- Events elicited from the subject by means of a general non-directive question. [Have you had any problems with your health since you were here the last time?] The use of a specific question allows the sponsor to standardize procedures across all sites. A non-directive question does not prompt a subject to answer in a specific way. Asking subjects about specific events [Have you had any headaches?], although appropriate in some studies, will lead to a higher reporting rate for the specific event than a non-directive question.
- Events spontaneously volunteered by the study subject. [You know, Doc, ever since I started taking these pills, I have had an upset stomach.]
- Laboratory, EKG or other test results that meet protocol requirements for classification as adverse events. [example: laboratory values more than 10% outside the normal range.

**Event collection periods.** The study periods during which adverse events will be collected should be specified. Some protocols require adverse events to be collected during a pre-treatment period as baseline data, while others only require collection during active treatment. It is also quite common to collect AEs during a post-treatment follow-up period. Adverse events are always collected during the entire period that a subject is on, or could be on (in the case of blinded trials), the investigational product or study drug.

**Diaries and other data collection instruments.** Whenever data collection instruments are used that may elicit information about adverse events (e.g., quality of life questionnaires, patient diaries), the methods for handling these events should be specified in the protocol. Although they certainly have a place in data collection, instruments such as diaries can complicate the orderly collection of adverse events. The problem is that subjects may write comments in diaries that refer to potential adverse events, and there is often no orderly way to officially collect the pertinent information. There is an example of a patient diary with a written comment about a potential event in Table 2.

Notice that this patient was filling in the times she took her investigational medication, but she also added some additional information—the migraine headache. Certainly, the study site personnel would want to know about the migraine, but this is not the place for it to be recorded. The study coordinator will need to ensure that this event is recorded on the appropriate adverse event case report forms, and not missed.

---

**Table 2: Example: Patient Diary**

ACMEPHARMA STUDY 1234                                    Patient Diary—Week 4

Name: _____*Betsy Smith*_____

Each day, please enter the time you took your study medication. Remember, you should always take one pill just before breakfast (about 8:00 am) and two pills before dinner (about 6:00 pm).

Sunday        Date: _____*2/2/09*_____
              Morning dose time _____am
              Evening dose time _____pm

Monday        Date: _____
              Morning dose time _____am
              Evening dose time _____pm

Tuesday       Date: _____
              Morning dose time _____8__ am
              Evening dose time _____6__ pm    *migraine - felt dizzy*

---

**Unresolved adverse events.** Sometimes adverse events that occur during a study are unresolved at the time the subject's study participation ends. The protocol should state what is to be done in this case. Usually serious AEs are followed to resolution, that is, until they resolve, disappear or become stable.

There is often a time period during which any events that are ongoing at the end of the study are followed. Thirty days is a frequently used time period, but it varies depending on the compound, its half-life, the amount of time the subject was in the trial and the complexity of the diagnosis and protocol.

**Exposure *in utero*.** If women of childbearing potential are allowed entry into the trial, then the protocol should include instructions for reporting exposure *in utero* and the subsequent outcome of the pregnancy. In general, the investigator will be required to follow up on any cases of pregnancy that occur during the study until the child is born or the pregnancy is terminated. There is usually no requirement for interim visits throughout the pregnancy, just an assurance that the subject will be contacted periodically to determine the outcome.

**Timely notification.** The sponsor will want to be notified of serious events by the investigator in a timely manner, usually within 24 hours. It is extremely important that the investigator notify the sponsor of each serious adverse event as soon as possible, even if all the details are not yet available. Additional details can be reported as they become available; the initial report should never be delayed while awaiting more information.

An investigator may not know about an event for some time after it has occurred, especially if he or she is not the subject's primary physician. The study site may not know about the event until the subject comes in for his or her next appointment, or fails to show up for the appointment because of the event. However, the investigator should inform the sponsor of the event as soon as he or she becomes aware of it.

Non-serious adverse events are also reported to the sponsor. This reporting is done by way of the case report form and regular data collection process. Final reporting is done within a reasonable time following completion of the study (usually within three months). There are no FDA requirements for expedited reporting of non-serious events.

## Investigator Reporting Responsibilities

Investigators are required to collect, assess and report all the adverse events that occur during a trial. The following information is usually gathered for each event: onset (date/time), duration, severity (mild, moderate, severe), relationship to the study drug, and whether or not it is serious. All events are to be recorded on the CRF. In addition, if an event is serious, the investigator is usually expected to report it to the sponsor very quickly (e.g., within 24 hours).

Not only must the investigator report adverse events to the sponsor, but he or she also has a requirement for reporting these events to the IRB, in the manner in which the IRB has requested. As with sponsors, some IRBs will want notification of all serious events, while others will want to hear only about events that are serious and related, or only those that are serious, related and unexpected. The IRB will let the investigator know what is expected, and what the report timing and mechanisms are. It is important that the investigator notify the IRB according to the rules the IRB has established.

It is a regulatory requirement that the investigator notify both the sponsor and the IRB of adverse events.[3]

The investigator may receive IND Safety Reports (discussed in the next section) from the sponsor. Whenever one is received, the investigator must forward the information to the IRB.

## Sponsor Responsibilities

Sponsors are required to review safety data throughout a trial. This is so appropriate adjustments can be made if there are any relevant safety issues. For example, the protocol might be amended, or, if there are serious safety concerns, the trial might be stopped. Remember that the sponsor is the only entity that has access to all the safety data for a drug; investigators and IRBs only see safety data from the site or sites with which they are involved. Therefore, the burden is on the sponsor for prompt and thorough review of safety information as it is generated.

Sponsors have the responsibility of reporting adverse events that are serious, related and unexpected to the FDA within the expedited reporting time frames, as was discussed earlier.

Sponsors have an additional reporting requirement for serious adverse events in clinical trials; they must also inform all investigators who are currently working with the drug of any serious, related, unexpected adverse event. The investigators need to receive the same information as that sent to the FDA and within the same fifteen-day time period. These reports are called IND Safety Reports. Note that IND Safety Reports are sent to all investigators working with the compound, not just those doing the same protocol. The requirements for IND Safety Reports are found in 21 CFR 312.32.[6]

There may be rare instances where an adverse finding or a series of adverse events indicate that the drug has a safety issue that is so serious that the continued use of it in clinical trials is unacceptable. If this occurs, the sponsor must notify the FDA and all investigators who ever participated in a clinical trial with the drug immediately of that decision. This includes all investigators who ever studied the drug, not just those with currently active clinical trials. The investigators of open trials must then, in turn, immediately notify their IRBs of the trials' discontinuation for reasons of safety.

## Differences Between Clinical Studies and Clinical Practice

One of the most important tasks of a CRA is training and working with investigative sites on adverse event reporting. One reason that adverse event reporting is fraught with problems stems from the fact that clinical practice and clinical research are not the same thing, and it is easy to get the two confused when it comes to safety reporting. It is often difficult for investigators to understand that the definitions used for adverse event reporting in trials are regulatory definitions, not clinical definitions. A good CRA understands the definitions and reporting requirements, and takes the time to thoroughly train each site on the requirements before subjects are enrolled. In this section, we will discuss some ways the CRA can help sites with the proper reporting of adverse events.

First, the CRA should discuss with his or her sites the differences between clinical practice and clinical research. In studies, the investigator has a dual role as a physician and an investigator. It is a physician's duty to act in the best interest of the patient, while at the same time, it is the duty of the investigator to perform good research. These duties are not necessarily in conflict, but there are differences in the roles that must be understood.

Some examples that a CRA may want to discuss with site personnel are the following:

- Concomitant medications that might normally be prescribed for a patient may not be allowed under the protocol.
- Treatment periods may be longer or shorter under the protocol than are usual in general practice.
- Adverse events that are "normal" for the disease must usually be reported under study rules.

A worsening or progression of the disease may or may not be reported as an adverse event. For example, a worsening of anxiety in an anxiety trial would usually require reporting, while a progression of Alzheimer's disease in an Alzheimer's trial might not be reported, as this is a progressive disease.

Occasionally investigators do not understand the importance of reporting adverse events if they do not seem to be connected with the trial or the study medication, or if they are commonly seen with the disease under study. An investigator may say something on the order of "we see that all the time in this disease…" or "it's not connected to the trial…" or "that isn't of any importance…." These remarks signify a misunderstanding of the differences between clinical practice and research. As a CRA, you will want to be attuned to this type of misunderstanding and aware of the need for additional explanations and training.

Sometimes it helps to remind the investigator and staff that the study is being done to find out about the investigational drug, including safety as well as efficacy. That is why studies are done—we never really know what we will learn about a drug or device when it is under investigation.

The investigator may also need to be reminded of his or her regulatory responsibilities with respect to doing trials. He or she is also bound by the contract with the sponsor, and most contracts require the investigator to report adverse events as mandated by the regulations.

## Assessing the Relationship of an
## AE to the Study Drug

Investigators are usually asked to assess the relationship between an adverse event and the investigational product by picking the term that best characterizes the relationship of the adverse event to the investigational product. The choices are commonly on the order of: not related, probably not related, possibly related, probably related, definitely related. Because not much is known about the product, investigators are often uneasy about making this decision. Here are some aids a CRA might use when training investigators to make these decisions.

### Temporal relationship

Does the timing of taking the investigational drug make sense in relationship to the timing of the event? For example, assume that the subject takes the drug, comes in two days later and is diagnosed with a cancer. The cancer is probably not related, because it occurred too soon after taking the study drug. Or, assume that a subject has been taking the study drug without problem but develops an adverse event just after the dose was titrated upward; in this case, the event might well be related to the drug.

### Known patterns of reaction

Assume that the study drug causes a distinctive rash, and a study subject develops that type of rash. Chances are good that the rash is related to the study drug.

### Other potential cause

Is there something else that would explain the occurrence of the event? For example, assume that the subject is allergic to chocolate, but couldn't resist that piece of devil's food chocolate birthday cake last night. He ate some and ended up with hives. The hives are probably not related to the study drug, but to the chocolate.

### Does it make sense?

Assume that a study subject suffers from regular migraines, takes the study drug and has a migraine. It's probably not related. However, assume that the subject usually has one or two migraines a month, but ever since starting the study drug, she has them every two or three days. They are probably related to the study drug. This might, in fact, be reported as an exacerbation of a previously existing medical condition, e.g., a change in severity.

### Dechallenge/rechallenge

In this scenario, the subject has an adverse event. The study drug is stopped (the dechallenge), and the event stops. The study drug is restarted (rechallenge), and the event occurs again. It is probably related to the drug under study. This is a very definitive test, but may not be done unless allowed in the protocol. Although an investigator may stop a study drug (dechallenge) at any time it is deemed appropriate, he or she may not restart it (rechallenge) unless allowed by the protocol or after discussion with and agreement by the sponsor.

## Common Reporting Problems

There are a number of common misunderstandings that result in incorrect adverse event reporting. Many of these errors can be avoided if the CRA takes time to explain them to site personnel in advance. One of these misun derstandings involves symptoms vs. a syndrome. Usually sponsors want a syndrome reported rather than the individual symptoms, for example, flu vs. cough, sniffles and sore throat all reported separately.

Another common error is the reporting of a procedure, as opposed to reporting the disease/condition that resulted in the procedure. An example of this is reporting a coronary bypass as the event, instead of reporting the heart condition that necessitated the bypass.

Changes in severity are frequently reported incorrectly, or not at all. The general convention is that if an event worsens in severity, it is reported as a new event, even if the event is in the pre-study history for the subject. Some protocols also require the reporting of changes in events when the change is for the better.

Although it was mentioned earlier in this chapter, it is critical for the CRA to ensure that his or her sites understand the distinction between the terms "serious" and "severe" where the "severe" refers to the intensity of an event, without regard to whether or not it meets the criteria for being classified as "serious."

In case of exposure *in utero*, it is a good idea for a CRA to make a note to follow up with the investigator on any cases of pregnancy. It is easy to forget to do this when the subject is not being seen on a regular basis.

### Dealing with problems

If a CRA is having trouble with appropriate adverse event reporting at a site, the first step is to discuss the situation with the site personnel, and do additional training, including a discussion of both the protocol and the regulations as they pertain to adverse events. If training and retraining do not help the situation, the CRA should discuss the situation with his or her supervisor and/or the study medical monitor.

At times, the sponsor will send people from the quality assurance/ auditing group to assess the problem. This will usually get the attention of the investigator, as audits tend to be somewhat frightening for most people. If the problems do not resolve, the sponsor may need to take more drastic action and actually stop the trial at the problem site. [Note: In this case, you will not want to use the site again for another trial.] Stopping the trial for this reason is quite rare, as investigators usually become compliant earlier in the process. Most people want to do a good, appropriate job when doing a study and simply need the help of a knowledgeable CRA to keep things running smoothly and well.

Everyone who is involved in clinical trials must recognize that clinical trials differ from clinical practice and that subject safety is paramount. A CRA must have expert knowledge of the adverse event rules and regulations in order to help study sites remain compliant in this endeavor. Helping sites report adverse events appropriately is one of the most difficult and most important tasks of a CRA.

## Key Takeaways

- Subject safety is paramount in clinical trials.
- There are differences between clinical practice and clinical trials when it comes to reporting adverse events.
- The definitions used in adverse event reporting are regulatory definitions, not clinical definitions.
- Adverse events that are serious and related and unexpected require expedited reporting to the FDA.
- All investigators working with an investigational drug must be informed of any event with the drug that is serious, related and unexpected. The sponsor sends an IND Safety Report to each investigator for any adverse event meeting these criteria.
- The investigator must inform his or her IRB of any IND Safety Report received from a sponsor.
- Serious adverse events must be reported to the sponsor of the study within a very short time period (usually 24 or 48 hours).
- Protocols should contain explicit directions for collecting, assessing and reporting adverse events.
- CRAs must train their sites in proper reporting of adverse events.

**References**

1. ICH Guideline for Good Clinical Practice, as published in the Federal Register May 9, 1997. Part I. Glossary.
2. ICH Guideline for Good Clinical Practice, as published in the Federal Register May 9, 1997. Section 4.11.
3. 21 CFR 312.64, 66.

# 12

# Recruitment, Retention, and Compliance

In this chapter, we will cover three of the most difficult aspects of doing clinical trials: recruitment of subjects into the trial, retention of subjects after they have been entered and subject compliance with the protocol throughout the study.

## Recruitment of Study Subjects

Finding, enrolling and retaining study subjects are some of the largest and costliest challenges facing clinical research professionals today.[1] Enrollment will undoubtedly continue to be problematic in the future. Between government and industry, more than 20,000 study sites a year in the United States are involved in carrying out research based on 5,000 to 6,000 unique protocols. More than one million volunteer subjects will complete these trials.[2]

In 2002, pharmaceutical and biotechnology companies are expected to spend more than $10 billion on clinical research, including more than $4 billion in grants to investigators for clinical studies.[3] The average cost of developing one new drug has increased over the past ten or so years from $230 million to over $800 million, and the development process time from the pre-clinical stage to approval by the FDA averages about ten years.[4] Given the enormous development costs, it is obvious that companies want to speed up the process as much as possible, allowing for more marketing time before their patent protection for the product expires. The timely enrollment of appropriate subjects into trials is critical to managing the timelines for a development program.

## Lasagna's Law

Knowing the patient population and being able to accurately estimate the number of subjects that can be enrolled are critical to completing a trial in the given time period. Before a study actually starts at an investigative site, there always seem to be more than enough potential subjects waiting in the wings. For some reason, however, it frequently happens that as soon as the trial starts, these potential subjects disappear. This is known as Lasagna's Law,[5] and can be shown visually in Figure 1:

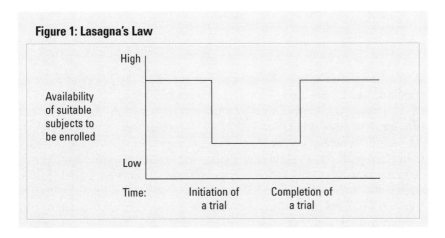

Figure 1: Lasagna's Law

Lasagna's Law is like a corollary to one of Murphy's laws, namely, "whatever can go wrong, will." In the case of Lasagna's Law, when the study is over, there seems, again, to be plenty of suitable subjects.

## Estimating Enrollment Potential at Sites

One of the most important pre-study activities a CRA has is to help sites accurately estimate the number of subjects that they can reasonable expect to enroll in each trial. Investigators frequently overestimate the number of potential subjects they have. This is often due to the fact that they are looking only at the number of potential subjects who match the overall diagnosis, for example, depression. However, there are a number of other factors that must be weighed and taken into account, including the protocol inclusion criteria and the subjects themselves.

Protocol considerations include the inclusion and exclusion criteria, activities and logistics. The largest constraints on enrollment are usually the inclusion and exclusion criteria for study entry. These criteria delineate the specific characteristics of the population to be enrolled. They will include demographic parameters, such as age, sex, disease and diagnostic criteria, and study-specific requirements. In a study of depression, for example, the following (simplified) inclusion/exclusion criteria might be found:

- Age 18 to 65 years
- Men, and women who are post-menopausal, surgically sterile or using acceptable birth control
- Depression lasting at least 6 months, but no longer than one year
- No previous depressive episodes before current episode
- No previous treatment with anti-depressive medications
- Not taking any other medications that might interfere with the study medication (list provided)
- Able to read and comprehend the informed consent document
- Willing to sign the informed consent
- Able to swallow pills
- Able to make weekly visits to the clinic site for three months

Now let's look at how these criteria might affect the ability of a site to enroll subjects.

The upper age limit of 65 may limit enrollment from sites that treat a large geriatric population. Depression is a disease that tends to recur in people over time, so the criterion that disallows previous depressive episodes would be a problem. The criterion disallowing previous treatment with anti-depressants will be a big factor because if these subjects are already in the care of the investigator, many of them will already be on anti-depressive therapies. Willingness and ability to make weekly clinic visits are apt to interfere with a potential subject's life situation, especially when working. On top of these problems, many people are just not willing to participate in research, especially if the protocol requirements are burdensome and they do not see much potential value to themselves for participation.

How can these factors influence the ability to enroll? As discussed in Chapter 8, if a CRA takes the number of subjects a physician has in his or her practice that meet the diagnosis for the study (depression), then halves that number for each major inclusion/exclusion criteria, the number that remains is apt to be close to the number of subjects that will actually be enrolled. If we assume in our example that the site does not see many geriatric patients, then the four main criteria we need to be concerned with are: no previous episode, no previous treatment, no current medications for depression and willingness to sign a consent form. Let us also assume that the investigator says there are about 400 patients in the practice that suffer from depression. Take 400 and divide it in half for each of four major inclusion/ exclusion criteria.

$$400 \rightarrow 200 \rightarrow 100 \rightarrow 50 \rightarrow 25$$

The CRA can assume that the site is probably going to be able to enroll about 25 subjects into the study, in total. This number may be acceptable, but the rate of enrollment needs to be factored in as well. [Note that if a site regularly does research similar to the protocol in question, they may be able to estimate enrollment much more exactly, based on their recent experience. In this case, there should be hard data about recent past trials, including the inclusion and exclusion criteria, numbers of subjects enrolled and rates of enrollment to back up the estimate.]

The CRA must help the investigator analyze the requirements for the rate of enrollment. The sponsor may expect, for example, two patients to be enrolled every week, for the total of 25. Two patients a week does not seem too onerous, but remember that we have a three-month study, and that subjects are seen on a weekly basis. Let's look at what happens as the site begins enrolling. (See Figure 2) At week one, they enroll two subjects. During the second week, they enroll two more, for a total of four subjects on study. By week six, they are up to twelve subjects, and by week ten, they have 20 subjects on study. Since this is a three-month study, all these subjects are still being seen on a weekly basis, and there are still five more to enroll. (We will assume no dropouts for the purpose of this example.) The site must determine, with the CRA's help, if they are able to see and manage that many study subjects within a given week. Assessments must be made that include the investigator's available staff and space, as well as the ancillary help needed for such things as scheduling visits and calling the subjects to remind them of their visits and other study responsibilities. Unfortunately, most sponsors and investigators do not look at the cumulative workload as the study progresses. This is an area where a good CRA can make a significant difference in accurate assessments of enrollment and study load capacities. Before starting a study, the investigator should feel confident that his or her site could manage the enrollment rate and number of subjects appropriately.

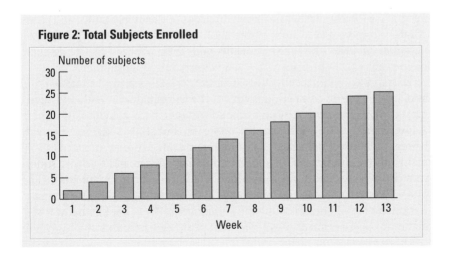

**Figure 2: Total Subjects Enrolled**

It is especially important for a CRA to help new sites, those with no or very little study experience, to estimate the potential workload. Understanding what will be required in terms of time, staff and space throughout the trial will add to the overall chance of success.

## Other Factors That Influence Enrollment

Another major factor influencing enrollment is that of competing studies. CRAs need to be aware of the enrollment problems that can result from having a competing study at an investigative site. Competing studies automatically reduce the resources available to your study, including the pool of available subjects. Even if the study is not competing for the same subject population, too many studies at a site can be a problem; they will compete for the other resources, including coordinator and investigator time, and space.

There can also be a significant impact from other studies within the same community. These studies may be trying to enroll the same type of subjects, and will draw from the same community pool of potential subjects. For example, in the early 1990s, there were more than 150 different AIDS study sites in San Francisco. The AIDS activists had a web site and a toll-free number that listed all of the studies, plus the main inclusion/exclusion criteria for each and contact names and numbers. The people interested in these studies were very well informed, and knew which ones had the most to offer in terms of potential benefit to subjects. Those studies with the newest and potentially best drug were meeting enrollment targets. Enrollment in the others languished. If a sponsor did not have an exciting compound, it was almost impossible to enroll sufficient numbers of subjects.

General interest in the trial, both on the part of the potential subjects and the investigator and staff, can have a major impact on enrollment. CRAs will want to remember that both investigators and subjects have a choice when it comes to participating in a clinical trial; the more exciting the trial and the compound, the more interest there will be in participating. It also helps if the CRA keeps the trial in the forefront of the investigator's and coordinator's minds; if they are thinking about the trial, they will be looking for potential subjects when they see patients in their regular practice. Regular phone calls and visits from a CRA can help encourage enrollment.

It is important for a CRA to consider the available staff and space at a site, even if there are no competing studies. If the coordinator and other involved personnel do not have sufficient time to conduct study activities, or if there is not room to store study supplies and carry out study activities, they will be loath to enroll subjects. Sites sometimes underestimate the staff, space and time requirements for doing a study; the CRA can help them realize what is involved and needs to be done to complete a successful study. The best way for a CRA to assess these things is to look around—check for organization, a relaxed attitude and happy employees. Think about what you see, and make an assessment of whether it appears that an additional study will create a workload problem.

## Advertising for Study Subjects

Sometimes advertising for study subjects is planned right from the start of a study. In general, advertising planned from the start is used when it is expected that subjects will be difficult to find and enroll, when the timeline for enrollment is extremely ambitious, or when a site routinely advertises for all their studies. In other cases, it becomes necessary to advertise for study subjects when enrollment targets are not being met as the study progresses, i.e., there is already an enrollment problem. However, the goal of advertising is the same no matter when it begins—to find and enroll suitable subjects into a trial.

The FDA has deemed that advertising for potential study subjects is not objectionable. In general, advertising is anything that is directed toward potential study subjects with the goal of recruiting them into the study. It may consist of radio or television spots, newspaper ads, posters on bulletin boards, flyers or any other items that are intended to directly reach prospective subjects. For example, one large general practice that does studies has multiple copies of a notebook in their waiting room. Each study they are doing has a brief explanatory page in the notebook that gives basic details about the study and whom to contact for further information. These notebooks count as advertising.

The FDA considers advertising for study subjects to be the start of the informed consent process.[6] Consequently, all advertising must be reviewed and approved by the IRB before use. Note that advertising may not be needed until later in the study, when it is apparent that enrollment goals are not being met. It does not matter that advertising materials were not submitted to the IRB when the study was first reviewed and approved; they simply must be approved before they may be used.

There are some items that do not count as advertising under FDA rules. Not included as advertising are:

> *"(1) communications intended to be seen or heard by health professionals, such as "dear doctor" letters and doctor-to-doctor letters (even when soliciting for study subjects), (2) news stories and (3) publicity intended for other audiences, such as financial page advertisements directed toward prospective investors."[7]*

Investigators must keep in mind, however, that ads written like news stories are still not news stories, but more akin to "infomercials" or "advertorials"—ads with a newsy feel or element. They are still ads. All ads need to be approved by the IRB.

Somewhat confusing is the fact that there is a certain class of Internet advertising that also does not need prior IRB review. Quoting from the same guidance document:

> *"IRB review and approval of listings of clinical trials on the internet would provide no additional safeguard and is not required when the system format limits the information provided to basic trial information, such as: the*

*title; purpose of the study; protocol summary; basic eligibility criteria; study site location(s); and how to contact the site for further information. Examples of clinical trial listing services that do not require prospective IRB approval include the National Cancer Institute's cancer clinical trial listing (PDQ) and the government-sponsored AIDS Clinical Trials Information Service (ACTIS). However, when the opportunity to add additional descriptive information is not precluded by the database system, IRB review and approval may assure that the additional information does not promise or imply a certainty of cure or other benefit beyond what is contained in the protocol and the informed consent document."*[8]

Submitting all advertising to the IRB for review and approval is the best course. That eliminates all doubt and the need to make the determination of what is and is not appropriate material for the general public.

Advertising is reviewed by the IRB to ensure that it is not coercive and that it does not make promises about a cure or favorable outcome, or promise things other than what appears in the protocol or the consent. This is especially important if the study involves subjects who are likely to be vulnerable to undue influence, such as children, prisoners and economically or educationally disadvantaged people.[9]

For written advertisements, such as those designed for use in newspapers, the IRB will want to see finished copy so that they can evaluate the whole ad, including type size and any visual effects. For audio and video advertising (radio, television), the IRB will review both the written text and the audio version. Most IRBs will advise the investigator to submit the text first to be sure it is acceptable before the actual audio- or videotaping is done.

Advertising must not make any explicit or implicit claims that the investigational drug, biologic or device is safe and effective or that it is equivalent or superior to any other product. Remember that the reason the trial is being done is to determine these things; they are not yet known. The ads must explain that the test article is investigational or experimental. Using a term such as "new treatment" implies it is a proven and approved product and is not appropriate.

---

# New Treatment For The
# Common Cold!!!

### Cut your sniffle time in half!!!
### Get paid $1,000 after only 7 days

Study subjects needed. Three shots a day for 4 days. Call Success Clinical at 1-800-999-9999

---

Advertisements may say that subjects will be paid for participating in the study, but the payments should not be emphasized by big, bold type or other methods.

On the previous page is an example of an unacceptable advertisement. Note that it says "new treatment," promises to cut the time of the cold in half and emphasizes the overly high payment amount.

A more appropriate advertisement might look like this:

---

### Research Study

**Subjects needed for a study to investigate the effects of an experimental medicine on lessening the symptoms of the common cold.**

Subjects must be seen by the second day of the cold
and must be at least 18 years old.

For details, contact Shirley Williams at Eastside Clinic. (222) 222-2000

---

What information should go into an advertisement? In general, the information should be limited to what prospective subjects need to know to determine whether or not they might be interested in and eligible for the study. These may include the following items, although the FDA does not require that they all be included:

1. Name and address of the investigator or research facility;
2. Condition under study and/or purpose of the research;
3. Summary of the criteria for study eligibility;
4. Brief list of benefits (e.g., no-cost health examination);
5. Time or other subject commitment; and
6. Contact information.[10]

CRAs should be familiar with the information in the guidance document about advertising so that they may better assist investigators in the proper development and use of advertising materials. The CRA should review all ads to make sure they are IRB-approved prior to use.

## Other Recruitment Methods

Although advertising comes immediately to mind when discussing recruitment for study subjects, there are several other methods for finding subjects. The starting place for most sites is their own clinical/medical records. Many sites have their patients in a computer database that allows them to search based on diagnostic criteria. After they have found patients with an appropriate diagnosis, they are able to contact them to ascertain their interest and suitability for the trial. In the case of studies in chronic diseases, such as diabetes or hypertension, most subjects will probably come from the investigator's own practice. In the case of acute diseases, such as pneumonia and other infectious diseases, searching the records from the investigative site may not be particularly useful.

According to CenterWatch, two out of three patients refer themselves to clinical trials.[11] Many potential subjects hear about a trial by word of mouth, perhaps from a friend who is in the trial. Sites that do a number of trials often have "free advertising" from current or past study subjects spreading the word. Subjects also find clinical trials by talking to people, contacting organizations, including disease-related support groups and pharmaceutical companies and doing web searches.

There are many web sites available to potential study subjects that list trials that are in progress or about to start. CenterWatch, for example, has an online database listing of clinical trials that is easily accessible (www.centerwatch.com). There are other web sites, particularly through the NIH, that list active trials with information for potential subjects. For an example of one of these, sign on to www.cancer.gov/clinical_trials.

Advocacy groups for various diseases, such as AIDS, are sources of information about trials; sites may receive interested subjects from these groups or from people who have been in contact with them.

Frequently, other physicians or healthcare professionals will refer potential subjects to a trial. Investigators often contact other physicians in the community to inform them of the trial, and ask that it be mentioned to suitable subjects. The investigator may make these contacts by phone or may send letters to other healthcare professionals in the community.

Usually finding subjects for a trial is accomplished by a combination of methods. The more difficult it is to enroll, the more variety there will be in the methods used to attract potential subjects. The important things for a CRA to do are to monitor enrollment and enrollment rates right from the start of each study and to make suggestions of ways to enhance enrollment before it becomes a major problem. It is usually much easier to help when things are just starting to look like there may be trouble, than to wait until there is no question that a major problem has occurred. For enrollment problems, the way to fix things is often by implementing several small ideas and suggestions; not everything works in each case, and a single change is frequently not sufficient.

## Payments to Research Subjects

It is quite common for subjects to be paid for participating in clinical trials, especially in the early phases of development. When subjects are paid, however, it is viewed by the FDA as a recruitment incentive, not as a study benefit. All payments schedules must be approved by the IRB in advance of the study, or in advance of being used. The IRB will look at both the payment amounts and the timing of the payments, to be sure they are not coercive and would not present an undue influence on the subject's trial-related decisions.[12] The payment amount must be included in the informed consent.

Subjects are usually paid on a regular basis throughout the trial, most commonly for each completed visit. It is rarely appropriate to pay subjects only if they complete the entire trial; this might encourage them to continue with the trial even if they would have normally discontinued due to side effects or other reasons. The FDA does allow a small payment as an incentive to finish the study, as long as it is not coercive. However, the IRB must determine that this bonus payment is reasonable and not so large that it would influence subjects to stay in the trial when they would otherwise withdraw.

The amount of payments to subjects varies with respect to the complexity of the study and the involvement of the subjects. Payments usually are designed to cover any costs the subjects might incur by participating, such as transportation costs, parking, lunch and childcare. Payments must not be so large as to be coercive; that is, the subjects should not be entering a trial only because of the compensation. Before approving subject payments, the IRB will also take into account where the study is being done and the patient population. Payments of $25 per visit may be no enticement at all to people in some neighborhoods, but may constitute a great deal of money and enticement to subjects in other areas.

The exception for payments is Phase I trials where normal healthy volunteers are the subjects. In this case, there are no real benefits for participating in the trial, so subjects are usually paid more. The amounts are not exorbitant, but are more than in other trials, and generally compensate the subjects for the greater amount of time required, such as overnight stays in the testing facility. Note that in the FDA's Guidance for Institutional Review Boards and Clinical Investigators, it states that "It is not uncommon for subjects to be paid for their participation in research, especially in the early phases of investigational drug, biologic or device development. Payment to research subjects for participation in studies is not considered a benefit, it is a recruitment incentive. Financial incentives are often used when health benefits to subjects are remote or non-existent."

Some sites routinely pay subjects for participating in trials, while others never pay study subjects at all. Either is acceptable. The important things to remember about payments to study subjects are that they must not be coercive or present undue influence, and that they must be pre-approved by the IRB.

## Incentive Payments to Healthcare Professionals

There are two types of incentive payments, those paid by the investigator to other professionals to encourage them to find study subjects, and bonus payments by study sponsors to investigators and their staffs to enhance enrollment.

Incentive payments to healthcare professionals by an investigator for the referral of study subjects are known as referral fees or finder's fees. Examples are payments made to a coordinator or nurse, resident or intern physicians or other local physicians for each subject referred and entered into a study. These payments are usually not acceptable and may compromise the integrity of a trial. They may also be in violation of regulations or institutional policies.

Some states have laws that prohibit referral fees. For example, the California Health and Safety Code § 445 clearly prohibits referral fees. It states:

> *"No person, firm, partnership, association or corporation, or agent or employee thereof, shall for profit refer or recommend a person to a physician, hospital, health-related facility, or dispensary for any form of medical care or treatment of any ailment or medical condition."*[13]

Also, the American Medical Association has stated in its Code of Medical Ethics that referral fees for research studies are unethical. Section 6.03 of the code, Fee Splitting: Referrals to Health Care Facilities, states:

> *"Offering or accepting payment for referring patients to research studies (finder's fees) is also unethical."*[14]

Many IRBs have taken a firm stand on the issue of finder's fees, and will not permit them.

Incentive payments to healthcare professionals also include bonus payments by the study sponsor to investigators and coordinators for enhanced (faster or more) enrollment. True bonus payments are usually not acceptable because they may encourage the enrollment of "borderline" subjects, subjects the investigator would not otherwise recruit. This creates a conflict of interest and should be avoided.

There is no problem, however, with a sponsor covering true extra costs for enrollment procedures. These payments might be for additional people to help with the screening of potential subjects, advertising costs or other direct costs borne by the investigative site. This is frequently decided upon before the study starts, even though not implemented unless necessary to increase enrollment or to speed the rate of enrollment. For example, a sponsor may be willing to pay a per-screen amount for the pre-screening of study candidates. In this case, there is usually a limit on the number of pre-screens allowed in relation to the number of subjects actually entered into the trial. This ensures that the site is actually looking for and pre-screening suitable candidates. The CRA will usualy act as the liaison between the site and the sponsor on questions of appropriate support for enrollment.

If site personnel are not sure whether or not a payment plan is appropriate, they should contact their IRB for an opinion before implementation.

**Figure 3: Venn Diagram Showing Stages of Enrollment for a Clinical Trial**

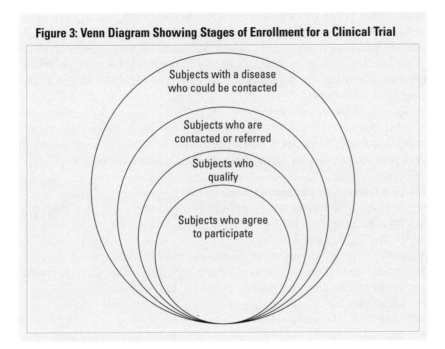

Subjects with a disease who could be contacted

Subjects who are contacted or referred

Subjects who qualify

Subjects who agree to participate

## Summary

Timely and appropriate recruitment and enrollment of subjects into clinical trials are essential for a drug, biologic or device development program. CRAs must be aware of the regulations regarding recruitment and have an understanding of the potential problems and solutions for enrollment. It is important to remember that at each step from initial screening to actual study enrollment, the number of potential subjects decreases. The Venn diagram in Figure 3, patterned after one developed by Bert Spilker,[15] shows this in graphic form.

The CRA plays a significant role in subject enrollment by acting as an advisor to sites, by being aware of the rules and regulations regarding recruitment and by being the liaison between the sponsor and the site for managing enrollment concerns.

# Retention of Study Subjects

Once subjects are enrolled in a trial, it is important that they stay in the trial until it is complete, if at all possible. CRAs should be familiar both with the reasons that subjects drop out and how retention can be enhanced. The CRA should be the expert for helping sites with retention problems. In this section, we will explore the reasons that subjects leave trials and what can be done to increase retention.

## Reasons that investigators or sponsors discontinue subjects

Before discussing reasons that subjects choose to discontinue their participation in clinical trials, it is important to differentiate between subjects who choose to drop out on their own and subjects who are discontinued by the investigator or sponsor.

Investigators and sponsors may discontinue a subject for a number of reasons. Some of these reasons are medical, some are based on the patient's compliance and cooperation and some are trial-related. Some of the more common reasons for discontinuing a subject are listed below.

### Medical reasons for discontinuation:
- Failure of the investigational drug to be effective
- Intolerable adverse events
- Patient's condition deteriorates
- Patient's condition improves (eliminates need to continue)
- Patient develops an intercurrent illness (an illness other than the one under study but occurs during the course of the trial)
- Pregnancy
- Abnormal laboratory values
- Did not meet original entry criteria (discovered after study entry)

### Patient compliance and cooperation reasons:
- Unacceptable compliance with protocol activities
- Unacceptable compliance in taking the study medication
- Not keeping appointments
- Not cooperating with study staff and/or study procedures
- Use of non-approved concomitant medications
- Moved out of the area
- Died

### Trial-related reasons:
- Trial was terminated by the sponsor due to safety concerns
- Benefit so great trial is no longer ethical
- Business reasons
- Investigator no longer to continue the trial (retired, died, moved)
- Investigator did not meet enrollment targets in a timely fashion or did not comply with the protocol
- Investigator had other problems or was put on the debarred list by the FDA

Since it was either the investigator or the sponsor who decided to discontinue patients or the trial for these reasons, we will not discuss them further. The main concern for CRAs is helping sites retain subjects who would have decided to drop out of the study on their own.

## Reasons that subjects drop out of trials

There are many reasons that study subjects decide to stop participating in a trial. Some of them are valid medical reasons, such as intolerable adverse reactions or a worsening of the disease. These cases are usually discussed with and agreed to by the investigator.

There are, however, other reasons that subjects drop out, which are not so compelling and could perhaps be avoided. This is where the CRA can help site personnel understand what causes some of the problems and how they might prevent them from occurring. The key for the CRA is catching problems, or patterns of problems, early so that they can be fixed. The CRA wants to ensure that losses do not become the standard and that they do not exceed what would normally be expected during a study. Some reasons subjects drop out are:

- The subject does not understand the importance of remaining in the trial, even when the disease condition has improved.
- The study requirements are too burdensome.
- The subject loses interest in the trial.
- The medication is unpleasant to take.
- The subject does not like some of the study staff or finds people at the investigative site unfriendly (which could be anyone, including the receptionist).
- The subject has to spend too much time at the clinic.
- Transportation, childcare, or time off work difficulties.
- The subject is upset about some aspect of the trial.
- Friends or family are unhappy about the subject's participation.
- The subject has a change in his or her personal life.

## Maximizing retention in clinical trials

The secret to subject retention in clinical trials is easy. It's not really a secret at all, but is just plain common sense. All site personnel have to do is be nice, treat subjects well, spend time with them, listen carefully to what they are saying and communicate openly and often.

Investigators and study coordinators are very busy people. They get rushed and behind on things, have good and bad days and experience all the problems the rest of us do. Nevertheless, if a study is to go well, they must be able to set aside their concerns and problems when study subjects are in for their visits. Study subjects want to feel that their contribution is important, and during their time with the investigator and/or coordinator, want to be the sole focus of attention.

When a study subject comes in for a clinic visit, he or she wants to be able to discuss what has happened since the last visit, to have any study concerns allayed, to be praised for doing well, to have questions answered and to be treated like an important partner in the study venture. In short, a study subject wants to be appreciated. It is his or her time and body. After all, there are risks in becoming part of a study, there is no guaranteed outcome and it is voluntary … no one has to participate at all. People who volunteer for studies are special people, and they should be treated that way.

Given the premise of wanting to be treated well, there are many things, and they are frequently small things, that can make subjects decide that trial participation may not be worth the effort. Some of these things are:

- Having to wait when coming in for an appointment
- Not being treated nicely and with respect
- Not seeing the investigator or the coordinator, but being seen by a "substitute" that they don't know
- Not seeing the same person at each visit (developing a one-on-one relationship)
- Being rushed and hurried through the appointment.
- Feeling that the investigator/coordinator doesn't really want to see them
- Not being asked about how they feel and how the study is going for them
- Not having the opportunity to ask questions
- Being afraid to ask study-related questions
- Being made to feel dumb or silly when asking questions
- Being berated for doing something wrong
- Having the investigator or coordinator disparage the study

There are also situations where a subject does not return and is lost to follow-up, or where a subject drops out but refuses to give a reason, other than personal choice, which is the subject's right—he or she doesn't have to give a reason. But that doesn't help site personnel understand if there is a more pervasive, underlying problem. These situations are difficult to prevent, so the investigative site cannot do much about them.

If there are many of these cases at a center, however, they should serve as a wake-up call. Chances are that the real reasons are in the list above, but the subject just doesn't want to say anything about them to site personnel.

These problems are all fixable, but first they need to be recognized and acknowledged. It's critical to catch them early. Some problems are easy to fix. For example, if a subject has a logistics problem, such as transportation to the investigative site, a solution may be to pay for a taxi to transport the subject back and forth. If childcare is a problem, perhaps the visit time can be adjusted to an evening or weekend time so that the subject can come in when a spouse is home to stay with the children. Questioning the subject about problems and being willing to help with arrangements or adjustments may allow the subject to continue participating. Subject payments in any form (cash, goods or services) should be reviewed by the IRB. It is fine to vary payments according to subjects' needs (taxi fare for one, but not another), but it would usually be stated as "payment for (actual) transportation costs," for example. Since these are actual costs to subjects, they would not be considered coercive. Coercion normally implies a sum of money above costs, with no purpose other than to entice people to enter the trial.

Some successful investigative sites have very clever ways of making their study subjects feel happy, important and wanted. Some of the ideas and little things that have added to retention success for sites are:

- Giving each volunteer a special study tee shirt
- Mugs, tote bags, gym bags for a study where there was exercise testing
- Separate waiting room with coffee, tea and doughnuts—and current magazines and newspapers
- Reminder calls the day before each visit
- Sending a cab to pick someone up if transportation is a problem
- Thank you notes from the coordinator after a few weeks on a study
- Thank you notes at the end of the subject's participation (leads to repeat volunteering)
- Balloons
- Birthday cards

For new investigative sites especially, though it will be beneficial for most sites, it helps if the CRA meets with the investigator and coordinator at the beginning of the trial and plans out a strategy to help retain subjects. Many sponsors are willing to foot the bill for little extras (mugs, tee shirts) that may encourage subjects to feel good about their participation and remain in the trial until completion.

Any time there is a pattern of more-than-expected dropouts at an investigative site, the CRA should discuss the situation with the investigator and coordinator. Each case should be analyzed. Perhaps the reasons are clear-cut and recognizable, perhaps not. It may be time to reflect on the atmosphere at the site, and to take a hard look at how subjects are being treated. The site personnel might even want to talk with subjects about their perceptions of how the study is going, how they feel when they come in for visits, and if there are ways in which the investigative site could improve the study process.

Difficult as it is, site personnel must also take an honest look at their interactions with study subjects. Sometimes it helps to think about how you would feel if you were in the study, or how you would feel about having one of your loved ones participating.

## Summary
Retention of subjects in clinical trials is critical to the completion of an informative, sound clinical trial. Site personnel should help subjects understand that a successful trial is a partnership between the subjects and the investigative staff. Respect, courtesy, honesty and open communication on the part of both subjects and investigators will increase the chances of successfully completing a study.

# Subject Compliance

Clinical trials are conducted in order to assess the safety and efficacy of an investigational drug. To be able to accurately assess safety and efficacy, however, study subjects must take the medication as it is prescribed. Unfortunately, subjects do not always do this. In this section, we will look at compliance, what can go wrong and how to increase the probability of good compliance.

Undetected poor compliance can lead to invalid study results. Lack of compliance in one subject may affect only that particular subject; if several subjects are noncompliant, however, it can invalidate the entire study. Noncompliance can have the following results:

- An effective medication may look ineffective. This can mean that a medication that would be effective, and that would be of benefit to patients, never makes it to the marketplace. This is an unfortunate result for the sponsor company that has made the development investment in the investigational drug, and even more unfortunate for those people who would have received benefit from it.
- An ineffective medication looks effective. This result is worse than the one above, because, once marketed, the medication will be relied on to effect a cure and will not be effective in doing so.
- Failure to detect serious adverse events.
- Inappropriate dosage labeling. Depending on the noncompliance, the drug labeling could recommend either too high or too low a dose. This is not good in either direction—patients could be taking too little to be an effective treatment, or more than they need, which could lead to an excess of adverse reactions.

The effects of the investigational drug in noncompliant subjects cannot be extrapolated to compliant subjects. It is very important that all study subjects are as compliant as possible during their involvement in clinical trials.

## Reasons for Noncompliance

Sometimes study subjects are noncompliant for disease-related reasons. One reason is a lack of symptoms, or what can be called the "antibiotic effect." As many of us know from personal experience, it is hard to remember to take medications when you feel better and have very few or no remaining disease symptoms. A prime example of this is the standard 10-day course of treatment with many antibiotics. After five or six days, when the patient appears to be over the disease, it is very common to stop taking the pills. The subject has become noncompliant with the medication schedule; this happens in trials as well as in general practice.

There are also compliance problems with people suffering from terminal diseases. When someone knows they are going to die soon anyway, they do not have the same incentive for taking a course of medications that they might have otherwise.

There are many other reasons subjects are not compliant when it comes to taking medication. Sometimes they just forget to take their pills. Sometimes there is a lack of belief in the treatment—"it isn't going to work anyway, I'm sure I'm on the placebo...." If the medication is unpleasant to take, such as not tasting good or pills that are so big they are hard to swallow, compliance may be poor.

Noncompliance can result from the way the drug is packaged. Think about using safety containers (childproof lids) in an arthritis study, for example. The subjects may not be able to open the containers without help, which will surely affect compliance. Sometimes study drug is packaged in large blister packs containing several days' worth of drug and with each day's drug clearly marked as to when it should be taken. At first glance, it appears this would help compliance, but think about it a bit more. What happens when a subject has to go to work? Most people do not want to carry a large blister pack to work with them and have other people asking about it. Consequently, subjects might take the day's drug out of the package and just carry it in a pocket, not knowing that the ordering of the pills for the day is important—they become noncompliant.

Sometimes subjects just do not understand the dosing scheme, especially if it is complicated. "Oh, it's two white ones and one pink one? I thought it was two pink ones and one white one. That's why I ran out of pink ones last week." Sometimes it is the regimen that is confusing, with too many pills, too many different times per day to take them or confusion about the times and/or doses. It may also be the duration of the study, as subjects can lose interest over time.

Subjects may also become noncompliant because of adverse reactions. If a subject becomes nauseated after taking the medication, or thinks it is causing headaches, he or she may not take it as often as required, if at all. A subject may not take medication appropriately because of mistrust, either in the medication or in the physician. A subject may be influenced by family or friends in ways that affect compliance also; if people important to the subject do not want him or her to take the pills, or be in the study, this may affect compliance.

Other ways in which subjects may be noncompliant that are related to the study medication are by prematurely discontinuing the drug or by sharing the drug with other people. Some of the other reasons subjects may become noncompliant include:

- Taking other medications at the same time, when the other medications are not allowed by the protocol.
- Using alcohol or other disallowed substances such as marijuana while in the study.
- Changes in their living situations that have an impact on when and how the study drug is taken.

- Their mental conditions have an unfavorable effect on their ability to follow protocol instructions.

There are other compliance issues in studies that are not related directly to the medication. Subjects may also be noncompliant by missing visits or not coming in for visits within the visit windows. They may not adhere to other study requirements, such as special tests (eye exams, for example), dietary requirements or keeping diaries.

Sometimes compliance problems stem from investigator-related reasons. Subjects will be less compliant if it is difficult to schedule study visits, or if they are kept waiting when they come in for a visit. If study staff do not keep appointments, subjects are apt to do the same. Worst of all is a poor physician-patient relationship. In general, subjects want to please the physician and do things correctly, but if the relationship is poor, the subject is not as likely to care about complying with study requirements.

Unfortunately, there are many ways to be noncompliant, both on purpose and by mistake. The key is finding out about them and fixing the problem before it has a negative impact on the study.

## Managing Compliance

Study protocols should be designed to enhance compliance, as much as possible. They should also make it possible to monitor compliance.

CRAs should discuss compliance with site personnel and help them understand not only why it is important, but also how they can help to ensure compliance during the study. First of all, the CRA must help the investigator and coordinator understand that they need to work with their patients, both before and during the trial. There are certain things that study patients must be aware of and do during the study. Just as clinical trials are different than clinical practice for investigators, they are different for study subjects. The investigator and coordinator must ensure that potential study subjects are aware that if they are in the study, they must:

- Come in for all study visits on time and within the visit windows.
- Answer the questions truthfully, especially with respect to their medical histories and disease history.
- Cooperate fully with study procedures. This is one reason it is critical that the investigator fully explains the study to potential subjects.
- Allow tests to be done as appropriate, and on time.
- Take study medications as prescribed.
- Follow all study directions.
- Ask if something is not clear and inform the site of any problems.
- Report any new medications (OTC or Rx) before they take them or as soon as possible afterward.

The CRA should emphasize to the site that patients must be told how important it is to answer questions truthfully, especially about their compliance during the study. Patients need to know that it is better to let the investigator/coordinator know that they missed some doses than say nothing about it, and that they will skew the results of the study if they are not forthcoming with this information. A CRA should remind the site personnel that they must thoroughly question each subject about compliance at each visit. They should be sure to let subjects know that they should call if they are having any problems complying with study activities or are confused about what needs to be done.

There are a variety of ways of testing for compliance in studies. Every study will have some way of asking about and maintaining drug accountability. Usually a record is kept for each subject of the amounts and dates study drug is dispensed, and the amounts and dates of study drug returned. Subjects are told to bring back any unused medications at each visit. The returned study drug is counted and recorded by the coordinator. This is a reasonable way to assess compliance, but, unless the subject admits a problem, there is no way of knowing about the pill that fell down the drain or got swallowed by the dog. The person seeing the subject should also question him or her about whether or not all doses were taken.

Watching subjects take the pills in person would encourage good compliance, but studies are not usually set up in such a way that the subject is at the site each time a dose needs to be taken. This would work only if there is a single dose of medication being given, or if an IV drug is being administered, or something similar.

Subjects are sometimes asked to keep diaries and record when each medication dose was taken. This is probably a good solution for very compliant subjects, but for the others, it is as easy to forget writing in the diary as it is to forget to take the medication.

The "gold standard" for testing for compliance is to check blood levels. This is done in some studies, but mostly only the very early (phase I) studies. It is expensive and not feasible to do most of the time.

What can site personnel do to maximize compliance? First, it helps to know the subjects they enrolled. If an investigator and coordinator have worked with a subject before, they should have an idea of whether or not the person will be compliant. They should question subjects before entering the study on their willingness to comply with study activities, if they can swallow the pills, if they can come in for visits, etc.

The investigator and coordinator must pay attention to the signs of potential noncompliance. Does the patient show up for visits? On time? Did the subject complete all necessary pre-study activities? Is the person really interested in the study and aware of the requirements?

The coordinator should ask the subject about anything that may interfere with completing the study. Does the subject have a vacation planned during the time of the study? Does he or she understand what is involved in participating? Does the patient's lifestyle allow for complying with the study rules and activities?

In short, if site personnel know or think that a subject will not be a good, compliant patient, he or she should not be enrolled in the study.

## When Noncompliance Happens

If the site is aware that a subject has been noncompliant, either in taking the medication or other study activities, the site should call and inform the sponsor of the noncompliance issue. Details of any noncompliance situations should be documented both in the case report form and in a note to the investigator's study file. The coordinator should discuss the situation with the subject and do some re-training in study procedures. If the subject continues to be noncompliant, he or she may need to be dropped from the trial. Keeping subjects who are not compliant in a trial is not good for the subject or the trial. When subjects are dropped from a study for noncompliance, the relevant information must be recorded both in the case report form and in the subject's office chart or with a note to the investigator's study file.

By working closely with each potential subject before enrollment into a trial, and by working closely with the subjects throughout the trial, compliance can be maximized, and study results will be more reliable than if there had been major compliance problems.

Good study designs and protocols will anticipate noncompliance and give instructions for minimizing it and handling it if it occurs. If the CRA and the investigator do their jobs, both to minimize noncompliance and to detect and report it, the study should remain valid.

## Key Takeaways

### Recruitment

- Timely enrollment of subjects is critical to a drug, biologic or device development program.
- CRAs must help investigative sites accurately estimate the number of subjects they can expect to enroll in a study.
- Sites need to have the necessary personnel, time and space to handle the enrollment needed for each trial.
- Protocol requirements, especially the inclusion and exclusion criteria, are the primary limiting factors for enrollment.
- Assessment of the rate of enrollment is critical to managing a trial at the investigative site.
- Competing studies, both at the site and in the community, can have a significant impact on enrollment.
- Advertising for study subjects is allowed by the FDA, but must not be coercive or exert undue influence on potential subjects.
- All advertising must be approved by the IRB before use.
- Most study subjects refer themselves to clinical trials.

- Payments to study subjects must be approved by the IRB and must not be coercive or exert undue influence on study subjects.
- Finder's fees or referral fees are not acceptable and in some states are illegal.
- Sponsors will usually pay true extra costs for enrollment procedures.
- CRAs must be able to monitor enrollment and to suggest methods to increase enrollment if it lags behind expectations.

## Retention of Study Subjects

- Investigators may discontinue subjects from a trial for medical reasons, compliance or cooperation issues or because the sponsor is stopping the trial.
- Subjects have many reasons for dropping out of a trial, including medical reasons and logistics problems.
- Determining problems as early as possible is the first step to retaining subjects in trials.
- Respect and open communication are the biggest factors in subject retention.
- CRAs can help their sites achieve good retention.

## Subject Compliance

- Good compliance is critical for valid conclusions from clinical trials.
- Subjects need to be aware of the importance of compliance.
- Sites need to determine if potential study subjects are likely to be compliant, and not enroll subjects who probably will not be compliant.
- There are many different ways in which subjects may be noncompliant with study procedures.
- Site personnel need to be alert to compliance problems throughout the study.
- If noncompliance occurs, the site should notify the sponsor.

## References

1. "Sponsors Take On Patient Recruitment," CenterWatch, March 2002, Vol. 9, Issue 3, Deborah Borfitz.
2. Informed Consent, Kenneth A. Getz and Deborah Borfitz, CenterWatch, p. 22.
3. Ibid.
4. Tufts Center for the Study for Drug Development, 2002.
5. Guide to Clinical Trials, Bert Spilker, Lippincott-Raven, 1996
6. Guidance for IRBs and Clinical Investigators. FDA. Sept. 1998, p. 29.
7. Ibid.
8. Guidance for IRBs and Clinical Investigators. FDA. Sept. 1998, p. 29
9. 21 CFR 56.111 (a)(3) and 21 CFR 56.111 (b).
10. Guidance for IRBs and Clinical Investigators. FDA. Sept. 1998, p. 30
11. Informed Consent, Kenneth A. Getz and Deborah Borfitz, CenterWatch, 2002, p. 157.

12. Guidance for IRBs and Clinical Investigators. FDA. Sept. 1998, p. 31.
13. California Health and Safety Code § 445.
14. AMA Code of Medical Ethics § 6.03.
15. Guide to Clinical Studies and Developing Protocols, Bert Spilker, Raven Press, 1984, 237.

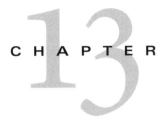

C H A P T E R

# Study Closeout

When a study is over at an investigative site, it must be officially closed. This is almost always the responsibility of the CRA. In this chapter we will look at the reasons studies are closed and what must be done to close a study.

## Reasons for Study Closeout

The primary reason to close a study is that it is complete and finished: enrollment has stopped, all subjects have completed their study-related activities and the data are complete and correct. This is, of course, the best and most desired outcome.

There are also reasons for closing a study before it is complete. Studies may be terminated early for both positive and negative reasons. Some of the reasons are listed below.

**Positive reasons for early study termination:**
- The investigational treatment is so beneficial that it would not be ethical to conduct a trial during which subjects might not be receiving the active treatment.
- Overall enrollment was met in the trial, so all sites are being closed even if they did not complete the site enrollment goal.

- Statistical stopping criteria were set up in advance (in the protocol), and those criteria were met. This means that the endpoint was reached (either positive for the investigational treatment or not), and the trial will end. Whether or not the outcome was the one hoped for, there is no reason to expend additional resources on the trial.

**Negative reasons for prematurely ending a trial:**
- The investigational treatment was found to be unsafe.
- The investigational treatment was not effective.
- It was not possible to find and enroll sufficient study subjects.
- The sponsor decided the potential product was not viable for marketing.
- Sponsor terminates the program for another reason.
- The company ran out of funds. (This is being seen more frequently in small startup companies that rely heavily on venture capital.)
- The protocol is too difficult to execute.
- An investigator loses interest in the trial.
- An investigator dies, retires, moves, etc., and there is no replacement investigator.
- Problems arise in the manufacturing or stability of the compound.
- Compliance or other problems at the site.

As might be suspected from the length of the two lists, more studies are terminated early for negative reasons than for positive ones.

A trial may be discontinued at all sites at the same time or at individual sites at different times. Whatever the timing, the activity is essentially a single-site activity, that is, it must be done at each site without regard to the activity at the other sites.

One cautionary note: if the study is stopped abruptly while subjects are still taking the study medications, there should be an orderly plan for discontinuing each subject. This plan will be formulated by the sponsor and communicated to each investigator. The CRA should be prepared to explain the plan to the site and ensure that it is followed correctly. The site must also be prepared to notify subjects promptly and assure them of appropriate therapy and follow-up outside of the trial.

Closing a study because it is finished and complete is the most common situation. It is also the easiest to handle. Site personnel are usually pleased that it was finished, hopeful of a favorable outcome and, frequently, hoping for additional studies from the sponsor in the future. In this case, the CRA is welcomed.

If a study was closed for a negative reason, it may affect all sites or just one. In this case, site personnel may not be happy about the closeout. Since the CRA is the sponsor's on-site representative, the CRA may be the recipient of the site's anger or unhappiness. This is the time for a CRA to use all of his or her tact and interpersonal skills. If at all possible, you want to leave the investigator and other site personnel as friends rather than enemies, even if they are unhappy friends.

No matter what the reason is for closing the study, the same procedures must be followed. In the rest of the chapter, we will discuss what needs to be done to close a study.

# Closeout Procedures

A CRA must be at the site to do a closeout visit. It would be extremely unusual to try to close out a site without being there in person. The main items to be addressed during a closeout visit are: case report forms, drug accountability, the investigator's study file and administrative items.

### Case report forms
If the case report forms have not already been reviewed, submitted and corrected, this must be done now. If the study has come to it's natural end, this activity has probably been done. If the study has been stopped abruptly or early, this may not be complete. It is always better not to do a final closeout visit until after the case report forms have been submitted and reviewed, in case final corrections need to be made.

The CRA should make sure that all the case report forms, as well as any corrections or query forms, are complete, in order and ready for storage.

### Drug accountability
If there are still study drug supplies at the site, the CRA should complete a final inventory at the closeout visit. The study drug should then be packaged for return to the sponsor, according to company policy. A copy of the drug inventory form should be placed in the investigator's study file.

Drug reconciliation should have been done throughout the study, rather than left to the end. In this case, it will be relatively easy for the CRA and the coordinator to finish the reconciliation. Otherwise, drug accounting could be the most time-consuming study closeout activity.

### Investigator's study file
The CRA must thoroughly check the investigator's study document file at this visit. It is wise to use a checklist (See Appendix C) to ensure that nothing is overlooked. All documents must be present, including appropriate re-approvals and correspondence from the IRB. If there were protocol amendments during the study, or amendments to the informed consent form, all versions should be in the file, including their dates of use.

Informed consent forms for each subject must be present. The CRA should double-check to be sure they were all signed and dated appropriately.

There should be documentation for any protocol variations, whether they were previously approved or not. The investigator brochure should be available in or with the file.

If any documents are missing from this file, the CRA should help the investigative site to obtain copies. Remember the suggestion that CRAs keep copies of important documents for each site in their own study files? Now is a time when this can be very beneficial. When the file is complete and in order, it is ready for storage.

## Investigator's final report to the sponsor and the IRB

The investigator is required to make a final study report to the sponsor.[1] This report should include an enrollment summary, including the numbers of subjects entered, those who completed, those who dropped out and their reasons for dropping out. It will also include information about adverse events and any other information relative to the trial at that site.

The investigator will also make a final report to the IRB. It will contain the information above, in addition to any other information specifically requested by the IRB.

The investigator must also notify the institution that the study is complete, if appropriate.

The CRA should verify that these reports were done, collect copies for the sponsor, if appropriate, and ensure that the reports are in the investigator study file.

## Administrative issues

Since this is probably the last visit the CRA will make to the investigative site for the trial, any outstanding business or issues should be resolved before the study closeout is complete. Any loose ends should be resolved and taken care of before the site is completely closed.

The CRA should verify that all appropriate grant monies have been paid or requested. Be sure that the amounts are in agreement between the investigator and the sponsor.

If there are unused study materials at the investigative site (case report forms, unused laboratory kits, etc.), they should be returned or disposed of according to the sponsor's direction.

Any outstanding issues from previous visits, or issues that arose during sponsor review, should be resolved before the study is closed out at the investigative site. If not documented elsewhere, a note detailing the resolution should be put in the investigator's study file.

The CRA should discuss record retention with the investigator. Not only do the records need to be stored and maintained, but also there must be a record of where they are stored. According to the regulations, records must be kept for two years after the NDA is approved for marketing, or, if an NDA is not filed or is disapproved, for two years after the investigation is discontinued and the FDA notified.[2] However, most sponsors expect the investigator to retain all study records until notified by the sponsor that they may be disposed of; this will usually be in the contract that the investigator signed before starting the study. The CRA must be sure that the investigator and site personnel are aware of and understand the retention period. This was also discussed in Chapter 8 under "Investigator Responsibilities."

Investigative sites do not always keep study records as long as they should. Years go by, and things happen—they run short of storage space, or move to a new facility or just don't think they need to "keep all that old stuff" around any longer. Unfortunately, these records may be needed years after the study is over. For example, the sponsor may decide to file a new application based in part on old studies; when the FDA visits investigative sites as part of the NDA review process, they will expect to see all the documents in place, even if the study was done many years previously. It will be an embarrassment to the investigator if he or she has thrown them away, and it may have a negative impact on the sponsor's NDA.

CRAs need to impress upon their sites that record retention is important and not something to be taken lightly, along with the reasons for keeping everything. The records must be kept until the sponsor has informed the site in writing that they may be destroyed. It is recommended that the boxes be labeled on the outside "DO NOT DESTROY," with the names of both the investigator and the sponsor as contacts for questions about them. If there is some reason that a site can no longer maintain the records, the site should contact the sponsor. In most cases, the sponsor will arrange storage for these materials so that they are not destroyed.

This is also the time to remind the investigator of any publication terms for the study and to notify the sponsor of any impending FDA audit. When everything is complete and accounted for, the CRA should thank the site for their participation, being sure to include everyone who worked on the study. It is nice to follow up with a written letter of thanks.

### Final visit report

The CRA must complete a visit report after this site visit, as for any other visit. Many companies have a special visit report for the closeout visit. This report documents that the study was officially closed.

In the final report, the CRA should verify that everything was checked, found complete and prepared for storage. If there were any outstanding issues from previous visits, the resolution of those issues should be documented in this visit report. The CRA should be sure that the report is clear and does not leave any unresolved loose ends.

## Key Takeaways

- Studies can be stopped because they are complete, or for a variety of other reasons—both positive and negative.
- The CRA is the person who will do a study closeout at an investigative site.

- All study documents, including case report forms, informed consent forms, drug accountability and study regulatory documents must be complete and filed at the end of the study.
- All study drug and other supplies must be returned to the sponsor or otherwise disposed of at the end of the study.
- The investigator must prepare a final study report to the sponsor and to the IRB at the end of the study.
- The investigator must be aware of record retention requirements at the end of the study.
- The CRA must verify in a final visit report that the study was properly closed.

**References**

1.  21 CFR 312.64c.
2.  21 CFR 312.62c.

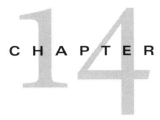

C H A P T E R

# Audits

During the clinical development process, the U.S. Food and Drug Administration (FDA) may conduct audits (also called inspections) of investigative sites. Sponsors and IRBs may also conduct their own audits of investigative sites. The FDA also audits sponsors and IRBs. In this chapter we will discuss these different types of audits, as well as the CRA role in each kind of audit. We will start with audits conducted by sponsors and institutional or independent review boards (IRBs) but will concentrate primarily on those audits done by the FDA, as they are the most critical to the drug approval process and to the CRA.

## Sponsor Audits of Investigative Sites

There are two main purposes for a sponsor to audit an investigative site. The first, and most common, reason is to ensure that a site is complying with the regulations and protocol when doing a study and that everything is in order in case of an FDA audit. These are referred to as routine audits. The second reason is because there is evidence that the site is out of compliance, and the sponsor wants to either verify the problem or be reassured that no problem exists. These are called for-cause audits.

A sponsor's right to audit a site is based on both the regulations and (usually) on the contract between the investigator and the sponsor. The contract will usually state that the investigator agrees that the sponsor may conduct audits of the site. The regulations under which sponsor audits are loosely covered are found in 21 CFR 312.56(a)(b), which states:

*(a) The sponsor shall monitor the progress of all clinical investigations being conducted under its IND, and (b) A sponsor who discovers that an investigator is not complying with the signed agreement (Form FDA—1572), the general investigational plan, or the requirements of this part or other applicable parts shall promptly either secure compliance or discontinue shipments of the investigational new drug to the investigator and end the investigator's participation in the investigation.*[1]

Sponsor audits are usually carried out by the sponsor's quality assurance (QA) department, if it has one. The CRA may or may not accompany the audit team but usually does not assist in the actual audit. If the sponsor company is too small to have a QA department, or if the QA department does not have the resources to do an audit, the sponsor may contract with a contract research organization (CRO) to do the work for them. In general, a sponsor may contract out routine audits, but will usually do for-cause audits itself.

**Routine audits**

If the sponsor knows or suspects that a site will be audited by the FDA, a routine audit may be done, either while the study is in progress or after it has been completed and during the new drug approval (NDA) review period. The sponsor knows that the FDA will inspect some sites during its review of the NDA, so the sponsor will focus on the sites that are logical for the FDA to pick: those where enrollment was the highest or where multiple studies contributed to the NDA.

For a routine audit the sponsor will send in an audit team, who will follow the same inspection plan used by the FDA. This inspection plan can be found in the FDA Compliance Program Guidance Manual for Clinical Investigators (Program 7348.811) or can be found on the Internet at www.fda.gov/oc/gcp/compliance.html.

A written report of sponsor audit results is usually not given to the investigator. This is because FDA inspectors do not have routine access to sponsor audit reports, and sponsors do not want to have these reports freely circulating, either at the investigative site or internally. If a written report is sent to an investigator, the sponsor will usually ask that it be destroyed after corrective action is taken.

If any problems are found during the audit, the CRA will most likely be asked to work with the site to remedy them, with the goal of ensuring that the site is ready for an FDA audit. The CRA will report back on the final status at the site; this is sometimes done in a formal audit response, which is kept with the original audit report. Audit reports and responses are usually maintained in and by the QA department, and any other copies are to be destroyed.

---

### Nightmare Audit

*I had a nightmare FDA audit two years ago that lasted more than two weeks. The one thing that kept me going was that I had personally done a good job from my end. I had no control over what was done to CRFs or source docs after the study was closed, and things were done. I learned that early on I gave the site too many chances without documenting that there were problems; I had not wanted to "tell on them" without giving them a chance to fix things.*

*Document, document, document. Having to fax the FDA auditor my visit reports (with my company's blessing) was quite a learning experience. I wished, of course, that there was more on my reports about the problems that I was aware of and had addressed with the site. I had communicated all the problems to the project manager on the phone, but not in writing, except for too briefly on visit reports. This site had enrolled too quickly— 60 patients when the average everywhere else was about eight.*

*—A CRA Friend*

---

## For-cause audits

For-cause audits of investigator sites by a sponsor may be handled somewhat differently. These are audits done because of suspected noncompliance at a site, either with the regulations or with the protocol. They have the potential for being much more serious, both for the sponsor and ultimately for the investigator. The sponsor is unlikely to tell the investigator it is a for-cause audit; the CRA will probably know, since the information about the suspected problems was most likely reported to the sponsor by the CRA. The audit team will look at most of the things they would inspect for any audit, but will pay particular attention to the area of the suspected noncompliance.

### Depending on the results of the audit, a number of things could happen:

- If everything appears to be in compliance, the results will be handled in the same way as they would be for any routine audit.
- If the problem was not found but is still suspected, another group may be sent to look. Or the sponsor might inform the FDA and ask them to inspect the site.
- If problems were found, they will either be rectified, or enrollment may be put on hold pending further investigation, or the study may be stopped at the site. In this case the FDA will be informed, if appropriate. If so, this will be done by the QA department, probably in conjunction with the medical monitor for the study and the sponsor's regulatory group.

closed. These are not pleasant situations to be in, and the CRA will need a lot of tact and diplomacy in working through the problems.

## IRB Audits of Investigative Sites

IRBs also visit or audit sites upon occasion. A central or independent IRB may visit sites simply because they are not located nearby, and they want to be assured that the site is managing studies correctly. These are routine audits.

An IRB may also make for-cause visits if there is reason to think that the site has ethics or compliance violations. IRBs are required to report to the FDA any instances of unanticipated problems involving risks to human subjects, serious or continuing noncompliance with the regulations or IRB requirements or any suspension or termination of IRB approval.[2]

CRAs will not be involved in IRB audits. Of course the CRA would be involved in closing the study at a site if approval was withdrawn.

## FDA Audits

The FDA's Bioresearch Monitoring Program (BIMO) includes visits to investigators, sponsors, IRBs, CROs and animal labs. All FDA-regulated products are involved, including drugs, biologics, devices, radiological products, foods and veterinary products. Although the BIMO programs vary somewhat from product to product, they all have the same goals:

1. To ensure the quality and integrity of the information submitted to the FDA
2. To protect human research subjects

**The FDA compliance program has three parts, including:**
- Clinical Investigators (Program 7348.811)
- Sponsors, Contract Research Organizations and Monitors (Program 7348.810)
- Institutional Review Boards (Program 7348.809)

Copies of the FDA Compliance Program Guidance Manuals for Inspections (the three programs listed above) are available through the Freedom of Information Act and can be requested by writing to:

Freedom of Information Staff (HFI-35)
Food and Drug Administration
5600 Fishers Lane
Rockville, Maryland 20857

The information is also available through the FDA's web site: www.fda.gov. It would be useful for a CRA to read these documents, as they delineate the particular items an FDA inspector will concentrate on.

The FDA can make inspection visits to sponsors and to IRBs at any time, with the purpose of determining compliance to the regulations and the organizations' own standard operating procedures (SOPs). CRAs will not be involved in IRB inspections and would only rarely be involved in sponsor inspections, so there is no need to discuss these any further. However, we will discuss FDA audits of clinical investigators in detail, as CRAs have a decided role and impact on this process.

## FDA audits of investigative sites

The FDA conducts three types of inspections at clinical investigator sites: study-related, investigator-related, and bioequivalence study. Bioequivalence study inspections are conducted when one study is the sole basis for a drug's approval; we will not discuss these here. The other two types are important for a CRA to be aware of. For either study- or investigator-related audits, the purpose is threefold:

1. To determine the validity and integrity of the data
2. To assess adherence to regulations and guidelines
3. To determine that the rights and safety of the human subjects were properly protected

We will take a detailed look at both study and investigator audits.

### Study-related audits

Study-related audits/inspections are almost always done on the studies that are important to an NDA or biological license application that has been submitted to the agency. These studies are the primary efficacy studies on which a sponsor relies for showing that the product works and should be approved for marketing.

The sites picked are usually those that contributed the most data to the application, either by high enrollment or by doing multiple studies. Because of this, sponsors usually have a reasonable idea of which sites have a high probability of being audited. The sponsor also knows that studies will be inspected during the NDA review time, which is currently six months or less for a Track A product, and one year or less for all others, from the date the FDA receives the application.

The primary efficacy studies are closed at this point, as the trials are complete and analyzed before being submitted in the NDA; in fact, they may have been closed for quite some time. Sometime early in the NDA review process, CRAs are often sent to the sites with high probability of being audited in order to ensure that all the study materials are available and organized for FDA review. (Note that a site will usually inform the sponsor of an FDA scheduled audit, in which case the sponsor may send the CRA in to help the site prepare.) If the CRA finds missing documents or other problems, the site may be able to remedy the situation before an FDA audit occurs.

### Investigator-related inspections

Investigator-related inspections are initiated for a variety of reasons, many of which are listed below:

- Investigators have done a large number of studies or have done work outside their specialty areas.
- An investigator has done a pivotal study that is critical to a new product application and it merits extra attention.
- The safety or efficacy findings of an investigator are inconsistent with the results from other investigators working with the same test product.
- The sponsor or IRB has notified the FDA about serious problems or concerns at the site.
- A subject has complained about the protocol or subject rights violations at the site.
- There were an unexpectedly high number of subjects with the diagnosis under study, given the location of the study.
- Enrollment at the site was much more rapid than expected.
- The study and investigator were highly publicized in the media.
- Any other reason that piques the curiosity of the agency.

Unless a sponsor alerted the FDA to problems at a site, the sponsor will probably not know in advance about an investigator-related inspection. (If the sponsor did alert the FDA, then it has probably already done its own QA audit.) Consequently, a CRA is rarely, if ever, involved in these audits.

### Site preparation

The best preparation for an audit is for the site to have done things correctly to begin with, in which case an audit will reveal no problems. However, once an audit is scheduled, the site should prepare by amassing all the study documents in one easily accessible place, and by reviewing them to be sure everything is accounted for, complete and well organized. The study documents that should be available for review include all informed consent forms, patient charts and other source documents, case report forms and the study regulatory file. When an inspector asks to see a document, the site should be able to retrieve it easily and quickly. Sometimes, although this is seen most often when the FDA audits non-U.S. sites, the FDA may ask the site to send them a letter of availability of records; this letter certifies that all study records will be available for FDA review upon their arrival.

If there is time, and travel schedules allow, the CRA often goes to the site and assists in the audit preparation; if not, the CRA should at least be available by telephone to answer any questions the site may have, or to send copies from the sponsor study file of any missing documentation. Sometimes a CRA can lend moral support by telling the site what to expect during the audit, how to interact with the inspector and what the process is. No one from the sponsor will be present during the audit; the audit is between the investigator and the FDA.

## The audit process

The audit process begins with the notification of the site. The inspector usually contacts the site by telephone to arrange a mutually acceptable time for the audit visit. Sites are usually given about two weeks' notice; it is acceptable to negotiate a delay in the visit date, as long as the investigator has a good reason and the time is not lengthened too much. If the audit is investigator-related, and if the FDA has concerns about subject safety or compliance, the time between the notification and the visit will probably be very short, and delays will not be acceptable. If there are serious concerns, the FDA could just appear at the site without advance notice. Most sponsors ask and expect their investigators to let them know immediately about an impending audit.

The role of the investigator in the audit is to be present, to provide the inspector with a quiet, comfortable place to work, to assemble the necessary documents and to answer questions. The investigator should be polite, courteous, cooperative and reasonable when interacting with the FDA inspector; antagonism is inappropriate and will undoubtedly be regretted later. The investigator should provide all the materials/documents the investigator requests, but should never give the inspector free access to the files. All questions should be answered, but extra information should not be volunteered. The inspector knows what he or she is asking for and will continue to question until the needed information is obtained. The investigator should not offer the inspector anything beyond a cup of coffee; offering even a meal may be misconstrued. At this time, the FDA is not privy to grant information or to sponsor audit results, so if the inspector asks for this information, the investigator should politely refuse to answer. If the inspector is treated politely, the audit will be more pleasant for everyone. The CRA should go over these suggestions on conduct with the investigator and staff before an audit occurs.

When the inspector arrives at a site, he or she will present credentials (a photo ID) and a Notice of Inspections Form (482) to the clinical investigator. If the inspector does not present these credentials, the investigator should ask for them. The investigator should check the date on the inspector's credentials to be sure it is still valid and note the inspector's badge number. During the inspection, the inspector will meet with study staff and will review study documents. If people who played a substantial role in the study are no longer at the site, the investigator should be able to contact them, if at all possible, during the audit if the inspector wishes to talk with them. There are two main aspects of the study that will be looked at during the inspection: study conduct and study data. According to the FDA Guidance for IRBs and Investigators, the conduct of the study will be considered by reviewing the following items:

- who did what
- the degree of delegation of authority
- where specific aspects of the study were performed
- how and where data were recorded
- how test article accountability was maintained
- how the monitor communicated with the clinical investigator
- how the monitor evaluated the study's progress.[3]

Notice that the monitor (CRA) is mentioned in two of these bullets. A CRA must communicate carefully with the investigator throughout the study and may want to make use of written communications to reiterate the points discussed during a monitoring visit. These communications should be kept in the investigator's study file, and copies should also be kept in the sponsor's file. At the very least, the monitor should sign a study visit log at each monitoring visit to verify that the site was actually visited. (There is an example of a study visit log in Appendix C.) This also underscores the need for complete monitoring visit reports, which were discussed in Chapter 10.

When the inspector audits the study data, he or she will compare the data that were submitted to the agency with the site records that support the data, i.e., investigator copies of the case report forms and all the available source documents, including patient charts, laboratory reports, other test reports, and so forth. Sometimes the inspector will also have copies of the case report forms from the sponsor, and will compare all three versions. The inspector will pay close attention to:

- the diagnosis
- whether the patients were properly diagnosed based on their past history
- whether or not the subjects met the protocol inclusion/exclusion criteria
- concomitant medications, especially those that were not allowed
- appropriate follow-up of adverse events

The inspector may look at data for only a sampling of subjects, or, if there appear to be problems, he or she may look at the data from all subjects. All informed consents are usually reviewed.

An FDA audit usually takes one to two weeks, although it depends on the amount of data to review, the findings and the amount of time the inspector has available for the audit. The days may not be consecutive for the entire period, but rather a day or two at the site at one time until the review is complete.

At the end of the inspection, the inspector will meet with the investigator to review the audit findings. During this meeting, the investigator may ask questions about anything that is not understood, and may clarify things that the inspector has interpreted incorrectly. Sometimes a misunderstanding or negative finding of the inspector can be explained satisfactorily at this point. If there are significant findings, the inspector may issue a Form FDA-483 (Notice of Observations) to the investigator. This form will detail the findings from the audit that may constitute compliance violations.

Most sponsors ask that an investigator call them after the inspector leaves and let them know the results of the audit. If the investigator has received a 483 form, the sponsor will help the investigator formulate his or her reply (a written reply is mandatory).

## After the audit

After the audit is completed, the FDA inspector prepares an Establishment Inspection Report (EIR). This report goes through FDA compliance channels, and a classification is assigned to it. The investigator will receive a copy of the report approximately four months after the audit. The report is also available through the Freedom of Information Act, and most sponsors will request copies for their files.

### The EIR classifications are:
- No action indicated (NAI). This is the best outcome, and means that no significant deviations from the regulations were found. The clinical investigator is not required to respond to this report.
- Voluntary action indicated (VAI). This report will provide information about findings of deviations from the regulations and good clinical practice. The letter may or may not require a response from the investigator. If a response is required, the letter will specify what is necessary. A contact person will also be listed for any questions.
- Official action indicated (OAI). This is the worst result to receive and is known as a warning letter. It identifies serious deviations from the regulations that require prompt action from the investigator. For OAIs, the FDA may also inform the sponsor and the IRB. The FDA may also inform the sponsor if the agency feels that monitoring of the study was deficient (beware, CRAs). In addition to issuing the warning letter, the FDA may take other action, such as regulatory and/or administrative sanctions against the investigator.[4] All in all, this is a very unpleasant process and should be avoided at all cost.

## Consequences

The consequences of problems found during audits can be significant, especially when they have an impact on a large amount of the data for a pivotal trial. The study at a particular site may be invalidated, especially if sufficient source documents were not available, if there were significant unreported concomitant therapies, or if there was a failure to follow the protocol. If the site was a high enroller and generated a significant amount of data in support of the sponsor's NDA, these problems could delay the NDA or result in a disapproved application. A sponsor may even have to repeat a study, which could add years to the drug development cycle.

There are also significant consequences for the investigator in these cases. An investigator may be disqualified or restricted from conducting clinical trials. This puts them on the infamous "black list," known more formally as the List of Disqualified and Restricted Investigators.[5] An investigator can be added to the list through a court hearing or through a consent agreement; he or she can be disqualified from ever doing clinical studies, or may have other restrictions placed on him or her, such as only doing studies as a sub-investigator, or not doing more than one study every two years, etc. Once on the list, the investigator stays on the list forever, even if corrective actions are taken.

It does not happen often, but in the worst cases an investigator can be fined and/or sentenced to prison. For example, let's look at the case of Dr. Richard Borison, a psychiatrist, and Dr. Bruce Diamond, a pharmacologist. They were conducting schizophrenia trials for eight years using resources at the Medical College of Georgia, but pocketing the proceeds. They also encouraged psychotic patients to enter trials by giving them money and cigarettes and had untrained staff doing study procedures, including blood draws. These abuses were discovered when a disgruntled employee told the university what was going on. The two doctors were fined and jailed in 1997 and were ordered to pay back millions of dollars to the university.

## Results from FDA audits of investigative sites

The Center for Drug Evaluation and Research (CDER) is a branch of the FDA. The CDER conducted 259 investigator-specific inspections in 2007, which represents the majority of site inspections conducted that year. (See Figure 1.) These complaints have added to the Department of Health and Human Services' (HHS) and FDA's resolve to tighten compliance in clinical trials. The most common site inspection results were distributed as shown in Figure 2. Notice that protocol violations and inadequate and incorrect records are the two most common citations.

There have also been several large institutions where studies have been temporarily suspended, primarily due to problems with their IRBs, including informed consent noncompliance, poor record keeping and problems with continuing review of active studies.

It is clear from the problems cited that the compliance system is stretched. We are seeing more training requirements for all clinical

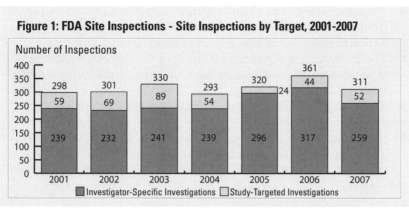

**Figure 1: FDA Site Inspections - Site Inspections by Target, 2001-2007**

Source: CenterWatch Analysis, 2009; CDER Department of Scientific Investigations, 2009

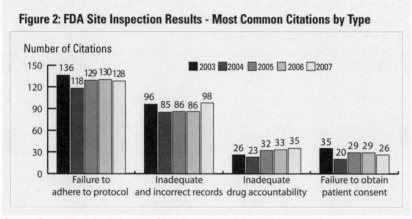

**Figure 2: FDA Site Inspection Results - Most Common Citations by Type**

Source: CenterWatch Analysis, 2009; CDER Department of Scientific Investigations, 2009

researchers. CRAs can help by educating themselves and by training site personnel to be compliant and perform research according to good clinical practices.

# Key Takeaways

- Sponsors audit investigative sites for studies that contribute highly to their development programs. They also audit sites where it appears that there may be compliance problems.
- IRBs can also audit sites, especially if they suspect ethics violations.
- The FDA performs both study-related and investigator-related audits.
- The best preparation for an audit is to do the study correctly.
- CRAs should help their sites understand the audit process and prepare for audits.

- There are three classes of Establishment Inspection Reports that result from an FDA inspection: no action indicated (NAI), voluntary action indicated (VAI) and official action indicated (OAI).
- The consequences of noncompliance are great and can result in delays in an NDA, and/or in disqualification and other penalties for investigators.
- There has been an increase in compliance problems during the past few years.
- CRAs must be educated about the correct procedures for clinical trials and must watch their sites closely to ensure compliance.

### References

1. 21 CFR 312.56(a)(b).
2. 21 CFR 56.108(b).
3. FDA Guidance for IRBs and Investigators, FDA inspections of clinical investigators, p. 75.
4. www.fda.gov/oc/gcp/compliance.html
5. www.fda.gov/ora/compliance_ref/bimo/dis_res_assur.htm.
6. CDER

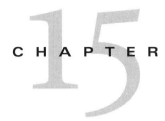

# Errors, Misconduct, and Fraud

In this chapter, we will discuss some serious situations CRAs face, namely errors, misconduct and fraud. Our discussion will be limited to the occurrence of these unfortunate events at investigative sites, and we will focus primarily on the CRA's role in detecting and coping with these problems. We will start by defining each term and then look at the impact of each on a clinical trial and on the CRA.

## Definitions

If you consult a dictionary, you will find the following definitions for error, misconduct and fraud:

> *Error: an act involving an unintentional deviation from truth or accuracy.*

> *Misconduct: intentional wrongdoing.*

> *Fraud: intentional perversion of truth in order to induce another to part with something of value or to surrender a legal right.*[1]

As you can see, these are listed in increasing severity, and the same is true of their impact on a clinical trial and on the CRA. We'll consider each category in detail.

# Errors

If you think about the definition of an error, it contains two key ideas. The first is that an error is a deviation from truth or accuracy, and the second is that it is unintentional. There is no doubt that a CRA will see errors when monitoring studies; in fact, the CRA can expect to see some errors at every study site he or she monitors, assuming the sites enroll any subjects at all. The errors that CRAs will most commonly see are those in case report forms, although these are not the only errors that can occur during a study. Errors may also occur in drug dispensing, study documents, protocol conduct or any other aspect of study performance.

We will now look at some of the errors that may occur during a study, starting with case report forms (CRFs). Types of errors commonly seen on CRFs result from omissions (missing values), inconsistencies, incorrect entries, out of range entries, illogical entries and undecipherable entries.

As an example, we will use one of the standard questions that is asked in almost every study and see how it can be answered (on a CRF) to meet the error types listed above. The question is:

Sex:   Male ☐   Female ☐

It looks very straightforward and should be easy to answer this question without making an error. Here is the error of omission:

Sex:   Male ☐   Female ☐

Notice that neither box is checked—the question was not answered.

An error of inconsistency would be, in this case, that the subject was listed as a male in one place and as a female in another. Most CRFs will not ask this question directly more than once, but there may be other questions where the sex is implied by the answer. One common question in the inclusion/exclusion criteria is one that asks if the subject, if female, has had a pregnancy test. Assume the answer was "Yes," but then the entry for our example is:

Sex:   Male X   Female ☐

We have an inconsistency between the two entries.

An incorrect entry is easy—the wrong box was checked.

For this question, out-of-range entries would probably not be seen. An out-of-range happens when an answer is supposed to fall between two values, and doesn't. For example, when the answer to "Rate the subject's pain on a scale of 1 to 10" is recorded as "12." An illogical entry for this same question would be "Better" or "D." Neither entry makes sense, given the question and the way it is worded.

Undecipherable entries are sometimes illegible answers, those that cannot be read because of the handwriting. They may also be entries like:

Sex:    Male X    Female X

Overall, errors run the gamut from small discrepancies to glaring inconsistencies.

Because errors are unintentional, there is hope of eliminating, or at least reducing, their occurrence, over the course of a study. In Chapter 10, we discussed different ways in which the CRA can help lessen or eliminate errors at sites. We also discussed the impact of errors and the cost of errors. It is important to realize that the CRA can make a significant contribution to studies by working with his or her sites to eliminate errors made on case report forms.

In general, errors are easy to find and easy to fix. Although it depends on the parameter, the impact of errors on the study is usually quite low, since they are fixable. If the CRA is doing a good job, the error rate should go down as the study progresses. The following are some things the CRA can do to help decrease or eliminate errors:

- Review the first patient or two very soon after enrollment. Do a very thorough review. Quick feedback to the site can do more than anything else to eliminate future errors. Many errors, especially at the beginning of a study, are due to misunderstandings on the part of the study coordinator and other site personnel. If these problems are found and corrected early, they will usually not occur in the future.
- Look for systematic errors and instruct the site on the correct way to record the data. Systematic errors are also usually due to misunderstandings and can be eliminated by quick feedback. For example, the CRF may have a question that reads: Have there been any changes in concomitant medications since the last visit? The site may be recording only new or stopped medications, rather than including changes in dosage for medication during the study. Once this is clarified, these systematic errors should not continue.
- Train your sites well in the beginning, and retrain them if:
  - There are misunderstandings
  - New personnel are added
  - The study or procedures change in any way.
- Demand good work, nicely. This is especially important when there are errors due to carelessness. One of the techniques that a CRA may find

helpful here is to remind the site of the high cost, in both time and money, of correcting errors. Chapter 10 has details about this, but an estimate of the cost of each error for a site is about $20 and 15 minutes of time.

The CRA also has a great influence when it comes to eliminating other errors in studies, such as those that occur in drug dispensing, study documents, protocol conduct and other aspects of study performance. Remember that the CRA is the sponsor representative who visits the site most often, and may, in fact, be the only sponsor representative that ever goes to an investigator's site. No one else will have a better opportunity to eliminate errors in a study than the CRA who monitors it. It is the responsibility of the CRA to:

- Be aware of problems that might occur
- Be aware and vigilant in looking for problems
- Instruct the site personnel in how to handle problems if they occur
- Train site personnel to decrease and/or eliminate problems in the future

To summarize, most errors are caused by misunderstanding or inattention. The impact of errors on study results is generally low, as they are usually correctable once they are caught. They can be eliminated, or at least reduced in number, by training, including feedback. The dual role of the CRA is checker and trainer; actual error correction must be done by site personnel.

## Misconduct

Misconduct is a degree more serious than error. Misconduct implies that someone knowingly did something that was wrong. In studies, some of the more commonly seen types of misconduct are enrolling subjects who "almost qualify" without permission, guessing at vital signs and easing things into compliance, examples of which can be found later in this section.

Investigators are under enormous pressure to enroll subjects quickly into clinical trials. The pressure has increased even more over the last year or two with the widespread use of "competitive enrollment." Competitive enrollment usually means that sponsors will sign up more investigators than they expect to need for a trial and will allow enrollment of subjects to continue only until the necessary number of subjects is reached. If investigators enroll quickly, they will remain investigators for the trial; if they enroll slowly, they may have very few subjects entered when enrollment is halted, or even none, which would result in their being dropped from the trial. Knowing that some study-related activities must take place at a site before subjects can be enrolled, it is possible that an investigator can even lose money on a study if he or she has no, or low, enrollment when the enrollment period is closed.

Given this enrollment scenario, it is easy to understand why an investigator would use all means to find suitable subjects. As some of the inclusion and exclusion criteria for studies have measurements that are somewhat imprecise or could lend themselves to differing interpretations, such as blood pressure readings or rating scales such as the Hamilton Rating Scale for Depression (HAM-D), it can be tempting, and fairly easy, to ease these readings or ratings into compliance. For example, if a subject in a hypertension study was supposed to have an initial diastolic blood pressure of between 90 and 100 mmHg and the person being evaluated for the study is perfect in every way, except that his initial diastolic blood pressure is 88 mmHg, who would know if the investigator recorded it as 90 or 91? No one, as long as the office chart and the case report form match. But if it is incorrect and was done on purpose; it is an example of misconduct.

Another example from actual experience was a case where subjects were to read an eye chart from a distance of fifteen feet. Each subject, and there were many, did this at every visit. It wasn't until a new and astute CRA measured the distance that it was found to be only thirteen feet, rendering the data unusable. The investigator knew he didn't have a fifteen-foot span to use, but figured it was "close enough" and that no one would measure. The investigator was aware of the discrepancy, but didn't really think it made any difference, so he never mentioned it and continued to use the shorter span. This is misconduct.

Misconduct can have a more pronounced effect on studies than errors, simply because it may not be discovered, or it may be unfixable if it is found. In the eye exam example above, the misconduct was discovered, but the data for about 25 subjects were unusable, and it was in a very difficult study where every subject enrolled was critical. When misconduct is not discovered, it can, depending on the magnitude of the problem, affect the results of a study. It could make an investigational drug look effective or safe when it is not, or vice versa; neither is a good outcome for consumers.

It is much more difficult for a CRA to root out misconduct than errors. A CRA must be vigilant in performing source document review, particularly when it comes to verifying the inclusion and exclusion criteria for a subject. Sometimes site personnel may change things slightly in the case report form to make the subject fit the study, but do not think about past entries in an office chart. The CRA must also be aware of the pressures to enroll and be cognizant of enrollment that seems a little too good to be true. (Things that seem to be too good to be true often are.)

CRAs also need to think about what is needed in a study and should not be afraid to verify that they are correct. What a difference it could have made if the original CRA on the eye study had measured the 15-foot distance before subjects were enrolled.

# Fraud

Fraud is the most serious offense of the three and the most difficult to discover. Fraud is willful deception. The impact of fraud on a study is apt to be very great, but can only be measured if it is discovered. It is a nightmare for the sponsor(s) involved, and for the CRA. A CRA will not often see cases of fraud. We will discuss some publicized cases of fraud later in this chapter.

Fraud can manifest in various ways. Some of the more common ways are the use of fictitious trial subjects and/or fictitious data, faked test results and fraudulent study documents. Fraud is usually committed in order to increase revenue from the trial—either by enrolling more subjects, faster enrollment or cutting actual costs. After discussing some examples of fraud, we will talk about what a CRA can do to lessen the chances of fraud, how to look for fraud and what can be done when it is discovered.

Fraud is difficult to discover. The perpetrator of fraud is usually careful to do as much as possible to keep the deception hidden. However, there are some techniques that a CRA may find useful when reviewing data that may point to situations that should be investigated further. It is important to keep in mind that the incidence of fraud in clinical trials is very low, and most CRAs will not encounter fraud at all. Still, it is important for CRAs to remain vigilant and aware of the potential for fraud.

## Real-life examples of fraud

In a study at one investigative site, everything looked fine. The study went well, enrolled well, and no one suspected that things were not done correctly. It was only during a routine FDA inspection during the NDA review that a problem was found. The FDA inspector took all the informed consents, stacked them up and fanned through them looking at the signatures. What he saw looked something like this:

It became apparent to the inspector as he riffled through them that all the consent forms were signed by only three different people. The names were different, but the handwriting was the same. As it turned out in this case, they had been signed by the investigator and two research nurses. Study subjects did not exist at all, but were part of a carefully laid plan to collect the grant without actually enrolling subjects. The subjects were fictitious, as were the data. It was cleverly done and might not have been discovered at all, except for the savvy inspector who looked at the consents all together.

Why didn't the CRA find the consent problem? Because the consents were only checked individually, as each subject was enrolled. Each one was signed and dated before the subject was entered into the study. The consents were each kept with the individual study chart and case report form, not altogether in one place. It never occurred to the CRA to pull them out and fan through them. It is a good practice for CRAs to look at all the consents together occasionally, rather than only individually as each subject is enrolled.

Since this investigator had contributed heavily to the data submitted for approval of this drug, the sponsor company was required to re-analyze all the data without including this investigator. It was an enormous job and cost the company dearly in terms of time and resources.

In another case, the investigator had subjects, but didn't want to take the time to have their blood drawn. Instead, he drew blood from his own staff in greater quantities, divided it up, and labeled it with subject initials. This way it could all be done at one time and stored ready to ship.

In this study, all the blood samples were shipped to the sponsor. They were batched and sent every two or three months. The problem at this site was discovered when the samples for August and September came in, and the vials were marked for October—someone had grabbed the wrong ones by mistake. The CRA went in to investigate, checked the freezer, and there they all were, neatly labeled and stored for months in advance. Needless to say, the data were not usable either. Would this have been caught during routine monitoring? Probably not, unless the CRA just happened to look in the freezer and saw them. Had the site known the freezer would be checked, the samples probably would have been moved or disguised. One thing, though, that might have caught the notice of that CRA beforehand is the site's lack of "busy-ness." If you don't see many subjects during your monitoring visits, it may be time to suspect fraudulent practices.

## Do subjects really exist?

People who revert to fraud are usually quite clever at disguising their fraudulent practices, making them difficult to discover. However, there are some things a CRA can do when monitoring an investigative site that can help to uncover signs of potential fraud. The first thing is to think about whether or not subjects actually exist. When you are at an investigative site, look for signs that point to the existence of actual subjects/patients being seen. Do you see patients in the waiting room? Is the practice bustling? Are the phones ringing? Do you hear appointments being scheduled?

When the CRA is reviewing source documents, particularly office charts, there are things you would expect to see. Office charts usually contain the patient's name, address, phone number, social security number, date of birth and insurance information. If it is not there, where is it? Does the chart look like most office charts, with entries done over time, in different handwriting, with different pens? Are lab reports available in the chart? The CRA should think about whether or not the patient charts look like standard office charts in most medical practices.

Look at the dates of study visits and compare them with a calendar. Are people coming in on appropriate days of the weeks, or are there a lot of weekend and/or holiday visits? What you will need to look for are things that you would not expect to see. A site may see study patients on a Saturday, or even in the evenings, but you would not expect to see Sunday visits, or visits on holidays (Thanksgiving, Easter Sunday, July 4th, etc.).

Think about the accrual rate of subjects into the trial. Is it much faster than expected or than other sites? How can this site enroll well if others can't? If there is no explanation, a wise CRA will thoroughly check the source documents and look closely at the data. Also look at screen failure rate. Is it similar to other sites' or lower than expected?

## Numeric data

There are also things to look for when reviewing numerical data, such as blood pressure readings. Look at the blood pressure readings listed below:

| | | | | |
|---|---|---|---|---|
| 120/80 | 120/85 | 115/80 | 120/75 | 110/70 |
| 120/80 | 110/70 | 115/80 | 120/90 | 110/70 |
| 120/85 | 110/80 | 120/80 | 120/80 | 110/65 |
| 120/80 | 110/80 | 120/80 | 120/85 | 115/80 |

The first thing you should notice about these numbers is that they all end in either "0" or "5." You would not expect all blood pressure readings to end in 0 or 5, when presumably they could end in any digit. Unless the instrument used is calibrated only in increments of five, this will not happen.

With numerical data, look for other digit preferences, as well as 0 and 5. You should expect to see a pretty random distribution of the last digits; you would not expect to see mostly "7" or "3," for example. Look also for other invented patterns of numbers (lots of "77"s or "123"s, for example), and for more duplicate numbers than you would expect.

Look also for too few or too many outliers (outliers are the data values that lie outside the range you would normally expect to see). If you are dealing with a population of subjects whose blood pressures are "normal," as opposed to a hypertension study, for example, you will expect to see some people with higher than normal pressures and a few with lower than normal pressures. If you are seeing too many that are outside the normal range, you may want to investigate further. The same is true if you see no one outside the normal range. The data may be valid, but it is worth checking the source documents for verification, or asking about it.

## Commonly chosen data for fabrication

According to Iber, Riley and Murray in their book *Conducting Clinical Trials*,[2] the data points that are commonly chosen for fabrication, with comments in italics added by us, are:

**Entry criteria:**
- Known disqualifying factors are suppressed. *Such as taking a non-allowed medication prior to entry.*
- Birth date altered to meet eligible age range; weight or height altered. *It's more difficult to alter the birth date in source documents, since it appears in many places. Since weight is variable and may change from time to time, this is more likely to be changed.*
- Dates of prohibited medication use altered or suppressed. *Example: no previous treatment with an antibiotic allowed in an infectious disease trial. The subject was treated, but it was not put in his chart or on the CRF.*
- History of drug or alcohol abuse or mental illness suppressed. *If this information already appears in the chart, it is difficult to suppress. If it is a new patient, however, this information can just be omitted from the chart when the history is taken.*

**Safety checks:**
- Reports *of procedures* from previous visits or from other patients are used for the current visit. *Laboratory reports, ECGs, etc.[3] are either from a previous visit of the subject, or might be from a completely different person as in the example of the blood samples discussed previously.*
- Blood and urine samples substituted from other patients. *This can happen when the subject doesn't qualify. A sample from someone who does qualify might be split and relabeled with the subject's identifiers.*

**Visit data:**
- Visit dates altered to fit permitted windows. *This keeps the patient in compliance and the visit from being missed.*
- Visits fabricated. *This can be especially easy to do with phone visits, or visits where laboratory tests, ECGs, etc. are not done.*
- Medication counts falsified, with tablets discarded so inventories match false reports. *This makes things look like they are in compliance when they are not. It can also cover up incorrect dispensing on the part of site personnel.*
- Diaries fabricated. *Note that the handwriting on diaries can be checked in the same manner as the writing on consents—look at them all together, both for a single subject and for all subjects.*

## Suspicion of misconduct or fraud

When a CRA suspects that things may not be quite right at a site, there are a number of things that can be done. The first thing to do is thoroughly monitor everything, doing more than you might do under normal circumstances. Be thorough when doing source document review, taking time to check all variables. Check carefully across visits, thinking about whether the new data seems consistent with the older data in light of what you know about each subject. Are you seeing differences in the data that appear odd or unusual?

The CRA can also check the laboratory reports and other test results. Be sure the patient identifiers are consistent (name, age, sex, social security number, date of birth, etc.). If someone is falsifying information, they are apt to make mistakes on the small, non-essential information rather than the primary information. If you notice discrepancies, ask the study coordinator or the investigator about them and listen carefully to the explanations they give you.

If you have checked carefully and your suspicions remain, call in some help. Ask your supervisor or another (senior) CRA to monitor with you and see what one of them thinks. If there still appears to be cause for concern, ask your Quality Assurance (QA) group to send someone in to do an audit. The investigative site does not need to know at this point that you are concerned about misconduct or fraud. It is probably better that they do not know, as you would not want them to try to cover their tracks, and if there is no misconduct or fraud, it won't be appreciated if they know you suspected them of it. Remember that you need to continue working with them.

If your company has determined that there is probably fraud, it must be reported to the FDA. In this case, the FDA will most likely do a for-cause audit of the investigative site, which we discussed in the previous chapter.

## Consequences of fraud

The consequences of fraud can be disastrous for a sponsor. The data from the fraudulent site will probably not be usable, which may result in losing a complete study. This can delay the NDA or cause the FDA to declare it as "unfileable." This can set a development program back by several years or may cause the program to be completely halted. At the very least, a sponsor will probably need to re-analyze the data, eliminating all data from the questionable site.

The consequences for investigators who have participated in fraud are also severe. They may be placed on the FDA List of Disqualified and Restricted Investigators[3] or they may be barred from participating in clinical research. In the worst cases, they may also be fined and/or sent to prison.

There can be consequences for a CRA, also, if fraud has been found at his or her site. If the CRA found the problem through diligence and good monitoring, and found it early, he or she will probably be credited with a job well done. Given that fraud can be very difficult to detect, a CRA might not have found it even if doing a superb job of monitoring; in this case, there are not likely to be any tangible repercussions for the CRA. There may be intangible repercussions, however; memories are long when it comes to remembering cases of fraud. Even if the fraud was cleverly perpetrated and disguised and even if there was no blame placed on the CRA, it's not pleasant to have to explain (for years) what happened at "your" site. Of course, if the CRA did not find problems because of not monitoring appropriately, the outcome won't be as rosy. CRAs can be severely reprimanded, or even lose their job, in this situation.

The best things a CRA can do to minimize the potential for fraud at a site, or to detect it if it is present, are:

- Monitor carefully and thoroughly. Don't cut corners. Ask questions if you are seeing discrepancies.
- Think about what you are seeing and doing. Does it make sense?
- Pay attention to small signs and problems. Be aware of what is going on around you. Pay attention to your "gut feelings."
- Listen. Be approachable. Many times fraud is uncovered because an employee tells someone else about it.
- Bring in another set of eyes. The site does not have to know why you have someone else with you—it can just be a joint monitoring visit or a training session.
- If you see potential problems, share them with your supervisor. The problems will not just take care of themselves.

## Current Findings by FDA

Starting in 1999, the FDA began seeing a very large increase in the number of complaints filed with the agency against investigators. The FDA's Division of Scientific Investigations (DSI) has been promoting the importance of filing complaints, due in part to some of the abuses seen in clinical trials in the pasts few years. DSI tracks the complaints that come in very closely and has instituted an aggressive follow-up program for investigating them.

Complaint inspections find noncompliance at sites in far greater numbers than unsolicited inspections; in fact, during 1999 and 2000, approximately one in every four complaint inspections resulted in an Official Actions Indicated (OAI) inspection rating[1] (See Chapter 14).

The complaints to the agency come from many sources, including disgruntled employees, sponsors, IRBs and others. Complaints coming from sponsors often originate with CRAs, as CRAs are in the best position to determine what is occurring at study sites. In fact, in the June 2001 issue of *CenterWatch*, Stan Woollen, then acting director of the DSI's Office of Medical Policy, expected CRAs to be a valuable ally in detecting noncompliance at investigative sites. He said, "The efforts of study monitors have a system-wide effect. If the industry is out there monitoring what is happening with investigative sites, and that monitoring could be enhanced, we could certainly leverage our impact in improving the quality of data."[4]

# Conclusion

Errors will always happen during clinical trials. They are usually fairly easy to find and fix, and will usually decrease in number as the trial progresses. Since they are fixable, the impact on trial results is usually not significant.

The difference between misconduct and fraud is really only one of degree, since in both cases there is intention to do things incorrectly. Both can be difficult to detect, especially fraud, as it is often cleverly perpetrated on a large scale. In general, fraud is committed for personal gain, while misconduct is committed for expediency. Both can have a major impact on a trial.

# Key Takeaways

- Errors are unintentional, usually due to misunderstanding or carelessness, and can be fixed. They usually have a low impact on a trial.
- Early detection of errors by the CRA and close cooperation with site personnel will generally reduce errors in a study.
- Misconduct and fraud are intentional wrongdoing, are much more difficult to detect and can have a major impact on a trial.
- Fraud is usually committed for personal gain, while misconduct is often committed for expediency.
- The CRA is the first line of defense against errors, misconduct and fraud.
- Good monitoring and awareness can help in preventing and in detecting misconduct and fraud.
- The FDA is relying on help from CRAs to discover noncompliance at investigative sites.

### References

1.  Webster's Ninth New Collegiate Dictionary. Merriam, Webster. Springfield, MA. 1990
2.  Conducting Clinical Trials, Iber, Frank L.; Riley, W. Anthony; Murray, Patricia J., Plenum, 1987
3.  www.fda.gov/ora/compliance_ref/bimo/dis_res_assur.htm.
4.  "FDA Complaints Against Investigative Sites Still Rising" CenterWatch, June 2001, Vol. 8, Issue 6, Valerie Gamache, p. 14.

CHAPTER

# The Future for CRAs

In this chapter, we will discuss the oft-repeated prediction that technology will ultimately replace the role of the study monitor. That has yet to happen. Instead, technology has helped expand and change the CRA's role in clinical research for both regional and central monitors. CRAs have seen their role shift due to the nearly universal adoption of the regional field monitor structure among major pharmaceutical companies.

Clinical research associates, who have long had an essential role in ensuring the quality and integrity of clinical trial data, increasingly are finding their responsibilities grow beyond traditional monitoring duties.

Although specific approaches differ widely by company, drug sponsors are beginning to rely on CRAs to help build stronger local relationships with investigative sites. Increasingly, sponsors give study monitors additional responsibility for site management activities, such as evaluating patient enrollment plans or participating in site selection. In addition, CRAs often are relied upon to act as counselors and resolve site problems that could adversely impact a study, such as angry or overworked staff.

As adoption of electronic data capture (EDC) to record clinical trial data becomes more widespread, CRAs have begun to see change in where their work is done. CRAs are now able to identify problems, answer questions and make necessary corrections remotely before a site visit. The technology also gives CRAs a better ability to analyze information and to query data directly with the sites, making source verification activities more efficient.

As their role and responsibilities continue to grow, CRAs are becoming even more critical to the success of a clinical trial. Investigative sites consistently have rated the quality of CRAs as one of the top five most essential factors contributing to study success. For the sponsor or CRO, the study monitor is the person who can make or break the study. More often now this means not only monitoring data and ensuring investigator compliance, but also solving day-to-day problems at sites and acting as a liaison between the drug sponsor and the investigator.

## Shifting Responsibilities

CRAs have seen their role shift, in part, due to the nearly universal adoption of the regional field monitor structure among major pharmaceutical companies. At least 80% of the top 15 drug companies use this approach as opposed to sending CRAs from a centralized office to far-flung investigative sites. This regional structure has allowed drug companies to cut travel costs and also has led to improved job satisfaction and turnover rates of their CRAs. At the same time, drug sponsors have begun to realize another benefit to a regional study monitor structure: Regional monitors, who repeatedly visit the same sites and spend many hours with investigators and coordinators, have become an invaluable source of information about site operational issues, such as the professionalism of a site, the efficiency of the coordinator and how staff handle data. Study monitors also might notice other factors that could affect the success of a study, such as signs that the coordinator or ancillary staff are overworked or frustrated. They are the eyes and ears of the sponsor.

Since CRAs have this inside information, drug companies have begun to realize that they can use their study monitors in new ways and expand their duties beyond the traditional roles of checking to see that sites comply with regulations and verifying that source documents and other trial records are accurate and up-to-date.

More companies are empowering their regional monitors to be influential in site selection and to be a much better conduit for communication with investigators. While some sponsors already have their monitors conduct pre-study site visits, when they evaluate the investigator, staff, facility and lab, and then make recommendations about whether the site should participate in a study. But other drug companies still outsource the site selection process or have an employee other than the monitor perform the visit. Even when monitors are involved in these companies' pre-site visits, site selection decisions are made in the home office with little regard for the monitor's recommendation.

As drug company executives realize the importance of the information monitors have about the investigative sites they work with, they are allowing regional monitors to have more input into the site selection process. They are beginning to empower monitors to be far more influential in site selection and a much better conduit for communication.

In addition to the obvious cost benefits, since drug companies don't need to send two people to evaluate the site, involvement of regional monitors in the site selection process could result in more successful studies; the monitors, who work with investigative sites on a regular basis, know the quality—or lack of quality—of individual sites.

Allowing regional monitors more input into site selection could result in cleaner data and less monitoring during the study. Monitors will pick sites that they know are good. Sites that they don't have to babysit or teach the basics.

Job responsibilities for some study monitors have also been expanded to include evaluating enrollment plans before a study begins or helping solve patient recruitment problems. Some monitors now develop SOPs or work on study plans.

Monitors are also relied upon to identify and solve day-to-day problems at investigative sites, such as speaking to investigators about getting help for overworked staff, or noticing problems that could have an impact on data integrity.

While pharmaceutical companies are moving slowly in giving regional study monitors more site management responsibilities, industry experts say the concept is on the radar of all major pharmaceutical companies. And from their standpoint, investigators find this shift toward making monitors a stronger liaison between the site and sponsor a welcome trend.

## Coming Full Circle

The move to expand the role and responsibilities assigned to field monitors isn't a new trend. In fact, it's a return to practices prevalent when the clinical research and monitoring function began to evolve more than 25 years ago. When a CRA worked for a pharmaceutical company during the 1980s, the job likely included protocol development, case report form design, evaluation of sites, decision-making for site selection, study initiation, conducting investigator meetings, monitoring, problem-solving at sites, following up on data queries, development of analysis plans and writing clinical study reports. Their responsibilities were many.

Two factors narrowed the scope of the CRA's duties during the 1980s and 1990s: Pharmaceutical companies began forming specific units to handle administrative aspects of clinical research; some even developed special units to screen for investigators. At the same time, the growth of contract research organizations (CROs) during this period significantly changed the role and responsibilities of study monitors.

The recent growth of regional field monitor structures is the result of both cost controls and the desire of pharmaceutical companies to improve job satisfaction among their CRAs. A centralized structure resulted in a CRA traveling as much as 80% to 90% of the time. This constant travel, along with the fact that field monitors suffered from a lack of variety in their jobs and underutilization of their skills, often resulted in burnout and high turnover rates.

As the regional field monitor approach has become the primary structure adopted by nearly all major pharmaceutical companies and some CROs, the duties and responsibilities for CRAs has begun to shift. While these regional CRAs still perform traditional monitoring duties, they are now asked to take on additional duties during their site visits. The demands placed on these regional monitors, who work outside of their home office with minimal supervision, require a higher level of skill, experience and education than in the past. Many CRAs typically not only earn degrees in nursing or life sciences, but also study business, accounting, sociology or psychology.

Pharmaceutical companies have come to value the skills of their experienced CRAs. Pay and benefits have increased. And since travel requirements have been reduced and duties have expanded beyond ensuring the quality of data, job satisfaction has improved and the CRA position has become more of a career choice and less of a stepping stone to another job in clinical research.

## Improving Relationships with Investigators

Pharmaceutical companies now rely on regional study monitors to establish relationships with local investigators; some company job descriptions specifically require their field monitors to maintain contact with potential investigators to facilitate placement of future clinical trials. The monitor is often the first face representing the pharmaceutical company or CRO that the investigator or other site personnel may see, and the only such representative they may see on a regular basis.

When a study monitor has formed a strong relationship with an investigator, the result can be a better end-product. If, for example, a field monitor has gotten to know an investigative site, then helps select that site for a study, the investigator will work harder to make the study successful. Working with the same monitor on repeat studies also can help improve communication and expectations between investigators and field monitors.

Both sides benefit in these monitor-investigator relationships. Monitors may be able to alert investigators about potential studies in the pipeline, while investigators develop a sense of loyalty that extends to giving that drug sponsor preference when competing studies arise. At the same time, this mutual relationship can go a long way toward helping to solve problems that occur during a study.

# Impact of Technology

Since the mid-1990s, industry thought leaders have predicted that technology would ultimately replace the role of the study monitor. That hasn't happened and most likely won't. But technology has helped expand and change the CRA's role in clinical research for both regional and central monitors.

First and foremost, EDC has changed the nature of site visits. EDC allows field monitors to examine patient enrollment, look at actual data, review queries that have been generated, run reports and make sure the data entry is up-to-date before visiting a site. A recent survey of nearly 100 field monitors found that among the characteristics they liked best about EDC are the reduced numbers of queries and reduced time on site.

While EDC can improve a monitor's efficiency, it won't eliminate the need for source document verification, and monitors to do that work. Oversight will always be needed at the site for confirming that the source document matches the case report form.

# Conclusion

At a time when concerns about drug safety are growing industry-wide, CRAs will also find themselves on the front line of adverse event reporting. As the sponsor company's main representative at the investigative site, study monitors have the most direct impact on accurate reporting of adverse events in clinical trials. CRAs must make sure investigators both understand and comply with adverse event reporting requirements; often this involves initial training on adverse event reporting for investigators. Study monitors also review data to ensure accuracy and to detect potentially unreported adverse events.

In addition, CRAs are responsible for providing new information to investigators throughout the study and for making sure follow-up data for adverse events are reported when required. These responsibilities for adverse event reporting require a high level of education, experience and training for study monitors.

While some major pharmaceutical companies are giving their regional monitors increased responsibilities, many have not. Whether there will be an industry-wide move for drug sponsors to give regional study monitors more responsibilities for site management remains uncertain since big pharmaceutical companies are slow to change processes.

Another difficulty in giving regional monitors additional management responsibilities is the CRAs themselves. While turnover rates have dropped, the problem hasn't disappeared completely. And finding monitors with the skill, experience and education to take on these additional responsibilities can be difficult; the market for experienced monitors remains tight.

Ultimately, the concept of giving regional monitors increased responsibility will work only if a company has the right person in the right place.

## Key Takeaways

- EDC has changed the nature of site visits, allowing monitors to make sure data entry is up-to-date before visiting a site.
- Monitors are expanding their duties beyond checking to see that sites comply with regulations and verifying that source documents.
- Companies are empowering regional monitors to be influential in site selection and to help communication with investigators.

# A F T E R W O R D

We've covered a great deal of basic material in this book that we hope you will find useful and helpful as a CRA. Remember that it can be the little things that make a big difference and can make your job easier. There is no doubt about it—the job of CRA is not for the faint-hearted. It's an enormous amount of work and a lot of responsibility. It requires multiple skills, lots of travel and the ability to keep a lot of different balls in the air at one time. It's also fun and challenging, with numerous opportunities to learn new things, meet new people and have new experiences. If you enjoy this job as much as we did, you'll never regret having the chance to do it. We hope you have found this book useful and that you enjoy your CRA adventure. We'll leave you with some final key takeaways that will help you in this job and in your future.

## Key Takeaways

- Always know the protocol.
- Don't take job-related problems personally. It's just business.
- Never burn bridges. It's a small world.
- Keep educating yourself.
- Change is coming.
- Treat people as you like to be treated.
- Don't be afraid to admit you were wrong.
- Enjoy yourself.
- Be nice.
- Smile.

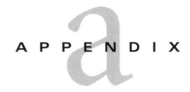

# A P P E N D I X

# Resources

## Books and Videotapes

*Acres of Skin: Human Experiments at Holmesburg Prison—A True Story of Abuse and Exploitation in the Name of Medical Science*
Allen M. Hornblum, 1998

*Bad Blood—The Tuskegee Syphilis Experiment*
James H. Jones, 1981

*Code of Medical Ethics*
American Medical Association, 150th Anniversary Edition, 1997

*Factories of Death—Japanese Biological Warfare, 1932-45, and the American Cover-up*
Sheldon H. Harris, 1994

*Guide to Clinical Trials*
Bert Spilker, Lippincott-Raven, 1996

*Human Radiation Experiments—(The) Final Report of the President's Advisory Committee*
Advisory Committee, 1996

*Nazi Doctors—(The) Medical Killing and the Psychology of Genocide*
    Robert Jay Lifton, 2000 (reprint)

*(The) Placebo Effect*
    Edited by Anne Harrington, 1997

*(The) Plutonium Files—America's Secret Medical Experiments in the Cold War*
    Eileen Welcome, 1999

*Protecting Human Subjects—A Series of Instructional Videotapes—Evolving
    Concern; Protection for Human Subjects* (3 videotapes)
    OPRR/OHRP

*Protecting Study Volunteers in Research—A Manual for Investigative Sites*
    Cynthia Dunn, M.D.; Gary Chadwick, Pharm.D. MPH, CIP 2002

*Tuskegee's Truths; Rethinking the Tuskegee Syphilis Study*
    Susan M. Reverby (Editor), 2000

## Agencies

**Center for Drug Evaluation and Research (CDER)**
**Clinical Investigator Information**
www.fda.gov/cder/about/smallbiz/clinical_investigator.htm

**FDA**
www.fda.gov

**International Conference on Harmonisation**
www.ich.org

**OHRP Site**
http://www.hhs.gov/ohrp

**World Medical Association**
www.wma.net
The World Medical Association (WMA) is the organization that issued the
Declaration of Helsinki and is responsible for its updates.

**Bioethics Resources on the Web**
http://bioethics.od.nih.gov
This site is maintained by the National Institutes of Health, and provides
links to a wide variety of bioethics resources on the web.

**Human Subjects Research and IRBs**
http://bioethics.od.nih.gov/irb.html

**ClinicalTrials.gov**
www.clinicaltrials.gov
The U.S. National Institutes of Health, through its National Library of Medicine, has developed ClinicalTrials.gov to provide subjects, family members and members of the public current information about clinical research studies.

# HIPAA References

## Background/Overview

**HHS HIPAA implementation process**
http://aspe.hhs.gov/admnsimp/kkimpl.htm

## Privacy

**The HHS Fact Sheet on final Privacy Rule**
http://aspe.os.dhhs.gov/admnsimp/final/pvcfact2.htm

# Other Information

**Department of Health and Human Services (HHS)
Protection of Human Subjects regulations. 45 CFR 46**
http://hhs.gov/ohrp

**Belmont Report**
www.hhs.gov/ohrp/belmontarchive.html

**FDA Forms**
www.fda.gov/opacom/morechoices/fdaforms/cder.html

**FDA Information Sheets**
www.fda.gov/oc/ohrt/irbs/default.htm

**Declaration of Helsinki**
www.wma.net/e/policy/b3.html

**Nuremberg Code**
http://ohsr.od.nih.gov/guidelines/nuremberg.html

**NIH Required Education in the Protection of
Human Research Participants**
http://grants.nih.gov/grants/guide/index.html

**Sources of Potential Investigators**
www.centerwatch.com
www.clinicalinvestigators.com

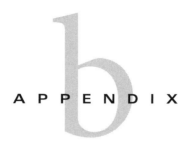

# Hints and Tips

## Travel Hints

### Planning

- Make your travel plans as far in advance as you can. You'll have better luck getting the flights and hotels you want. You will also have a better chance of getting the seat or type of hotel room you prefer. Early bookings are less expensive.
- Make sure you have your tickets and itinerary when you leave.
- Early morning flights don't have as many delays because the planes are often at the airport overnight.
- Carry an airline schedule with you in case you need to make changes along the way. It helps to know what is available.
- Two credit cards, an ATM card and a phone card are essential.
- Have some cash with you, but not an inordinate amount.
- Have some change with you for tolls and parking meters.
- Carry the 800 numbers for all the major airlines, hotels and car rental places with you when traveling.
- Cell phones are very useful when traveling, especially by car, but turn them off or to "vibrate" during meetings. Return calls after the meeting.
- Use a calendar that is sized for traveling well.

- Double-check with your sites before leaving for the airport to be sure they are expecting you.
- If you have an important meeting, go the day before to the city or town where it is being held. You can never count on getting there on time the same day.
- Wear comfortable shoes.
- Take all pertinent addresses and phone numbers with you.
- Obtain city maps for places you visit regularly.
- Ask your sites for suggestions about handy hotels, restaurants, etc.
- Take advantage of the cheaper fares by staying over Saturday night when you can. This gives you a chance to explore a new part of the country.

**Stress and health**
- Travel has the potential for being very stressful—try not to let it let it stress you too much.
- Take some time to relax when you travel. Read a book, do a crossword puzzle or find something else you like to do that will help relieve travel stress.
- Wash your hands frequently when traveling. This will help you avoid colds and other bad bugs. Also, carry some antibacterial hand cleaner with you. It comes in travel-size containers.
- Don't count on getting a meal on the flight. Take a sandwich with you if you'll miss meals during travel. It's bad enough to be tired from traveling, without being tired and hungry.
- Airplane air is very dry. Avoid getting dehydrated on long trips by drinking plenty of water. Alcohol, coffee and regular tea can further dehydrate you.
- Be careful about eating when traveling—it's easy to rely on fast food with tons of calories and fat. Try to include fruit and salads.
- A leftover bag of airline peanuts is not a meal. If you are arriving late and the hotel does not have room service, have the cab driver stop and let you pick up something on the way. Or, sometimes pizza places will deliver to the hotel, depending on the time of night.

**Luggage**
- Pack light. Never take more than you can carry comfortably by yourself. Remember that you may have case report forms to carry back with you, so allow some space for them.
- Find clothes that look professional but travel well. Check out travel catalogs that feature clothes especially made for traveling, comfortable clothes that don't wrinkle. Most hotels provide irons for quick touchups (if one is not in the room, call housekeeping and ask).

- Buy duplicate toiletries for a travel kit and keep your travel kit packed and ready to go. Replenish as needed. This is much easier than trying to remember and pack everything each time you leave.
- Many rooms have a small coffee maker. Pack a few cocoa packets or herbal tea, if you like them, so you can have some when you want.
- Carry a folding umbrella with you. Remember to take gloves if it will be cold at your destination.
- Carry your money, credit cards and important papers in a secure manner. Women: If you have a purse with a shoulder strap, put it across your chest and/or under your coat. Men: Don't carry a wallet in your back pants pocket. Make it difficult for pickpockets to see and acquire your things.
- Keep essential papers in your carry-on luggage/briefcase.
- Never check non-replaceable materials.
- You will lose checked luggage sometime.
- Your checked luggage will be delayed sometime.
- Mark your baggage in a distinctive way. Not only does this make it easier for you to see on the baggage carousel, it makes it less likely that someone else will think it is his or her bag. For example, many people have black suitcases that all look alike. Tie strands of colorful ribbon around the handle of yours. You'll be able to recognize that it's yours instantly, and others will realize it's not theirs.
- Watch for your suitcase on the carousel to be sure that someone else does not take it.
- If your bag does not appear on the baggage carousel, go as quickly as possible to the baggage place to report it. If you delay, you are apt to have a long wait in line.
- If your luggage does not arrive when you do, ask for an amenity kit from the airline. Many of them have small kits with a toothbrush and toothpaste, deodorant, etc., that can tide you over.

## Airlines
- Take advantage of airline, hotel and rental company frequent user programs. You can use the accrued points for vacations.
- Try to use one airline as much as feasible. You may travel enough to get a gold or platinum frequent flyer card, which gives you free upgrades to first class.
- Be very nice to airline counter attendants, hotel personnel, etc. You will deal with some of these people on a regular basis, and they can do nice things for you if they want to.
- Always be nice when problems arise. They are rarely the fault of the person you need to deal with, and these folks can either give you minimal service or go out of their way for you.

- At airline check-in security gates, do not place your bag on the x-ray conveyer until you are able to walk through. This is a common place for bags to be stolen.
- If you carry a laptop, PDA or floppy disks, be aware that x-ray machines can erase their contents. This can happen at the magnetic walk-through check as well. The guards will manually check your items if you ask. Note that you will be asked to take your laptop out of its case and may be asked to turn it on.
- Grab a pillow (and blanket) when you get on the plane. Better yet, bring your own if you can. These items can carry germs, if they're not individually sealed. Airplane seats do not fit all sizes, and a pillow can help. Plus you have one if you want to nap.
- The phones on airplanes are very expensive to use.
- Don't expect to get a lot of work done on the plane. They are usually so crowded it's hard to find space. And if the person in front of you puts his or her seat back, it's almost impossible to use a laptop or to work at the tray table.
- If you have a flight canceled or delayed, ask the airline for a phone card so that you can inform people of your delay. These are usually only good for about 10 minutes of call time, but it's better than nothing. They will not be offered if you don't ask.
- Also ask for a meal voucher when you have a long wait. These are valid in the airport. You'll probably have to ask for this also.
- Check the monitors regularly in the airport. Flights are often changed to other gates, and you may be hurrying to the wrong gate. Check occasionally even if you are at the gate.
- Be alert to the first signs of a canceled flight. This can put you near the front of the line for rebooking.
- If you are caught in a long line of people waiting to be rebooked from a canceled flight, it can be faster to call the airline's 800 number and make the changes over the phone.
- If your travel plans are flexible and you are caught up in weather delays, it can be easier and more efficient to get a hotel and wait until the next day to fly. You can get caught up on your paperwork in the hotel and avoid waiting and wondering in the airport.
- Airplanes can be cold. Be prepared with a sweater or jacket.
- If the trip is bumpy, order a club soda or water when the drinks cart comes by. They won't leave you with noticeable drips or stains, if you spill them on yourself.

**Transportation at your destination**
- Check the cab price from the airport to the hotel before you get in. Sometimes a limo service car costs no more but is much nicer.
- Sometimes it is less expensive to rent a car than to take cabs. Be sure you get a map and know where you are going.

- If you get a good cab (limo) driver, arrange for the same person to transport you while you are there and/or back to the airport.
- If you're taking a shuttle back to the airport, check with the hotel about needing to sign up for it in advance.
- When traveling regularly to the same city, find a rental car company you like and use it regularly. They will appreciate your repeat business, and you will have better service.
- Do the rental car paperwork while you wait for your luggage at the baggage claim.
- Be sure you have your driver's license with you and that it has not expired. You will not get a rental car otherwise.
- Some rental car companies have non-smoking cars.
- Fill up the rental car with gas before you return it—it's much cheaper than if the rental company does it.
- Two hours in a rental car costs as much as a whole day. Get the car back on time (or early) if you can to avoid the extra day charge.
- A rental car phone is very expensive to use.

## Driving to your sites
- Be sure you have good directions to the places you need to visit.
- A Global Positioning System (GPS) with a good map base can be very helpful.
- If you drive a lot, keep an emergency kit in your car for bad weather or other problems. Include a flashlight, flares, jumper cables, a small tool kit, a first aid kit, a blanket, umbrella, gloves and ice scraper. You can also keep a change of underwear, some toiletries, etc., in a car pack in case you can't make it back home because of bad weather. If the weather might be bad or you expect delays, pack a few granola bars, bottled water, etc.
- Be sure your car is dependable and serviced appropriately and that the tires are in good shape.
- An all-in-one tool is handy to keep in the car. So are pre-moistened wipes and antibacterial hand lotion.
- Never let your gas tank go below half full if you are in the country or not familiar with where the next gas station might be. Or in the winter, in case you get stuck somewhere.
- Keep a gallon of windshield washer fluid in the car.

## Hotels
- When traveling regularly to the same city, find a hotel you like and use it regularly. They will appreciate your repeat business, and you will have a familiar, comfortable place to stay. If you book in advance and ask for it, they may give you the same room each time.
- Use a hotel with guaranteed late arrival so that you don't lose your room if you are delayed.

- If you don't smoke, ask for a non-smoking room.
- If you get to the hotel and they don't have a room for you, ask them to call another hotel for you. Sometimes they will also have their shuttle take you to the alternate hotel.
- If you don't like your room, ask for a different one.
- If the hotel is dirty, don't go back. And tell them why.
- Use the hotel comment cards—for kudos as well as complaints.
- Check the hours for the hotel restaurant or room service when you arrive if you will need to depend on it later. Sometimes the hours and services printed in the hotel information in your room have changed.
- Don't be hesitant to dine at the hotel restaurant alone. They are used to having business travelers eat solo and will make you feel welcome. You can watch other people, chat with the waitperson and not feel cooped up in your room.
- On the other hand, room service can be great at the end of a long, tough day. Wearing your pajamas while watching TV and eating a club sandwich might really hit the spot. Most room service has a service charge and a tip already added in, so don't feel that you need to tip even more.
- Hotel breakfasts can be exorbitant, especially with room service. Look for a local breakfast place close to the hotel (ask the bell staff). Besides being much less expensive, a little fresh air is nice in the morning.
- Some hotels provide breakfast (Embassy Suites, for example), and sometimes snacks at night. This is especially useful if you are on a per diem for meals.
- If you are going to be in the same hotel for more than one night, unpack and use the drawers. It's easier than rummaging through your suitcase to find everything and easier to pack up again when you leave.
- If you need to work at the hotel, ask for a room with a desk.
- Many hotels offer easy laptop hookups. Some offer in-room faxes. If these are important to you, ask when booking your room.
- If it's too dark to read or work in your room, ask for another lamp or brighter light bulbs.
- If you like to exercise, inquire about the facilities when booking your hotel.
- Check with the hotel staff to be sure that the area is safe before going out to jog, etc., especially at night.
- Many hotels will extend the checkout time by a few hours if you ask.
- If you have to check out before the time you will be leaving, the hotel will hold your bags for you. Ask at the concierge desk or bell stand.
- If you need to meet with people at your hotel, the all suite hotels give you a place to meet that's not in the bedroom.
- Say "Thank you" when someone does something nice for you.

## Hints for Independent CRAs

As was mentioned in Chapter 1, many CRAs are currently self employed as independent contractors. There are advantages and disadvantages to working as an independent contractor. The advantages are that you are essentially your own boss. There will be someone at the sponsor company or CRO to whom you "report" for a specific job, but you are usually on your own as far as planning your schedule and hours. You are also able to work from your home, away from the hustle, noise and politics of a corporate office.

Probably the biggest hurdle for independents is finding work. You have to "market yourself," and this can be difficult and time consuming to do. Working as an independent also requires a significant amount of personal discipline. Many people prefer to work in an office environment with other people around to have coffee and lunch with, and with whom to discuss problems and job situations.

Because there are special considerations when working as an independent CRA, here are some helpful hints that may be of value in this situation.

- The IRS considers an independent CRA as a small business. Consequently, you must maintain your records and tax documents appropriately.
- Find yourself a good tax accountant/CPA. You will probably gain more than you spend to pay for this service.
- Always have a contract for the services you provide.
- You may want to discuss your company organization with an attorney. There are many kinds of small business organizations, and the appropriateness of each type varies according to personal situations and desires.
- You may also want the services of an attorney if you are not comfortable dealing with contracts.
- Build some structure into your workday, including break times for coffee and lunch.
- Save your household chores for the non-working times of the day.
- Keep yourself organized.
- Set up a good filing system, and keep current on your filing.
- Have a separate credit card that you use only for business.
- Keep a separate checking account only for business.
- Invest in a good computer program for tracking your financial information. There are several on the market. (Ask your accountant or CPA for advice.)
- Have business cards made. Since you may work for multiple companies, you might want to have a "generic" card that lists only your name and contact information.
- Develop a system for keeping track of your expenses. Be sure to write them down as they occur. This is important if you are being reimbursed, or for tax purposes if you are not reimbursed.

- Keep your receipts. File them in such a way that you can retrieve them when needed.
- Pay for most things using your credit card. This helps to track expenses.
- If you take someone out for a business meal, jot on the back or bottom of your receipt who was present and the reason.
- Maintain confidentiality. Never discuss one sponsor's program with another sponsor.
- If you are able to combine travel for multiple sponsors, let each sponsor know, and split the expenses appropriately.
- Many independent CRAs work on an hourly basis. Record your time honestly.
- Repeat business is critical. Do not do anything to jeopardize your reputation with a company.

### Maintaining ties with sites between studies
- Telephone them every couple of months to say hello.
- Know the coordinator's birthday and send her/him a card.
- If you see something written about the site (or any of the staff) in the paper, etc., drop them a note.
- If you happen to be in the vicinity and have time, drop by for just a minute to say hello. Keep the visit short so that it's not disruptive.
- When the drug they worked on is approved, drop them a note to tell them.
- Send a card (with a personal note) at the holidays.

### Home office work
- Make a separate folder for each protocol you are monitoring.
- Make a separate folder for each site you are monitoring.
- On the inside of the front folder cover, put the names and contact information for the site. Update it as soon as you become aware of a change.
- File the site folders in an order that works for you. Possibilities are by investigator name, by city or by protocol. You might file them by protocol during the trial and by investigator name when the trial is complete.
- Color code your investigator files by city. Then when you are preparing for a visit to Omaha, for example, you just pull all the yellow folders.
- Organize each folder in the same way, so you can easily find what you need.
- Label each folder clearly.
- File them. Don't let the filing pile up.
- File them in an organized manner.
- Always keep basic office supplies on hand—pens, paper, file folders, paper clips, labels, staples, mail supplies, etc. Get more before you run out.

- Keep an extra printer cartridge on hand.
- Use an uninterrupted power supply (UPS) with your computer. Don't forget to protect your computer's phone or network connection also; this is where the power problems frequently occur. A regular "surge suppresser" is practically worthless.
- Back up your computer regularly.
- Keep your calendar up to date.
- Don't forget to add regularly scheduled meetings, phone calls and reports to your calendar.
- Set aside some time each week to catch up on your paperwork.
- Complete your visit reports as soon as possible after each site visit, preferably on the same day that you make the visit.
- Use a tickler file so you won't forget important dates, etc.
- Clean your desk top off regularly. You'll be surprised at what you find on the bottom of the stack.
- Block out time and be on time for conference calls or other meetings.
- Keep basic office supplies for traveling in your briefcase.

## Hints for Monitoring

- If you aren't sure where the site is, scope it out the night before.
- Some computer sites that help you locate addresses are mapquest.com and expedia.com. You can also check with the local Chamber of Commerce.
- Don't be late.
- If you are going to be late, call the site to let them know.
- Do not expect site personnel to stay late for you because you were late in arriving. They have other commitments also.
- Don't spend your time at the site on the phone to other sites.
- Be polite. Good manners are important.
- Know the study you are monitoring. Be very familiar with the protocol. Never visit a site without reading the protocol first. Be sure you understand it—don't embarrass yourself by not being able to discuss it intelligently.
- Always use checklists.
- Carry a "Pocket Pharmacopoeia" by Tarascon with you.
- Use your own supplies. Don't expect them to be provided for you.
- Be careful about the language and phrasing in your monitoring reports, especially if they go to the site.
- If there is a problem to be dealt with, discuss it with the appropriate people while you are at the site. Don't hit them with it later.
- Document problems, but do it in a professional manner. Be sure to document the resolution to the problem.

- Be sure when you gather your papers to leave that you are not taking the site's copies of documents with you by mistake.
- Do not discuss grants and other financial information with anyone except the investigator without the investigator's permission.
- Be careful to leave things at a site in the same way you found them.
- Take some doughnuts or fruit in with you occasionally.
- Take the coordinator out for lunch once in awhile—especially if he or she is doing a wonderful job.
- Say thank you when someone makes your job easier.

## Tips for keeping the home fires burning (for travelers)

- Leave your itinerary, including flights and hotel information, where it can be seen (probably on the refrigerator).
- Call home every day—at least once. With children, perhaps in the morning and the evening. You can get very inexpensive calling cards now—between three and four cents a minute.
- Take home a little present. It doesn't have to be much, but shows your family they were in your thoughts. (Food works—a special pound of coffee, a loaf of sourdough bread, some salt-water taffy.)
- Try to schedule so that you can be home for important events—birthdays, the big soccer game, the school play.
- Don't plan to arrive just minutes before the big event—your plane will probably be delayed.
- If you're going somewhere interesting, and can, take your family with you on occasion. Maybe you can stay over a weekend for a mini vacation.
- Try to get home before bedtime.
- Remember that your travel is stressful for the ones left at home too.
- Send the kids a postcard or a letter when you travel. Carry a packet of stamps in your wallet.
- One traveler takes her daughter's small stuffed bear with her every time she travels. When the bear comes home, it reports everything about the trip to the daughter.
- Leave something special in the refrigerator for dinner. Suggest they order pizza one night for a treat.
- If you are in charge of groceries, don't leave the cupboard bare.
- Leave a treat once in awhile as a surprise.
- Leave notes (not instructions) to indicate you are thinking about them.
- If you are in charge of laundry, be sure it's done (or at least under control) when you leave.
- Put your travel dates on the family calendar.
- Don't forget important dates. Call your mother on her birthday.
- Be sure your bills are paid on time.

- Don't forget dentist appointments, etc.
- Say "Thank you."

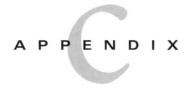

# A P P E N D I X C

# Sample Forms, Checklists, and Logs

Site Information Sheet
Elements of Consent
Activities for Preparation, Monitoring and Closeout of a Clinical Trial
Site Evaluation
Study Documents (based on ICH GCPs)
Study Closeout
Error Query/Correction
Query Resolution
Study Monitor Visit Log
Study Personnel Log
Study Subject Visit Tracking Log
Study Document File Verification Log
Site Visit Report
Investigational Drug Dispensing Record
Inventory of Returned Investigational Material

# Site Information Sheet

**Protocol** _____

**Investigator** _____

**Address** _____

_____

_____

**Telephone** _____ **Fax** _____

**Email** _____

**Directions to the site** _____

_____

**Coordinator** _____

**Telephone** _____

**Pharmacist** _____

**Telephone** _____

**Other personnel** _____

**Best days, times for**  _____
**monitoring visits**

**Other pertinent information** _____

_____

_____

# Elements of Consent

## Required elements

- ☐ Statement that the study involves research.
    - ☐ Explanation of the purpose of the research.
    - ☐ Expected duration of subject's participation.
    - ☐ Description of procedures to be followed.
    - ☐ Identification of any procedures that are experimental.

- ☐ Description of reasonably foreseeable risks and discomforts to subject.
- ☐ Description of benefits which may be reasonably expected.
- ☐ Disclosure of alternate procedures or treatment.
- ☐ Statement re confidentiality of records.
    - ☐ Statement that FDA may inspect the records.

- ☐ Statement re compensation for any research-related injury.
- ☐ Contact person for questions about the research and subject rights.
- ☐ Contact person in the event of research-related injury.
- ☐ Statement that participation is voluntary.
- ☐ Statement that refusal to participate will not result in the penalty or loss of any benefits to which the subject is otherwise entitled.
- ☐ Statement that the subject may discontinue at any time without penalty or loss of any benefits to which the subject is otherwise entitled.

## Additional elements (include as appropriate)

- ☐ Statement that the treatment may involve risks to the subject (or embryo or fetus) which are currently unforeseeable.
- ☐ Circumstances under which the subject's participation may be terminated by the investigator without regard to the subject's consent.
- ☐ Any additional costs to the subject.
- ☐ Consequences for withdrawal and procedures for orderly termination.
- ☐ Statement that significant new findings will be provided to the subject.
- ☐ Approximate number of subjects involved in the study.

# Activities for Preparation, Monitoring and Closeout of a Clinical Trial

Following is a list of activities from which personal checklists can be developed. Activities shown are generic and may vary from company to company.

## Study Planning Activities

### In-house
- ☐ Develop study timelines (IRB Approval, FDA-mandated waiting periods, bulk drug manufacturing, etc.)
- ☐ Update Investigator Brochure, when necessary (yearly or when changes are appropriate) Chemistry, Path/Tox, Pharmacology, and Clinical. (Date of last update _____)
- ☐ Obtain or assign unique protocol numbers
- ☐ Evaluate and finalize study budget(s)
- ☐ Determine if or which studies will be contracted to outside vendor and initiate, contract, or coordinate with CRO or company personnel according to company policy
- ☐ Provide CRAs or CRO with protocol summary to help identify potential investigators
- ☐ Order bulk drug supplies
- ☐ Prepare initial IND submission (if appropriate)
- ☐ Determine laboratory needs (central vs local)

### Field
- ☐ Interview potential investigators

## Pre-Study Activities

### In-house
- ☐ Circulate draft protocol for review or through review process
- ☐ Finalize and approve protocol (date of approval: _____).
- ☐ Update IND
- ☐ Get release from path/tox (e.g., all required pre-clinical activities are complete and no safety concerns exist)
- ☐ Submit request for investigational drug supplies
- ☐ Write informed consents
- ☐ Obtain investigator identifier numbers (if necessary)
- ☐ Request or design CRFs
- ☐ Send draft CRFs for review
- ☐ Finalize and order CRFs
- ☐ Obtain Use Patent Review
- ☐ Prepare Investigator/Study Coordinator Training Manuals, if appropriate

- ☐ Plan Investigator meeting, if appropriate
- ☐ Prepare randomization list
- ☐ Coordinate investigator meeting/start-up dates with field monitors
- ☐ Establish study files
- ☐ Design/set-up logs, tracking systems etc

### Field

- ☐ Evaluate and select investigators
- ☐ Final site evaluations (pre-study visit)
- ☐ Collect and submit all regulatory-/company-required documents
    - ☐ Signed protocol
    - ☐ 1572
    - ☐ Lab normal ranges and certification
    - ☐ CVs
    - ☐ IRB approval(s)
    - ☐ Informed consent approval
    - ☐ Letter of agreement/contracts
    - ☐ Ancillary Personnel/ Signature Form
    - ☐ Financial Disclosure information

## Study Initiation

### In-house

- ☐ Send study package(s) to field monitors (Protocol, Brochures, Consents, 1572, contracts/agreement letters, etc.)
- ☐ Submit appropriate documents to Regulatory Affairs and/or place in study file
- ☐ Submit initial grant payment request, if appropriate
- ☐ Send laboratory normal ranges to Biostatistician/Data Management
- ☐ Ship clinical supplies (notify field monitor (CRA) when drug is shipped)

### Field

- ☐ Conduct site initiation visits
    - ☐ Confirm receipt of clinical supplies with each site
    - ☐ Review protocol requirements
    - ☐ Review sponsor policy on CRF completion and correction
    - ☐ Confirm presence of all required documents
    - ☐ Ensure establishment of study files
- ☐ Establish monitoring visit frequency and communicate to site

## Study Monitoring

### In-house

- ☐ Assure all amendments or deviations are approved and filed with regulatory affairs, the investigators and internal study files
- ☐ Assure IRB approval was received for changes/amendments
- ☐ Monitor grant payments/adjustments
- ☐ Document and file annual IRB approvals
- ☐ Assure receipt and filing of CVs for investigators/subinvestigators added after study initiation
- ☐ Assure 1572s are updated as required
- ☐ Assure annual IND update is completed
- ☐ Assure Investigator Brochure is updated annually or as needed and that revisions are sent to all investigators
- ☐ Monitor site visit reports for any required action
- ☐ Maintain current study enrollment and progress data according to company SOPs
- ☐ Assure all adverse events are reported according to regulation and company policy
- ☐ Provide field monitors with current study status prior to site visits

### Field

- ☐ Check with in-house colleagues to review site status prior to visit
- ☐ Visit sites as scheduled/required
- ☐ Review protocol compliance, especially inclusion/exclusion requirements
- ☐ Assure required corrections are made
- ☐ Review CRFs and compare to source documents
- ☐ Review drug accounting, storage, dispensing
- ☐ Check for new adverse events
- ☐ Collect any outstanding data from previously reported adverse events
- ☐ Assure that any safety update letters sent to site have been sent to the IRB
- ☐ Review study files for extraneous documents and to insure required documents are present
- ☐ Meet with investigator and study coordinator to review study status, answer questions, etc.
- ☐ Document visit on written report
- ☐ Confirm date of next visit with site
- ☐ Written report of visit findings to investigation (optional)

## Study Termination

### In-house

- ☐ Notify regulatory department when all patients are off drug and study is terminated

- [ ] Send randomization sheets to investigators, if appropriate (only after all study documents are in-house)
- [ ] Send clinical data and statistical summary to investigators, if appropriate
- [ ] Prepare final study reports

### Field
- [ ] All CRFs collected, corrected and in-house
- [ ] No outstanding data for serious adverse events, deaths, or pregnancies
- [ ] Drug collected, inventoried and returned to sponsor
- [ ] Investigator files complete and investigator instructed regarding storage
- [ ] Drug reconciled from inventory and shipping invoices
- [ ] Investigator briefed on procedure if notified of FDA audit
- [ ] IRB notified of termination
- [ ] Study file complete and ready for audit

# Site Evaluation

CRA should evaluate each item below, making notes.

### Investigator
- ☐ Qualifications
- ☐ Licensure
- ☐ Specialty
- ☐ Clinical trial experience
    - ☐ Number of previous trials
    - ☐ Number of similar trials
    - ☐ Enrollment in previous trials (numbers, time to enroll)
- ☐ FDA audits

### Staff
- ☐ Study coordinator
- ☐ Other specialized personnel
- ☐ Training and licensure
- ☐ Experience
- ☐ Turnover
- ☐ General interest and attitude

### Facility
- ☐ Appropriate for trials
- ☐ Ample storage for study supplies
- ☐ Appropriate drug storage
- ☐ Special storage equipment available (freezer, etc.)
- ☐ Special equipment available
- ☐ Active practice
- ☐ Tour offered, taken

### IRB
- ☐ Local IRB available
    - ☐ Frequency and timing of meetings
    - ☐ Average time to approval
    - ☐ Responsiveness
- ☐ Use central IRB

### Laboratory/Tests
- ☐ Local lab available
- ☐ Necessary tests can be done
- ☐ Timeliness
- ☐ Certification
- ☐ Have experience with central lab

**Protocol feasibility**
- ☐ Experience with similar studies
- ☐ Interest level
- ☐ Availability of potential subjects
- ☐ Competing studies (in practice and in community)
- ☐ Timing appropriate
- ☐ Study coordinator availability
- ☐ Can attend investigator meeting

# Study Documents
## (based on ICH GCPs)

**Protocol** _____

**Investigator** _____

## Pre-Study
- ☐ Investigator Brochure
- ☐ Signed protocol and amendments (if any)
- ☐ Informed consent form
  - ☐ Any other information to be given to subjects
  - ☐ Any advertising materials for recruitment
- ☐ Dated, written IRB approvals for:
  - ☐ Protocol                          [Date:            ]
  - ☐ Amendments, if any                 [Date:            ]
  - ☐ Consent and any other material to  [Date:            ]
    be given to subjects
  - ☐ Advertising, if any                [Date:            ]
  - ☐ Subject compensation, if any       [Date:            ]
- ☐ CVs for investigator, subinvestigators
- ☐ Laboratory certification and normal ranges
- ☐ Study manual, if available
- ☐ Shipping records
- ☐ Decoding procedures for blinded trials
- ☐ Financial disclosure sheets
- ☐ Contract
- ☐ Sponsor-specific documents

## During the conduct of the trial
- ☐ Investigator Brochure updates
- ☐ Protocol amendments and/or revisions
- ☐ Consent revisions
- ☐ Dated, written IRB approvals of:
  - ☐ Protocol amendments               [Dates:           ]
  - ☐ Revised consents                   [Dates:           ]
  - ☐ New or revised subject materials   [Dates:           ]
  - ☐ New or revised advertising         [Dates:           ]
- ☐ CVs for new investigators and/or subinvestigators
- ☐ Laboratory updates of certification and/or normal ranges
- ☐ Shipping documentation (receipt of trial materials)
- ☐ Monitoring visit log
- ☐ Communications with sponsor (letters, telephone reports, etc.)
- ☐ Signed consent forms
- ☐ Source documents

☐ Signed, dated, completed case report forms (CRFs)
☐ Documentation of CRF corrections
☐ Notification to sponsors and IRB of serious adverse events and related reports
☐ IND safety reports received from the sponsor
☐ Interim and/or annual reports to the IRB
☐ Subject screening log
☐ Subject identification code list
☐ Subject enrollment log
☐ Investigational product accountability
☐ Signature sheet (all persons making CRF entries or corrections)
☐ Record of retained body fluids and/or tissue samples, if any

**After study completion or termination**
☐ Drug (device) accountability
☐ Documentation of drug/device return or disposal
☐ Completed subject identification code list
☐ Final report to the IRB                [Date:                ]


**Comments** _____

_____

_____

Checklist should be kept in front of study file and updated as appropriate.

# Study Closeout

**Protocol** _____

**Sponsor** _____

**Investigator** _____

**Date** _____

☐ Study documents file is complete (refer to Checklist: Study Documents).

☐ Final report has been made to the IRB and the sponsor.

☐ All case report forms (CRFs) are complete and have been submitted to the sponsor.

    ☐ All CRF corrections/queries have been addressed.

    ☐ Any patient diaries, etc. have been submitted, as required.

    ☐ All adverse event follow-up is complete.

☐ All source documentation is in order.

    ☐ If not with study files, location of materials is noted in the document file.

☐ Study personnel form is complete.

☐ Subjects' signed informed consent forms are filed.

☐ Drug dispensing and disposition forms are complete.

☐ Study drug has been returned as per sponsor instructions.

☐ All other study materials (extra CRFs, etc.) have been returned to the sponsor.

☐ Investigator Brochure is filed with other study materials.

☐ All study materials are filed together as per archival procedures.

    ☐ Location of materials is noted in site records.

# Error Query/Correction

Protocol _____

Protocol date _____

Sponsor _____

| Patient | Visit | Page | Field | Problem | Correction | Initials |
|---------|-------|------|-------|---------|------------|----------|
|         |       |      |       |         |            |          |
|         |       |      |       |         |            |          |
|         |       |      |       |         |            |          |
|         |       |      |       |         |            |          |
|         |       |      |       |         |            |          |
|         |       |      |       |         |            |          |
|         |       |      |       |         |            |          |
|         |       |      |       |         |            |          |
|         |       |      |       |         |            |          |

**Query Resolution**

Protocol _____ Investigator _____ Subject Number _____

| Page No. | Field | Issue | Resolution | Date | Initial |
|----------|-------|-------|------------|------|---------|
|          |       |       |            |      |         |
|          |       |       |            |      |         |
|          |       |       |            |      |         |
|          |       |       |            |      |         |
|          |       |       |            |      |         |
|          |       |       |            |      |         |
|          |       |       |            |      |         |

# Study Monitor Visit Log

Protocol _____  Protocol date _____  Sponsor _____

| Name | Job Title | Date(s) of Visit | Signature | Study Coordinator Initials |
|------|-----------|------------------|-----------|---------------------------|
|      |           |                  |           |                           |
|      |           |                  |           |                           |
|      |           |                  |           |                           |
|      |           |                  |           |                           |
|      |           |                  |           |                           |

Use addional sheets as needed. Keep with study documents file.

# Study Personnel Log

Protocol _____

Protocol date _____

Sponsor _____

| Name | Job Title | Initials | Start Date of Study Responsibility | End Date of Study Responsibility | Signature |
|------|-----------|----------|-----------------------------------|----------------------------------|-----------|
|      |           |          |                                   |                                  |           |
|      |           |          |                                   |                                  |           |
|      |           |          |                                   |                                  |           |
|      |           |          |                                   |                                  |           |
|      |           |          |                                   |                                  |           |

Use additional sheets as needed. Update when personnel changes occur. Keep with study documents file.

# Study Subject Visit Tracking Log

Protocol _____    Sponsor _____

| Subject | Consent Date | Baseline | Week 1 | Week 2 | Week 4 | Final Status | Comments |
|---------|--------------|----------|--------|--------|--------|--------------|----------|
|  |  |  |  |  |  |  |  |
|  |  |  |  |  |  |  |  |
|  |  |  |  |  |  |  |  |
|  |  |  |  |  |  |  |  |
|  |  |  |  |  |  |  |  |
|  |  |  |  |  |  |  |  |
|  |  |  |  |  |  |  |  |
|  |  |  |  |  |  |  |  |
|  |  |  |  |  |  |  |  |

# Study Document File Verification Log

| Study Document File Review | Initial / / | Review / / | Review / / | Final / / |
|---|---|---|---|---|
| Signed, IRB-approved protocol or cover sheet | | | | |
| Signed, IRB-approved amendments ■ Amendment #, date ■ Amendment #, date ■ Amendment #, date | | | | |
| IRB-approved informed consent document | | | | |
| Signed, completed FDA 1572 form (Statement of Investigator) | | | | |
| IRB approval letter, verifying approval of both the protocol and consent document | | | | |
| IRB approval of advertising and subject recruitment materials, including any subject compensation | | | | |
| Investigator Brochure (or package insert, for marketed products) | | | | |
| Verification of laboratory certification and laboratory normal ranges | | | | |
| Study Manual, if available | | | | |
| Shipping records for investigation product | | | | |
| Decoding procedures for blinded trials | | | | |
| Financial disclosure forms | | | | |
| Sponsor-specific documents and communications | | | | |
| **Reviewer initials** | | | | |

Attach a separate sheet with comments if any problems found.

# Site Visit Report

**Person Making Report**_____ **Title**_____

**Reason for Contact** _____

**Method of Contact** ☐ **Phone** ☐ **Visit Date of Contact** _____

**Study (Protocol) Identification**_____

**Site (Investigator) ID**_____

**Site Persons Contacted**_____

| Facilities/Staff | Yes | No | N/A | Comments |
|---|---|---|---|---|
| Changes in Staff? | * | | | |
| Are the investigator and staff fulfilling study obligations? | | * | | |
| Changes in facilities/ Equipment? | * | | | |
| **Adverse Events** | **Yes** | **No** | **N/A** | **Comments** |
| Have any serious medical events occurred since last visit? | * | | | |
| If yes, were required forms completed and submitted? | | * | | |
| Any outstanding data or forms for this or previous events? | * | | | |
| Was the IRB informed, if required? | | * | | |

| Study Conduct | Yes | No | N/A | Comments |
|---|---|---|---|---|
| Are protocol requirements being followed? | | * | | |
| Consent for all patients available and signed prior to enrollment? | | * | | |
| **Site Conduct** | **Yes** | **No** | **N/A** | **Comments** |
| Were CRFs reviewed? | | * | | |
| Source documents reviewed? | | * | | |
| Were CRF problems discussed w/staff? | | * | | |
| Was patient eligibility confirmed? | | * | | |
| Is recruitment on schedule? | | * | | |
| Were corrections made? | | * | | |
| Were any protocol deviations noted? | * | | | |
| Is the investigator accessible during visits? | | * | | |
| Are changes, events, etc. being communicated to the IRB? | | * | | |
| Were all completed CRFs collected? | | * | | |
| **Drug Supplies** | **Yes** | **No** | **N/A** | **Comments** |
| Is investigational product stored properly? | | * | | |

| Drug Supplies | Yes | No | N/A | Comments |
|---|---|---|---|---|
| Are dispensing procedures satisfactory? | | * | | |
| Is investigational product being accounted for properly? | | * | | |
| Are study supplies adequate? | | * | | |
| **Documentation** | **Yes** | **No** | **N/A** | **Comments** |
| Signed protocol | | * | | |
| 1572 | | * | | |
| CVs for PI and sub-investigators | | * | | |
| Approved consent | | * | | |
| IRB approvals | | * | | |
| Agreements/contracts? | | * | | |
| Signed amendments | | * | | |
| Lab normals/accreditation? | | * | | |
| Current Investigator Brochure | | * | | |
| All pertinent correspondence on file? | | * | | |
| IRB Correspondence- Annual, SAEs? | | * | | |
| Any unresolved issues from previous visits? | * | | | |

| Administration | Yes | No | N/A | Comments |
|---|---|---|---|---|
| Were results of visit discussed with investigator and staff? | | * | | |
| Will findings be provided to site in writing? | | | | |
| Was appointment made for next visit? | | * | | |

* Requires a comment. Add additional pages if necessary.

**Comments** _____

_____

_____

_____

**Signed** _____

# Investigational Drug Dispensing Record

**Protocol Number** _____

**Protocol Title** _____

**Investigator** _____

**Subject Number/Initials** _____

**Treatment Code (if applicable)** _____

Complete the following information using a new line each time medication is dispensed or returned. Use a separate sheet for each subject.

| Date Medication Dispensed or Returned | Lot Number and Identification Code | Quantity Dispensed (Number of tablets) | Quantity Returned (Number of tablets) | Initials | Comments |
|---|---|---|---|---|---|
|  |  |  |  |  |  |
|  |  |  |  |  |  |
|  |  |  |  |  |  |
|  |  |  |  |  |  |
|  |  |  |  |  |  |
|  |  |  |  |  |  |
|  |  |  |  |  |  |
|  |  |  |  |  |  |
|  |  |  |  |  |  |
|  |  |  |  |  |  |
|  |  |  |  |  |  |

# Inventory of Returned Investigational Material

**Sponsor/Address**_____

_____

**Protocol Number** _____

**Protocol Title** _____

**Investigator/Address** _____

_____

**Contact Person/Telephone Number** _____

The following investigational material is being returned.

| Drug | Lot Number | Code Number | Full Containers | Partial Containers | Empty Containers | Total Containers |
|------|-----------|-------------|-----------------|--------------------|------------------|------------------|
|      |           |             |                 |                    |                  |                  |
|      |           |             |                 |                    |                  |                  |
|      |           |             |                 |                    |                  |                  |
|      |           |             |                 |                    |                  |                  |
|      |           |             |                 |                    |                  |                  |
|      |           |             |                 |                    |                  |                  |
|      |           |             |                 |                    |                  |                  |
|      |           |             |                 |                    |                  |                  |
|      |           |             |                 |                    |                  |                  |

**Comments** _____

_____

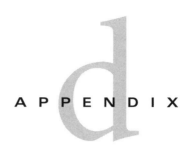

# Job Descriptions and
# Academic Programs

**CRA Job Summary**
**Clinical Research Associate (CRA)—Entry Level**
**Clinical Research Associate (CRA)—Advanced Level**
**Academic Programs**

# CRA Job Summary

This document describes two levels of CRA responsibilities. For simplicity, they are called CRA 1 (entry level) and CRA 2 (advanced).

| CRA 1 | CRA 2 |
|---|---|
| **Investigator Selection** | |
| ■ Will not be involved in this activity. Will work with Investigators/ CROs selected by the Sponsor | ■ In consultation with the Sponsor/CRO select investigators appropriate for the therapeutic area and protocol. Note: May also be involved in CRO evaluation/selection |
| **Pre-Study** | |
| ■ Meet with Investigator and staff and review study requirements (protocol, CRFs, sponsor policy and procedures, investigator responsibilities, staffing and patient recruitment) <br> ■ Conduct study initiation visit. <br> ■ Confirm appropriateness of the IRB. <br> ■ Collect and forward all required study documentation to Sponsor <br> ■ Document visit. | ■ Assess study site to ensure facility, patient population and staff are sufficient to support the protocol <br> ■ Negotiate study budget and/or indemnification agreement. <br> ■ Assist in planning and conducting Investigator Meeting and/or Start-up Meeting <br> ■ Meet with PI and staff and review study requirements (protocol, CRFs, Sponsor policy and procedures, investigator responsibilities, staffing and patient recruitment <br> ■ Conduct study initiation visit <br> ■ Confirm appropriateness of the IRB <br> ■ Collect and forward all required study documentation to Sponsor <br> ■ Document visit |

| CRA 1 | CRA 2 |
|---|---|
| **Study Monitoring** ||
| ▪ Conduct routine monitoring visits to include:<br>  – Review protocol compliance<br>  – Review CRF/source documents<br>  – Resolve questions/issues with Investigator/Staff<br>  – Check/inventory clinical supplies<br>  – Review communication with the IRB<br>  – Review drug accountability<br>▪ Confirm Informed Consent<br>▪ Correct previous errors<br>▪ Submit all collected documents and site visit report to Sponsor<br>▪ Log and track study progress | ▪ Conduct routine monitoring visits to include:<br>▪ Review protocol compliance<br>▪ Review CRF/source documents<br>▪ Resolve questions/issues with Investigator/Staff<br>▪ Check/inventory clinical supplies<br>▪ Review communication with the IRB<br>▪ Review drug accountability<br>▪ Confirm Informed Consent<br>▪ Correct previous errors<br>▪ Submit all collected documents and site visit report to Sponsor<br>▪ Log and track study progress |
| **Study Close Out** ||
| ▪ Review and collect remaining CRFs<br>▪ Retrieve clinical supplies and any other study materials.<br>▪ Review investigator's study file to insure that all documents are in order and ready for audit or inspection.<br>▪ Review file (document) retention schedule/policy.<br>▪ Submit documentation for study closeout.<br>▪ Arrange any final payments.<br>▪ Review publication policy/procedure<br>▪ Review any follow-up requirements that may be required (IRB notification, ongoing medical events). | ▪ Review and collect remaining CRFs<br>▪ Retrieve clinical supplies and any other study materials.<br>▪ Review investigator's study file to insure that all documents are in order and ready for audit or inspection.<br>▪ Review file (document) retention schedule/policy.<br>▪ Submit documentation for study closeout.<br>▪ Arrange any final payments.<br>▪ Review publication policy/procedure<br>▪ Review any follow-up requirements that may be required (IRB notification, ongoing medical events). |

# Clinical Research Associate (CRA)
## Entry Level

### Position Description

The Clinical Research Associate I will perform the following activities as directed by the Sponsor/CRO:

- Meet with Clinical Investigators and staff prior to study initiation to ensure all aspects of the study are understood by the investigator and staff, confirm the appropriateness of the IRB and ensure that all documentation required to initiate the study is complete.
- Monitor study progress to assure compliance with protocol requirements, FDA regulations and Good Clinical Practice by conducting site visits as directed by the Sponsor/CRO.
- Monitor and track patient enrollment and study progress
- Perform site audits to include source document review
- Ensure the timely accurate and complete collection and submission of study data
- Identify, address, and resolve issues and problems as they might occur.
- At study completion:
- Insure collection of all data and remaining study supplies for return to the Sponsor/CRO
- Insure that appropriate study documents are complete and properly filed
- Prepare the site for possible FDA inspection.
- Assist the Sponsor/CRO in problem solving and provide consultation on monitoring and study related activities.

This position requires 70% travel

### Educational Requirements

Must have a minimum of a Bachelors Degree in relevant biological or health science.

### Experience Requirements

This position requires a minimum of two years relevant clinical research experience that includes at least one year as a field monitor. Experience will include work in a clinical laboratory, clinic or pharmacy or as a member of a drug development team, or experience as a Study Coordinator or Research Nurse.

### Specialized Skills, Knowledge, Abilities

Excellent oral and written communication skills, interpersonal relationship skills, knowledge of scientific method, GCPs and regulations relating to clinical research. Must have a working knowledge of computer technology and its application to the clinical environment.

# Clinical Research Associate (CRA)
## Advanced Level

### Position Description

The Clinical Research Associate, independently or in consultation with the Sponsor/CRO will:

- Locate and select clinical investigators appropriate to the therapeutic area and phase of the study
- Assess potential study sites to insure the facility, staff and patient population are sufficient for study conduct
- Negotiate the study budget (grant) and any other contract agreements required by the Sponsor/CRO, if required
- Plan or assist in conducting study start-up meetings
- Meet with Clinical Investigators and their staff prior to study initiation to insure all aspects of the study are understood by the investigator and staff, confirm the appropriateness of the IRB and insure that all documentation required to initiate the study is complete
- Monitor study progress to assure compliance with protocol requirements, FDA regulations and Good Clinical Practice by conducting site visits as directed by the Sponsor/CRO.
- Monitor and track patient enrollment and study progress
- Perform site audits to include source document review
- Insure the timely accurate and complete collection and submission of study data
- Identify, address, and resolve issues and problems as they might occur.
- At study completion:
- Insure collection of all data and remaining study supplies for return to the Sponsor/CRO
- Insure that appropriate study documents are complete and properly filed
- Prepare the site for possible FDA inspection.
- Assist the Sponsor/CRO in problem solving and provide consultation on monitoring and study related activities.

This position requires 70% travel.

### Educational Requirements

Must have a minimum of a Bachelors Degree, preferably in a relevant biological or health science.

### Experience Requirements

This position requires a minimum of eight years of relevant clinical research experience, five years of which must have been as a working CRA or equivalent. Experience will include study design and field monitoring experience in drug/device development, or as a Study Coordinator or Research Nurse.

**Specialized Skills, Knowledge, Abilities**

Excellent oral and written communication skills, interpersonal relationship skills, negotiating skills, knowledge of scientific method, GCPs and regulations relating to clinical research. Must have a working knowledge of computer technology and its application to the clinical environment

# List of Academic Programs which train Clinical Research Professionals*

## United States

### Ph.D. Programs
Baylor College of Medicine, Houston, Texas
University of Colorado, Denver CO

### M.S. Programs
Albert Einstein College of Medicine, Yeshiva University, New York, NY
American Institute of Health Sciences, Los Angeles, CA
Campbell University, Research Triangle Park, NC
Duke University, Durham, NC
Massachusetts General Hospital, Institute of Health Professions, Boston, MA
Mayo Clinic, Rochester, MN
New York Medical College, Valhalla, NY
University of Louisville, Louisville, KY
University of Pittsburgh, Pittsburgh, PA
Virginia Commonwealth University, Richmond, VA

### Post-baccalaureate Certificate Programs
American Institute of Health Sciences, Los Angeles, CA
Boston University, Boston, MA
Duke University, Durham, NC
Eastern Michigan University, Ypsilanti, MI
Jefferson Medical College, Philadelphia, PA
LaSalle University, Philadelphia, PA
Massachusetts General Hospital, Institute of Health Professions, Boston, MA
Mayo Clinic, Rochester, MN
Medical College of Pennsylvania/Hahnemann University, Philadelphia, PA
Mercer County Community College, Trenton, NJ
University of California – San Diego, LaJolla, CA
University of California – Santa Cruz, Santa Cruz, CA
University of Chicago, Chicago, IL
University of Cincinnati, Cincinnati, OH
University of Louisville, Louisville, KY
Western Michigan University, Kalamazoo, MI

### B.S. Programs
George Washington University, Washington, DC
Campbell University, Buies Creek, NC

### Associate Degree Programs

Durham Community Technical College, Durham, NC
George Washington University, Washington, DC

## Outside United States

### Australia
Monash University, Sydney
University of Canberra, Canberra

### Canada
British Columbia Institute of Technology, Burnaby, British Columbia
Humber College, Toronto, Ontario
University of Western Ontario, London, Ontario

### United Kingdom
Institute of Clinical Research, Maidenhead, UK
John Moores University, Liverpool, UK
University of Leeds, Leeds, UK
University of Oxford, Oxford, UK

*Does not include K30 Programs designed for individuals with MD or PhD degree

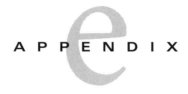

# A P P E N D I X

# ICH-FDA Comparison

| Activity | ICH Guidelines | 21 CFR |
|---|---|---|
| IRB | Requires the Investigator to furnish the IRB with a copy of the Investigator Brochure (4.4.2) | Requires the Sponsor to provide each Investigator with a copy of the Investigator Brochure (312.55a) |
| | Requires the Sponsor to obtain a statement from the IRB confirming that it is organized and operates according to GCPs and applicable laws and regulations ( 5.11.1b) Requires that the Subject be given a signed and dated copy of the consent form (4.8.11). | FDA does not require this statement. |

| Activity | ICH Guidelines | 21 CFR |
|---|---|---|
| Informed Consent | Requires the person administering the consent to sign the consent (4.8.8) | Requires a copy of the consent be given the subject. A signed copy is not required (50.27). |
| | Elements of consent differ between ICH and FDA. Does not have "optional" elements (4.8.10). | Requires only the Subjects signature and date (50.27) |
| | | Has "additional" elements that are optional. (50.25) |
| | Does not provide the option of using a "Short Form" and "Summary" for subjects who cannot read and are orally consented (4.8.9) | Provides the option of using a "Short Form" and "Summary" for orally consented subjects.(50.27) |
| Investigator Files/Records | Requires "all trial related records" be made available to the monitor, auditor, IRB/IEC, or regulatory authority (4.9.7) This includes financial records (8.2.4) | Does not require financial records be maintained in study files. |
| Protocol Deviations | ICH requires the investigator to document and explain all deviations | US regulations do not address this issue. |
| Protocol Signatures | ICH requires the sponsor and investigator to sign the protocol (5.6.3) | Is not required by regulation. Most sponsors require it. |

| Activity | ICH Guidelines | 21 CFR |
|---|---|---|
| Investigational Medication | ICH places responsibility for maintaining drug dispensing records and reconciliation of drug supplies with the clinical investigator (5.14.2) | FDA requires the return of unused supplies. |
| Study Documents | ICH places responsibility for ensuring that all study documents are available at the site (Study file) with the CRA ICH also requires the CRA to confirm the availability of the documents prior to closing the site. (8) | FDA holds the Investigator responsible complete, accurate study records. |
| Curriculum Vitae | ICH requires a CV for both the PI and any sub investigators (8.2.10) | FDA only requires CVs for principal investigators |
| Signature Sheets | ICH requires documentation of signatures and initials of all personnel authorized to enter and correct data on CRFs in both investigator and sponsor files (8.3.24) | FDA does not have this requirement. (Most sponsors, however, require it) |
| Site Visit (Monitoring) Reports | ICH requires the sponsor to document the review and follow-up of the site visit report filed by the CRA. (5.18.6d) | FDA does not have this requirement |

| Activity | ICH Guidelines | 21 CFR |
|---|---|---|
| Site Visit (Monitoring) Reports (continued) | ICH also requires a copy of the site visit report be placed in the investigator's study file. (8.2.20) | |
| Case Report Forms | ICH requires the CRA (study monitor) to ensure that all changes to CRFs are made properly (initialed, dated and explained if necessary) by the investigator or an authorized member of the site staff. The authorization must be documented. (5.18.4n) | FDA does not require that the authorization to make CRF changes be documented. |
| Notification of Subjects Physician | ICH recommends that the clinical investigator notify each study subject's primary care physician of his or her involvement in the study. (4.3.3) | FDA regulations do not address this issue |

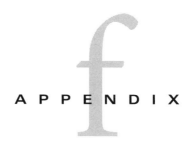

A P P E N D I X

# Harmonized Tripartite Guideline
# for Good Clinical Practice

## INTRODUCTION

Good Clinical Practice (GCP) is an international ethical and scientific quality standard for designing, conducting, recording and reporting trials that involve the participation of human subjects. Compliance with this standard provides public assurance that the rights, safety and well-being of trial subjects are protected, consistent with the principles that have their origin in the Declaration of Helsinki, and that the clinical trial data are credible.

The objective of this ICH GCP Guideline is to provide a unified standard for the European Union (EU), Japan and the United States to facilitate the mutual acceptance of clinical data by the regulatory authorities in these jurisdictions. The guideline was developed with consideration of the current good clinical practices of the European Union, Japan, and the United States, as well as those of Australia, Canada, the Nordic countries and the World Health Organization (WHO). This guideline should be followed when generating clinical trial data that are intended to be submitted to regulatory authorities. The principles established in this guideline may also be applied to other clinical investigations that may have an impact on the safety and well-being of human subjects.

# 1. Glossary

1.1 *Adverse Drug Reaction* (ADR). In the pre-approval clinical experience with a new medicinal product or its new usages, particularly as the therapeutic dose(s) may not be established: all noxious and unintended responses to a medicinal product related to any dose should be considered adverse drug reactions. The phrase responses to a medicinal product means that a causal relationship between a medicinal product and an adverse event is at least a reasonable possibility, i.e. the relationship cannot be ruled out. Regarding marketed medicinal products: a response to a drug which is noxious and unintended and which occurs at doses normally used in man for prophylaxis, diagnosis, or therapy of diseases or for modification of physiological function (see the ICH Guideline for Clinical Safety Data Management: Definitions and Standards for Expedited Reporting).

1.2 *Adverse Event* (AE). Any untoward medical occurrence in a patient or clinical investigation subject administered a pharmaceutical product and which does not necessarily have a causal relationship with this treatment. An adverse event (AE) can therefore be any unfavorable and unintended sign (including an abnormal laboratory finding), symptom, or disease temporally associated with the use of a medicinal (investigational) product, whether or not related to the medicinal (investigational) product (see the ICH Guideline for Clinical Safety Data Management: Definitions and Standards for Expedited Reporting).

1.3 *Amendment* (to the protocol). See Protocol Amendment.

1.4 *Applicable Regulatory Requirement*(s). Any law(s) and regulation(s) addressing the conduct of clinical trials of investigational products.

1.5 *Approval* (in relation to Institutional Review Boards). The affirmative decision of the IRB that the clinical trial has been reviewed and may be conducted at the institution site within the constraints set forth by the IRB, the institution, Good Clinical Practice (GCP), and the applicable regulatory requirements.

1.6 *Audit*. A systematic and independent examination of trial related activities and documents to determine whether the evaluated trial related activities were conducted, and the data were recorded, analyzed and accurately reported according to the protocol, sponsor's standard operating procedures (SOPs), Good Clinical Practice (GCP), and the applicable regulatory requirement(s).

1.7 *Audit Certificate*. A declaration of confirmation by the auditor that an audit has taken place.

1.8 *Audit Report.* A written evaluation by the sponsor's auditor of the results of the audit..

1.9 *Audit Trail.* Documentation that allows reconstruction of the course of events.

1.10 *Blinding/Masking.* A procedure in which one or more parties to the trial are kept unaware of the treatment assignment(s). Single-blinding usually refers to the subject(s) being unaware, and double-blinding usually refers to the subject(s), investigator(s), monitor, and, in some cases, data analyst(s) being unaware of the treatment assignment(s).

1.11 *Case Report Form* (CRF). A printed, optical, or electronic document designed to record all of the protocol required information to be reported to the sponsor on each trial subject.

1.12 *Clinical Trial/Study.* Any investigation in human subjects intended to discover or verify the clinical, pharmacological and/or other pharmacody-namic effects of an investigational product(s), and/or to identify any adverse reactions to an investigational product(s), and/or to study absorption, distri-bution, metabolism, and excretion of an investigational product(s) with the object of ascertaining its safety and/or efficacy. The terms clinical trial and clinical study are synonymous.

1.13 *Clinical Trial/Study Report.* A written description of a trial/study of any therapeutic, prophylactic, or diagnostic agent conducted in human subjects, in which the clinical and statistical description, presentations, and analyses are fully integrated into a single report (see the ICH Guideline for Structure and Content of Clinical Study Reports).

1.14 *Comparator* (Product). An investigational or marketed product (i.e., active control), or placebo, used as a reference in a clinical trial.

1.15 *Compliance* (in relation to trials). Adherence to all the trial-related requirements, Good Clinical Practice (GCP) requirements, and the applica-ble regulatory requirements.

1.16 *Confidentiality.* Prevention of disclosure, to other than authorized indi-viduals, of a sponsor's proprietary information or of a subject's identity.

1.17 *Contract.* A written, dated, and signed agreement between two or more involved parties that sets out any arrangements on delegation and distribu-tion of tasks and obligations and, if appropriate, on financial matters. The protocol may serve as the basis of a contract.

1.18 *Coordinating Committee.* A committee that a sponsor may organize to coordinate the conduct of a multicentre trial.

1.19 *Coordinating Investigator.* An investigator assigned the responsibility for the coordination of investigators at different centers participating in a multi-centre trial.

1.20 *Contract Research Organization* (CRO). A person or an organization (commercial, academic, or other) contracted by the sponsor to perform one or more of a sponsor's trial-related duties and functions.

1.21 *Direct Access.* Permission to examine, analyze, verify, and reproduce any records and reports that are important to evaluation of a clinical trial. Any party (e.g., domestic and foreign regulatory authorities, sponsor's monitors and auditors) with direct access should take all reasonable precautions within the constraints of the applicable regulatory requirement(s) to maintain the confidentiality of subjects' identities and sponsor's proprietary information.

1.22 *Documentation.* All records, in any form (including, but not limited to, written, electronic, magnetic, and optical records, and scans, x-rays, and electrocardiograms) that describe or record the methods, conduct, and/or results of a trial, the factors affecting a trial, and the actions taken.

1.23 *Essential Documents.* Documents which individually and collectively permit evaluation of the conduct of a study and the quality of the data produced (see 8. Essential Documents for the Conduct of a Clinical Trial).

1.24 Good Clinical Practice (GCP)
A standard for the design, conduct, performance, monitoring, auditing, recording, analyses, and reporting of clinical trials that provides assurance that the data and reported results are credible and accurate, and that the rights, integrity, and confidentiality of trial subjects are protected.

1.25 *Independent Data-Monitoring Committee* (IDMC) (Data and Safety Monitoring Board, Monitoring Committee, Data Monitoring Committee). An independent data-monitoring committee that may be established by the sponsor to assess at intervals the progress of a clinical trial, the safety data, and the critical efficacy endpoints, and to recommend to the sponsor whether to continue, modify, or stop a trial.

1.26 *Impartial Witness.* A person, who is independent of the trial, who cannot be unfairly influenced by people involved with the trial, who attends the informed consent process if the subject or the subject's legally acceptable representative cannot read, and who reads the informed consent form and any other written information supplied to the subject

1.27 *Independent Ethics Committee* (IEC). An independent body (a review board or a committee, institutional, regional, national, or supranational), constituted of medical professionals and non-medical members, whose responsibility it is to ensure the protection of the rights, safety and well-being of human subjects involved in a trial and to provide public assurance of that protection, by, among other things, reviewing and approving/providing favorable opinion on, the trial protocol, the suitability of the investigator(s), facilities, and the methods and material to be used in obtaining and documenting informed consent of the trial subjects. The legal status, composition, function, operations and regulatory requirements pertaining to Independent Ethics Committees may differ among countries, but should allow the Independent Ethics Committee to act in agreement with GCP as described in this guideline.

1.28 *Informed Consent.* A process by which a subject voluntarily confirms his or her willingness to participate in a particular trial, after having been informed of all aspects of the trial that are relevant to the subject's decision to participate. Informed consent is documented by means of a written, signed and dated informed consent form.

1.29 *Inspection.* The act by a regulatory authority(ies) of conducting an official review of documents, facilities, records, and any other resources that are deemed by the authority(ies) to be related to the clinical trial and that may be located at the site of the trial, at the sponsor's and/or contract research organization's (CRO's) facilities, or at other establishments deemed appropriate by the regulatory authority(ies).

1.30 *Institution* (medical) Any public or private entity or agency or medical or dental facility where clinical trials are conducted.

1.31 *Institutional Review Board* (IRB)
An independent body constituted of medical, scientific, and non-scientific members, whose responsibility is to ensure the protection of the rights, safety and well-being of human subjects involved in a trial by, among other things, reviewing, approving, and providing continuing review of trial protocol and amendments and of the methods and material to be used in obtaining and documenting informed consent of the trial subjects.

1.32 *Interim Clinical Trial/Study Report.* A report of intermediate results and their evaluation based on analyses performed during the course of a trial.

1.33 *Investigational Product.* A pharmaceutical form of an active ingredient or placebo being tested or used as a reference in a clinical trial, including a product with a marketing authorization when used or assembled (formulated or packaged) in a way different from the approved form, or when used for an unapproved indication, or when used to gain further information about an approved use.

1.34 *Investigator.* A person responsible for the conduct of the clinical trial at a trial site. If a trial is conducted by a team of individuals at a trial site, the investigator is the responsible leader of the team and may be called the principal investigator. See also Subinvestigator.

1.35 *Investigator/Institution.* An expression meaning "the investigator and/or institution, where required by the applicable regulatory requirements".

1.36 *Investigator's Brochure.* A compilation of the clinical and nonclinical data on the investigational product(s) which is relevant to the study of the investigational product(s) in human subjects (see 7. Investigator's Brochure).

1.37 *Legally Acceptable Representative.* An individual or juridical or other body authorized under applicable law to consent, on behalf of a prospective subject, to the subject's participation in the clinical trial.

1.38 *Monitoring.* The act of overseeing the progress of a clinical trial, and of ensuring that it is conducted, recorded, and reported in accordance with the protocol, Standard Operating Procedures (SOPs), Good Clinical Practice (GCP), and the applicable regulatory requirement(s).

1.39 *Monitoring Report.* A written report from the monitor to the sponsor after each site visit and/or other trial-related communication according to the sponsor's SOPs.

1.40 *Multicentre Trial.* A clinical trial conducted according to a single protocol but at more than one site, and therefore, carried out by more than one investigator.

1.41 *Nonclinical Study.* Biomedical studies not performed on human subjects.

1.42 *Opinion.* (in relation to Independent Ethics Committee). The judgement and/or the advice provided by an Independent Ethics Committee (IEC).

1.43 *Original Medical Record.* See Source Documents.

1.44 *Protocol.* A document that describes the objective(s), design, methodology, statistical considerations, and organization of a trial. The protocol usually also gives the background and rationale for the trial, but these could be provided in other protocol referenced documents. Throughout the ICH GCP Guideline the term protocol refers to protocol and protocol amendments.

1.45 *Protocol Amendment.* A written description of a change(s) to or formal clarification of a protocol.

1.46 *Quality Assurance* (QA). All those planned and systematic actions that are established to ensure that the trial is performed and the data are generated, documented (recorded), and reported in compliance with Good Clinical Practice (GCP) and the applicable regulatory requirement(s).

1.47 *Quality Control* (QC). The operational techniques and activities undertaken within the quality assurance system to verify that the requirements for quality of the trial-related activities have been fulfilled.

1.48 *Randomization.* The process of assigning trial subjects to treatment or control groups using an element of chance to determine the assignments in order to reduce bias.

1.49 *Regulatory Authorities.* Bodies having the power to regulate. In the ICH GCP guideline the expression Regulatory Authorities includes the authorities that review submitted clinical data and those that conduct inspections (see 1.29). These bodies are sometimes referred to as competent authorities.

1.50 *Serious Adverse Event* (SAE) or *Serious Adverse Drug Reaction* (Serious ADR). Any untoward medical occurrence that at any dose:

- results in death,
- is life-threatening,
- requires inpatient hospitalization or prolongation of existing hospitalization,
- results in persistent or significant disability/incapacity,

or

- is a congenital anomaly/birth defect

(see the ICH Guideline for Clinical Safety Data Management: Definitions and Standards for Expedited Reporting).

1.51 *Source Data.* All information in original records and certified copies of original records of clinical findings, observations, or other activities in a clinical trial necessary for the reconstruction and evaluation of the trial. Source data are contained in source documents (original records or certified copies).

1.52 *Source Documents.* Original documents, data, and records (e.g., hospital records, clinical and office charts, laboratory notes, memoranda, subjects' diaries or evaluation checklists, pharmacy dispensing records, recorded data from automated instruments, copies or transcriptions certified after verification as being accurate copies, microfiches, photographic negatives, microfilm or magnetic media, x-rays, subject files, and records kept at the pharmacy, at the laboratories and at medico-technical departments involved in the clinical trial).

1.53 *Sponsor.* An individual, company, institution, or organization which takes responsibility for the initiation, management, and/or financing of a clinical trial.

1.54 *Sponsor-Investigator.* An individual who both initiates and conducts, alone or with others, a clinical trial, and under whose immediate direction the investigational product is administered to, dispensed to, or used by a subject. The term does not include any person other than an individual (e.g., it does not include a corporation or an agency). The obligations of a sponsor-investigator include both those of a sponsor and those of an investigator.

1.55 *Standard Operating Procedures* (SOPs). Detailed, written instructions to achieve uniformity of the performance of a specific function.

1.56 *Subinvestigator.* Any individual member of the clinical trial team designated and supervised by the investigator at a trial site to perform critical trial-related procedures and/or to make important trial-related decisions (e.g., associates, residents, research fellows). See also Investigator.

1.57 *Subject/Trial Subject.* An individual who participates in a clinical trial, either as a recipient of the investigational product(s) or as a control.

1.58 *Subject Identification Code.* A unique identifier assigned by the investigator to each trial subject to protect the subject's identity and used in lieu of the subject's name when the investigator reports adverse events and/or other trial related data.

1.59 *Trial Site.* The location(s) where trial-related activities are actually conducted.

1.60 *Unexpected Adverse Drug Reaction.* An adverse reaction, the nature or severity of which is not consistent with the applicable product information (e.g., Investigator's Brochure for an unapproved investigational product or package insert/summary of product characteristics for an approved product) (see the ICH Guideline for Clinical Safety Data Management: Definitions and Standards for Expedited Reporting).

1.61 *Vulnerable Subjects.* Individuals whose willingness to volunteer in a clinical trial may be unduly influenced by the expectation, whether justified or not, of benefits associated with participation, or of a retaliatory response from senior members of a hierarchy in case of refusal to participate. Examples are members of a group with a hierarchical structure, such as medical, pharmacy, dental, and nursing students, subordinate hospital and laboratory personnel, employees of the pharmaceutical industry, members of the armed forces, and persons kept in detention. Other vulnerable subjects include patients with incurable diseases, persons in nursing homes, unemployed or impoverished persons, patients in emergency situations, ethnic minority groups, homeless persons, nomads, refugees, minors, and those incapable of giving consent.

1.62 *Well-being* (of the trial subjects). The physical and mental integrity of the subjects participating in a clinical trial.

## 2. The Principles of ICH GCP

2.1 Clinical trials should be conducted in accordance with the ethical principles that have their origin in the Declaration of Helsinki, and that are consistent with GCP and the applicable regulatory requirement(s).

2.2 Before a trial is initiated, foreseeable risks and inconveniences should be weighed against the anticipated benefit for the individual trial subject and society. A trial should be initiated and continued only if the anticipated benefits justify the risks.

2.3 The rights, safety, and well-being of the trial subjects are the most important considerations and should prevail over interests of science and society.

2.4 The available nonclinical and clinical information on an investigational product should be adequate to support the proposed clinical trial.

2.5 Clinical trials should be scientifically sound, and described in a clear, detailed protocol.

2.6 A trial should be conducted in compliance with the protocol that has received prior institutional review board (IRB)/independent ethics committee (IEC) approval/favorable opinion.

2.7 The medical care given to, and medical decisions made on behalf of, subjects should always be the responsibility of a qualified physician or, when appropriate, of a qualified dentist.

2.8 Each individual involved in conducting a trial should be qualified by education, training, and experience to perform his or her respective task(s).

2.9 Freely given informed consent should be obtained from every subject prior to clinical trial participation.

2.10 All clinical trial information should be recorded, handled, and stored in a way that allows its accurate reporting, interpretation and verification.

2.11 The confidentiality of records that could identify subjects should be protected, respecting the privacy and confidentiality rules in accordance with the applicable regulatory requirement(s).

2.12 Investigational products should be manufactured, handled, and stored in accordance with applicable good manufacturing practice (GMP). They should be used in accordance with the approved protocol.

2.13 Systems with procedures that assure the quality of every aspect of the trial should be implemented.

## 3. Institutional Review Board/Independent Ethics Committee (IRB/IEC)

### 3.1 Responsibilities
3.1.1 An IRB/IEC should safeguard the rights, safety, and well-being of all trial subjects. Special attention should be paid to trials that may include vulnerable subjects.

3.1.2 The IRB/IEC should obtain the following documents:
Trial protocol(s)/amendment(s), written informed consent form(s) and consent form updates that the investigator proposes for use in the trial, subject recruitment procedures (e.g. advertisements), written information to be provided to subjects, Investigator's Brochure (IB), available safety information, information about payments and compensation available to subjects, the investigator's current curriculum vitae and/or other documentation evidencing qualifications, and any other documents that the IRB/IEC may need to fulfil its responsibilities.

The IRB/IEC should review a proposed clinical trial within a reasonable time and document its views in writing, clearly identifying the trial, the documents reviewed and the dates for the following:
- approval/favorable opinion;
- modifications required prior to its approval/favorable opinion;
- disapproval/negative opinion; and
- termination/suspension of any prior approval/favorable opinion.

3.1.3 The IRB/IEC should consider the qualifications of the investigator for the proposed trial, as documented by a current curriculum vitae and/or by any other relevant documentation the IRB/IEC requests.

3.1.4 The IRB/IEC should conduct continuing review of each ongoing trial at intervals appropriate to the degree of risk to human subjects, but at least once per year.

3.1.5 The IRB/IEC may request more information than is outlined in paragraph 4.8.10 be given to subjects when, in the judgement of the IRB/IEC, the additional information would add meaningfully to the protection of the rights, safety and/or well-being of the subjects.

3.1.6 When a non-therapeutic trial is to be carried out with the consent of the subject's legally acceptable representative (see 4.8.12, 4.8.14), the IRB/IEC should determine that the proposed protocol and/or other document(s) adequately addresses relevant ethical concerns and meets applicable regulatory requirements for such trials.

3.1.7 Where the protocol indicates that prior consent of the trial subject or the subject's legally acceptable representative is not possible (see 4.8.15), the IRB/IEC should determine that the proposed protocol and/or other document(s) adequately addresses relevant ethical concerns and meets applicable regulatory requirements for such trials (i.e. in emergency situations).

3.1.8 The IRB/IEC should review both the amount and method of payment to subjects to assure that neither presents problems of coercion or undue influence on the trial subjects. Payments to a subject should be prorated and not wholly contingent on completion of the trial by the subject.

3.1.9 The IRB/IEC should ensure that information regarding payment to subjects, including the methods, amounts, and schedule of payment to trial subjects, is set forth in the written informed consent form and any other information to be provided to subjects. The way payment will be prorated should be specified.

### 3.2 Composition, Functions and Operations

3.2.1 The IRB/IEC should consist of a reasonable number of members, who collectively have the qualifications and experience to review and evaluate the science, medical aspects, and ethics of the proposed trial. It is recommended that the IRB/IEC should include:
a.  At least five members.
b.  At least one member whose primary area of interest is in a nonscientific area.
c.  At least one member who is independent of the institution/trial site.

Only those IRB/IEC members who are independent of the investigator and the sponsor of the trial should vote/provide opinion on a trial-related matter. A list of IRB/IEC members and their qualifications should be maintained.

3.2.2 The IRB/IEC should perform its functions according to written operating procedures, should maintain written records of its activities and minutes of its meetings, and should comply with GCP and with the applicable regulatory requirement(s).

3.2.3 An IRB/IEC should make its decisions at announced meetings at which at least a quorum, as stipulated in its written operating procedures, is present.

3.2.4 Only members who participate in the IRB/IEC review and discussion should vote/provide their opinion and/or advise.

3.2.5 The investigator may provide information on any aspect of the trial, but should not participate in the deliberations of the IRB/IEC or in the vote/opinion of the IRB/IEC.

3.2.6 An IRB/IEC may invite nonmembers with expertise in special areas for assistance.

### 3.3 Procedures
The IRB/IEC should establish, document in writing, and follow its procedures, which should include:

3.3.1 Determining its composition (names and qualifications of the members) and the authority under which it is established.

3.3.2 Scheduling, notifying its members of, and conducting its meetings.

3.3.3 Conducting initial and continuing review of trials.

3.3.4 Determining the frequency of continuing review, as appropriate.

3.3.5 Providing, according to the applicable regulatory requirements, expedited review and approval/favorable opinion of minor change(s) in ongoing trials that have the approval/favorable opinion of the IRB/IEC.

3.3.6 Specifying that no subject should be admitted to a trial before the IRB/IEC issues its written approval/favorable opinion of the trial.

3.3.7 Specifying that no deviations from, or changes of, the protocol should be initiated without prior written IRB/IEC approval/favorable opinion of an appropriate amendment, except when necessary to eliminate immediate hazards to the subjects or when the change(s) involves only logistical or administrative aspects of the trial (e.g., change of monitor(s), telephone number(s)) (see 4.5.2).

3.3.8 Specifying that the investigator should promptly report to the IRB/IEC:
a.  Deviations from, or changes of, the protocol to eliminate immediate hazards to the trial subjects (see 3.3.7, 4.5.2, 4.5.4).

b. Changes increasing the risk to subjects and/or affecting significantly the conduct of the trial (see 4.10.2).
c. All adverse drug reactions (ADRs) that are both serious and unexpected.
d. New information that may affect adversely the safety of the subjects or the conduct of the trial.

3.3.9 Ensuring that the IRB/IEC promptly notify in writing the investigator/institution concerning:
a. Its trial-related decisions/opinions.
b. The reasons for its decisions/opinions.
c. Procedures for appeal of its decisions/opinions.

### 3.4 Records

The IRB/IEC should retain all relevant records (e.g., written procedures, membership lists, lists of occupations/affiliations of members, submitted documents, minutes of meetings, and correspondence) for a period of at least 3 years after completion of the trial and make them available upon request from the regulatory authority(ies). The IRB/IEC may be asked by investigators, sponsors or regulatory authorities to provide its written procedures and membership lists.

## 4. Investigator

### 4.1 Investigator's Qualifications and Agreements

4.1.1 The investigator(s) should be qualified by education, training, and experience to assume responsibility for the proper conduct of the trial, should meet all the qualifications specified by the applicable regulatory requirement(s), and should provide evidence of such qualifications through up-to-date curriculum vitae and/or other relevant documentation requested by the sponsor, the IRB/IEC, and/or the regulatory authority(ies).

4.1.2 The investigator should be thoroughly familiar with the appropriate use of the investigational product(s), as described in the protocol, in the current Investigator's Brochure, in the product information and in other information sources provided by the sponsor.

4.1.3 The investigator should be aware of, and should comply with, GCP and the applicable regulatory requirements.

4.1.4 The investigator/institution should permit monitoring and auditing by the sponsor, and inspection by the appropriate regulatory authority(ies)..

4.1.5 The investigator should maintain a list of appropriately qualified persons to whom the investigator has delegated significant trial-related duties.

## 4.2 Adequate Resources

4.2.1 The investigator should be able to demonstrate (e.g., based on retro-spective data) a potential for recruiting the required number of suitable sub-jects within the agreed recruitment period.

4.2.2 The investigator should have sufficient time to properly conduct and complete the trial within the agreed trial period.

4.2.3 The investigator should have available an adequate number of qualified staff and adequate facilities for the foreseen duration of the trial to conduct the trial properly and safely.

4.2.4 The investigator should ensure that all persons assisting with the trial are adequately informed about the protocol, the investigational product(s), and their trial-related duties and functions.

## 4.3 Medical Care of Trial Subjects

4.3.1 A qualified physician (or dentist, when appropriate), who is an investi-gator or a sub-investigator for the trial, should be responsible for all trial-related medical (or dental) decisions.

4.3.2 During and following a subject's participation in a trial, the investiga-tor/institution should ensure that adequate medical care is provided to a sub-ject for any adverse events, including clinically significant laboratory values, related to the trial. The investigator/institution should inform a subject when medical care is needed for intercurrent illness(es) of which the investigator becomes aware.

4.3.3 It is recommended that the investigator inform the subject's primary physician about the subject's participation in the trial if the subject has a pri-mary physician and if the subject agrees to the primary physician being informed.

4.3.4 Although a subject is not obliged to give his/her reason(s) for with-drawing prematurely from a trial, the investigator should make a reasonable effort to ascertain the reason(s), while fully respecting the subject's rights.

## 4.4 Communication with IRB/IEC

4.4.1 Before initiating a trial, the investigator/institution should have written and dated approval/favorable opinion from the IRB/IEC for the trial proto-col, written informed consent form, consent form updates, subject recruit-ment procedures (e.g., advertisements), and any other written information to be provided to subjects.

4.4.2 As part of the investigator's/institution's written application to the IRB/IEC, the investigator/institution should provide the IRB/IEC with a current copy of the Investigator's Brochure. If the Investigator's Brochure is updated during the trial, the investigator/institution should supply a copy of the updated Investigator's Brochure to the IRB/IEC.

4.4.3 During the trial the investigator/institution should provide to the IRB/IEC all documents subject to review..

### 4.5 Compliance with Protocol

4.5.1 The investigator/institution should conduct the trial in compliance with the protocol agreed to by the sponsor and, if required, by the regulatory authority(ies) and which was given approval/favorable opinion by the IRB/IEC. The investigator/institution and the sponsor should sign the protocol, or an alternative contract, to confirm agreement.

4.5.2 The investigator should not implement any deviation from, or changes of the protocol without agreement by the sponsor and prior review and documented approval/favorable opinion from the IRB/IEC of an amendment, except where necessary to eliminate an immediate hazard(s) to trial subjects, or when the change(s) involves only logistical or administrative aspects of the trial (e.g., change in monitor(s), change of telephone number(s)).

4.5.3 The investigator, or person designated by the investigator, should document and explain any deviation from the approved protocol.

4.5.4 The investigator may implement a deviation from, or a change of, the protocol to eliminate an immediate hazard(s) to trial subjects without prior IRB/IEC approval/favorable opinion. As soon as possible, the implemented deviation or change, the reasons for it, and, if appropriate, the proposed protocol amendment(s) should be submitted:
a.  to the IRB/IEC for review and approval/favorable opinion,
b.  to the sponsor for agreement and, if required,
c.  to the regulatory authority(ies).

### 4.6 Investigational Product(s)

4.6.1 Responsibility for investigational product(s) accountability at the trial site(s) rests with the investigator/institution.
4.6.2 Where allowed/required, the investigator/institution may/should assign some or all of the investigator's/institution's duties for investigational product(s) accountability at the trial site(s) to an appropriate pharmacist or another appropriate individual who is under the supervision of the investigator/institution..

4.6.3 The investigator/institution and/or a pharmacist or other appropriate individual, who is designated by the investigator/institution, should maintain records of the product's delivery to the trial site, the inventory at the site, the use by each subject, and the return to the sponsor or alternative disposition of unused product(s). These records should include dates, quantities, batch/serial numbers, expiration dates (if applicable), and the unique code numbers assigned to the investigational product(s) and trial subjects. Investigators should maintain records that document adequately that the subjects were provided the doses specified by the protocol and reconcile all investigational product(s) received from the sponsor.

4.6.4 The investigational product(s) should be stored as specified by the sponsor (see 5.13.2 and 5.14.3) and in accordance with applicable regulatory requirement(s).

4.6.5 The investigator should ensure that the investigational product(s) are used only in accordance with the approved protocol.

4.6.6 The investigator, or a person designated by the investigator/institution, should explain the correct use of the investigational product(s) to each subject and should check, at intervals appropriate for the trial, that each subject is following the instructions properly.

**4.7 Randomization Procedures and Unblinding**
The investigator should follow the trial's randomization procedures, if any, and should ensure that the code is broken only in accordance with the protocol. If the trial is blinded, the investigator should promptly document and explain to the sponsor any premature unblinding (e.g., accidental unblinding, unblinding due to a serious adverse event) of the investigational product(s).

**4.8 Informed Consent of Trial Subjects**
4.8.1 In obtaining and documenting informed consent, the investigator should comply with the applicable regulatory requirement(s), and should adhere to GCP and to the ethical principles that have their origin in the Declaration of Helsinki. Prior to the beginning of the trial, the investigator should have the IRB/IEC's written approval/favorable opinion of the written informed consent form and any other written information to be provided to subjects.
4.8.2 The written informed consent form and any other written information to be provided to subjects should be revised whenever important new information becomes available that may be relevant to the subject's consent. Any revised written informed consent form, and written information should receive the IRB/IEC's approval/favorable opinion in advance of use. The subject or the subject's legally acceptable representative should be informed in a timely manner if new information becomes available that may be relevant to the subject's willingness to continue participation in the trial. The communication of this information should be documented.

4.8.3 Neither the investigator, nor the trial staff, should coerce or unduly influence a subject to participate or to continue to participate in a trial.

4.8.4 None of the oral and written information concerning the trial, including the written informed consent form, should contain any language that causes the subject or the subject's legally acceptable representative to waive or to appear to waive any legal rights, or that releases or appears to release the investigator, the institution, the sponsor, or their agents from liability for negligence.

4.8.5 The investigator, or a person designated by the investigator, should fully inform the subject or, if the subject is unable to provide informed consent, the subject's legally acceptable representative, of all pertinent aspects of the trial including the written information and the approval/favorable opinion by the IRB/IEC.

4.8.6 The language used in the oral and written information about the trial, including the written informed consent form, should be as non-technical as practical and should be understandable to the subject or the subject's legally acceptable representative and the impartial witness, where applicable.

4.8.7 Before informed consent may be obtained, the investigator, or a person designated by the investigator, should provide the subject or the subject's legally acceptable representative ample time and opportunity to inquire details of the trial and to decide whether or not to participate in the trial. All questions about the trial should be answered to the satisfaction of the subject or the subject's legally acceptable representative.

4.8.8 Prior to a subject's participation in the trial, the written informed consent form should be signed and personally dated by the subject or by the subject's legally acceptable representative, and by the person who conducted the informed consent discussion.

4.8.9 If a subject is unable to read or if a legally acceptable representative is unable to read, an impartial witness should be present during the entire informed consent discussion. After the written informed consent form and any other written information to be provided to subjects, is read and explained to the subject or the subject's legally acceptable representative, and after the subject or the subject's legally acceptable representative has orally consented to the subject's participation in the trial and, if capable of doing so, has signed and personally dated the informed consent form, the witness should sign and personally date the consent form. By signing the consent form, the witness attests that the information in the consent form and any other written information was accurately explained to, and apparently understood by, the subject or the subject's legally acceptable representative, and that informed consent was freely given by the subject or the subject's legally acceptable representative.

4.8.10 Both the informed consent discussion and the written informed consent form and any other written information to be provided to subjects should include explanations of the following:
a.  That the trial involves research.
b.  The purpose of the trial.
c.  The trial treatment(s) and the probability for random assignment to each treatment.
d.  The trial procedures to be followed, including all invasive procedures.
e.  The subject's responsibilities.
f.  Those aspects of the trial that are experimental.
g.  The reasonably foreseeable risks or inconveniences to the subject and, when applicable, to an embryo, fetus, or nursing infant.
h.  The reasonably expected benefits. When there is no intended clinical benefit to the subject, the subject should be made aware of this.
i.  The alternative procedure(s) or course(s) of treatment that may be available to the subject, and their important potential benefits and risks.
j.  The compensation and/or treatment available to the subject in the event of trial-related injury.
k.  The anticipated prorated payment, if any, to the subject for participating in the trial.
l.  The anticipated expenses, if any, to the subject for participating in the trial.
m.  That the subject's participation in the trial is voluntary and that the subject may refuse to participate or withdraw from the trial, at any time, without penalty or loss of benefits to which the subject is otherwise entitled.
n.  That the monitor(s), the auditor(s), the IRB/IEC, and the regulatory authority(ies) will be granted direct access to the subject's original medical records for verification of clinical trial procedures and/or data, without violating the confidentiality of the subject, to the extent permitted by the applicable laws and regulations and that, by signing a written informed consent form, the subject or the subject's legally acceptable representative is authorizing such access.
o.  That records identifying the subject will be kept confidential and, to the extent permitted by the applicable laws and/or regulations, will not be made publicly available. If the results of the trial are published, the subject's identity will remain confidential.
p.  That the subject or the subject's legally acceptable representative will be informed in a timely manner if information becomes available that may be relevant to the subject's willingness to continue participation in the trial.

q. The person(s) to contact for further information regarding the trial and the rights of trial subjects, and whom to contact in the event of trial-related injury.

r. The foreseeable circumstances and/or reasons under which the subject's participation in the trial may be terminated.

s. The expected duration of the subject's participation in the trial.

t. The approximate number of subjects involved in the trial.

4.8.11 Prior to participation in the trial, the subject or the subject's legally acceptable representative should receive a copy of the signed and dated written informed consent form and any other written information provided to the subjects. During a subject's participation in the trial, the subject or the subject's legally acceptable representative should receive a copy of the signed and dated consent form updates and a copy of any amendments to the written information provided to subjects.

4.8.12 When a clinical trial (therapeutic or non-therapeutic) includes subjects who can only be enrolled in the trial with the consent of the subject's legally acceptable representative (e.g., minors, or patients with severe dementia), the subject should be informed about the trial to the extent compatible with the subject's understanding and, if capable, the subject should sign and personally date the written informed consent.

4.8.13 Except as described in 4.8.14, a non-therapeutic trial (i.e. a trial in which there is no anticipated direct clinical benefit to the subject), should be conducted in subjects who personally give consent and who sign and date the written informed consent form.

4.8.14 Non-therapeutic trials may be conducted in subjects with consent of a legally acceptable representative provided the following conditions are fulfilled:

a. The objectives of the trial can not be met by means of a trial in subjects who can give informed consent personally.

b. The foreseeable risks to the subjects are low.

c. The negative impact on the subject's well-being is minimized and low.

d. The trial is not prohibited by law.

e. The approval/favorable opinion of the IRB/IEC is expressly sought on the inclusion of such subjects, and the written approval/favorable opinion covers this aspect. Such trials, unless an exception is justified, should be conducted in patients having a disease or condition for which the investigational product is intended. Subjects in these trials should be particularly closely monitored and should be withdrawn if they appear to be unduly distressed.

4.8.15 In emergency situations, when prior consent of the subject is not possible, the consent of the subject's legally acceptable representative, if present, should be requested. When prior consent of the subject is not possible, and the subject's legally acceptable representative is not available, enrolment of the subject should require measures described in the protocol and/or elsewhere, with documented approval/favorable opinion by the IRB/IEC, to protect the rights, safety and well-being of the subject and to ensure compliance with applicable regulatory requirements. The subject or the subject's legally acceptable representative should be informed about the trial as soon as possible and consent to continue and other consent as appropriate (see 4.8.10) should be requested.

### 4.9 Records and Reports

4.9.1 The investigator should ensure the accuracy, completeness, legibility, and timeliness of the data reported to the sponsor in the CRFs and in all required reports.

4.9.2 Data reported on the CRF, that are derived from source documents, should be consistent with the source documents or the discrepancies should be explained.

4.9.3 Any change or correction to a CRF should be dated, initialed, and explained (if necessary) and should not obscure the original entry (i.e. an audit trail should be maintained); this applies to both written and electronic changes or corrections (see 5.18.4 (n)). Sponsors should provide guidance to investigators and/or the investigators' designated representatives on making such corrections. Sponsors should have written procedures to assure that changes or corrections in CRFs made by sponsor's designated representatives are documented, are necessary, and are endorsed by the investigator. The investigator should retain records of the changes and corrections.

4.9.4 The investigator/institution should maintain the trial documents as specified in Essential Documents for the Conduct of a Clinical Trial (see 8.) and as required by the applicable regulatory requirement(s). The investigator/institution should take measures to prevent accidental or premature destruction of these documents.

4.9.5 Essential documents should be retained until at least 2 years after the last approval of a marketing application in an ICH region and until there are no pending or contemplated marketing applications in an ICH region or at least 2 years have elapsed since the formal discontinuation of clinical development of the investigational product. These documents should be retained for a longer period however if required by the applicable regulatory requirements or by an agreement with the sponsor. It is the responsibility of the sponsor to inform the investigator/institution as to when these documents no longer need to be retained (see 5.5.12).

4.9.6 The financial aspects of the trial should be documented in an agreement between the sponsor and the investigator/institution.

4.9.7 Upon request of the monitor, auditor, IRB/IEC, or regulatory authority, the investigator/institution should make available for direct access all requested trial-related records.

## 4.10 Progress Reports

4.10.1 The investigator should submit written summaries of the trial status to the IRB/IEC annually, or more frequently, if requested by the IRB/IEC.

4.10.2 The investigator should promptly provide written reports to the sponsor, the IRB/IEC (see 3.3.8) and, where applicable, the institution on any changes significantly affecting the conduct of the trial, and/or increasing the risk to subjects.

## 4.11 Safety Reporting

4.11.1 All serious adverse events (SAEs) should be reported immediately to the sponsor except for those SAEs that the protocol or other document (e.g., Investigator's Brochure) identifies as not needing immediate reporting. The immediate reports should be followed promptly by detailed, written reports. The immediate and follow-up reports should identify subjects by unique code numbers assigned to the trial subjects rather than by the subjects' names, personal identification numbers, and/or addresses. The investigator should also comply with the applicable regulatory requirement(s) related to the reporting of unexpected serious adverse drug reactions to the regulatory authority(ies) and the IRB/IEC.

4.11.2 Adverse events and/or laboratory abnormalities identified in the protocol as critical to safety evaluations should be reported to the sponsor according to the reporting requirements and within the time periods specified by the sponsor in the protocol.

4.11.3 For reported deaths, the investigator should supply the sponsor and the IRB/IEC with any additional requested information (e.g., autopsy reports and terminal medical reports).

## 4.12 Premature Termination or Suspension of a Trial

If the trial is prematurely terminated or suspended for any reason, the investigator/institution should promptly inform the trial subjects, should assure appropriate therapy and follow-up for the subjects, and, where required by the applicable regulatory requirement(s), should inform the regulatory authority(ies). In addition:

4.12.1 If the investigator terminates or suspends a trial without prior agreement of the sponsor, the investigator should inform the institution where applicable, and the investigator/institution should promptly inform the sponsor and the IRB/IEC, and should provide the sponsor and the IRB/IEC a detailed written explanation of the termination or suspension.

4.12.2 If the sponsor terminates or suspends a trial (see 5.21), the investigator should promptly inform the institution where applicable and the investigator/institution should promptly inform the IRB/IEC and provide the IRB/IEC a detailed written explanation of the termination or suspension.

4.12.3 If the IRB/IEC terminates or suspends its approval/favorable opinion of a trial (see 3.1.2 and 3.3.9), the investigator should inform the institution where applicable and the investigator/institution should promptly notify the sponsor and provide the sponsor with a detailed written explanation of the termination or suspension.

4.13 Final Report(s) by Investigator
Upon completion of the trial, the investigator, where applicable, should inform the institution; the investigator/institution should provide the IRB/IEC with a summary of the trial's outcome, and the regulatory authority(ies) with any reports required.

## 5. Sponsor

### 5.1 Quality Assurance and Quality Control
5.1.1 The sponsor is responsible for implementing and maintaining quality assurance and quality control systems with written SOPs to ensure that trials are conducted and data are generated, documented (recorded), and reported in compliance with the protocol, GCP, and the applicable regulatory requirement(s).

5.1.2 The sponsor is responsible for securing agreement from all involved parties to ensure direct access (see 1.21) to all trial related sites, source data/documents , and reports for the purpose of monitoring and auditing by the sponsor, and inspection by domestic and foreign regulatory authorities.

5.1.3 Quality control should be applied to each stage of data handling to ensure that all data are reliable and have been processed correctly.
5.1.4 Agreements, made by the sponsor with the investigator/institution and any other parties involved with the clinical trial, should be in writing, as part of the protocol or in a separate agreement.

### 5.2 Contract Research Organization (CRO)
5.2.1 A sponsor may transfer any or all of the sponsor's trial-related duties and functions to a CRO, but the ultimate responsibility for the quality and integrity of the trial data always resides with the sponsor. The CRO should implement quality assurance and quality control.

5.2.2 Any trial-related duty and function that is transferred to and assumed by a CRO should be specified in writing.

5.2.3 Any trial-related duties and functions not specifically transferred to and assumed by a CRO are retained by the sponsor.

5.2.4 All references to a sponsor in this guideline also apply to a CRO to the extent that a CRO has assumed the trial related duties and functions of a sponsor.

### 5.3 Medical Expertise
The sponsor should designate appropriately qualified medical personnel who will be readily available to advise on trial related medical questions or problems. If necessary, outside consultant(s) may be appointed for this purpose.

### 5.4 Trial Design
5.4.1 The sponsor should utilize qualified individuals (e.g. biostatisticians, clinical pharmacologists, and physicians) as appropriate, throughout all stages of the trial process, from designing the protocol and CRFs and planning the analyses to analyzing and preparing interim and final clinical trial reports.

5.4.2 For further guidance: Clinical Trial Protocol and Protocol Amendment(s) (see 6.), the ICH Guideline for Structure and Content of Clinical Study Reports, and other appropriate ICH guidance on trial design, protocol and conduct.

### 5.5 Trial Management, Data Handling, and Record Keeping
5.5.1 The sponsor should utilize appropriately qualified individuals to supervise the overall conduct of the trial, to handle the data, to verify the data, to conduct the statistical analyses, and to prepare the trial reports.

5.5.2 The sponsor may consider establishing an independent data-monitoring committee (IDMC) to assess the progress of a clinical trial, including the safety data and the critical efficacy endpoints at intervals, and to recommend to the sponsor whether to continue, modify, or stop a trial. The IDMC should have written operating procedures and maintain written records of all its meetings.

5.5.3 When using electronic trial data handling and/or remote electronic trial data systems, the sponsor should:
a. Ensure and document that the electronic data processing system(s) conforms to the sponsor's established requirements for completeness, accuracy, reliability, and consistent intended performance (i.e. validation).
b. Maintains SOPs for using these systems.

c. Ensure that the systems are designed to permit data changes in such a way that the data changes are documented and that there is no deletion of entered data (i.e. maintain an audit trail, data trail, edit trail).
d. Maintain a security system that prevents unauthorized access to the data.
e. Maintain a list of the individuals who are authorized to make data changes (see 4.1.5 and 4.9.3).
f. Maintain adequate backup of the data.
g. Safeguard the blinding, if any (e.g. maintain the blinding during data entry and processing).

5.5.4 If data are transformed during processing, it should always be possible to compare the original data and observations with the processed data.

5.5.5 The sponsor should use an unambiguous subject identification code (see 1.58) that allows identification of all the data reported for each subject

5.5.6 The sponsor, or other owners of the data, should retain all of the sponsor-specific essential documents pertaining to the trial (see 8. Essential Documents for the Conduct of a Clinical Trial).

5.5.7 The sponsor should retain all sponsor-specific essential documents in conformance with the applicable regulatory requirement(s) of the country(ies) where the product is approved, and/or where the sponsor intends to apply for approval(s).

5.5.8 If the sponsor discontinues the clinical development of an investigational product (i.e. for any or all indications, routes of administration, or dosage forms), the sponsor should maintain all sponsor-specific essential documents for at least 2 years after formal discontinuation or in conformance with the applicable regulatory requirement(s).

5.5.9 If the sponsor discontinues the clinical development of an investigational product, the sponsor should notify all the trial investigators/institutions and all the regulatory authorities.
5.5.10 Any transfer of ownership of the data should be reported to the appropriate authority(ies), as required by the applicable regulatory requirement(s).

5.5.11 The sponsor specific essential documents should be retained until at least 2 years after the last approval of a marketing application in an ICH region and until there are no pending or contemplated marketing applications in an ICH region or at least 2 years have elapsed since the formal discontinuation of clinical development of the investigational product. These documents should be retained for a longer period however if required by the applicable regulatory requirement(s) or if needed by the sponsor.

5.5.12 The sponsor should inform the investigator(s)/institution(s) in writing of the need for record retention and should notify the investigator(s)/institution(s) in writing when the trial related records are no longer needed.

### 5.6 Investigator Selection

5.6.1 The sponsor is responsible for selecting the investigator(s)/institution(s). Each investigator should be qualified by training and experience and should have adequate resources (see 4.1, 4.2) to properly conduct the trial for which the investigator is selected. If organization of a coordinating committee and/or selection of coordinating investigator(s) are to be utilized in multicentre trials, their organization and/or selection are the sponsor's responsibility.

5.6.2 Before entering an agreement with an investigator/institution to conduct a trial, the sponsor should provide the investigator(s)/institution(s) with the protocol and an up-to-date Investigator's Brochure, and should provide sufficient time for the investigator/institution to review the protocol and the information provided.

5.6.3 The sponsor should obtain the investigator's/institution's agreement:
a.  to conduct the trial in compliance with GCP, with the applicable regulatory requirement(s) (see 4.1.3), and with the protocol agreed to by the sponsor and given approval/favorable opinion by the IRB/IEC (see 4.5.1);
b.  to comply with procedures for data recording/reporting.
c.  to permit monitoring, auditing and inspection (see 4.1.4) and
d.  to retain the trial related essential documents until the sponsor informs the investigator/institution these documents are no longer needed (see 4.9.4 and 5.5.12). The sponsor and the investigator/institution should sign the protocol, or an alternative document, to confirm this agreement.

### 5.7 Allocation of Responsibilities

Prior to initiating a trial, the sponsor should define, establish, and allocate all trial-related duties and functions.

### 5.8 Compensation to Subjects and Investigators

5.8.1 If required by the applicable regulatory requirement(s), the sponsor should provide insurance or should indemnify (legal and financial coverage) the investigator/the institution against claims arising from the trial, except for claims that arise from malpractice and/or negligence.

5.8.2 The sponsor's policies and procedures should address the costs of treatment of trial subjects in the event of trial-related injuries in accordance with the applicable regulatory requirement(s).

5.8.3 When trial subjects receive compensation, the method and manner of compensation should comply with applicable regulatory requirement(s).

## 5.9 Financing

The financial aspects of the trial should be documented in an agreement between the sponsor and the investigator/institution.

## 5.10 Notification/Submission to Regulatory Authority(ies)

Before initiating the clinical trial(s), the sponsor (or the sponsor and the investigator, if required by the applicable regulatory requirement(s)) should submit any required application(s) to the appropriate authority(ies) for review, acceptance, and/or permission (as required by the applicable regulatory requirement(s)) to begin the trial(s). Any notification/submission should be dated and contain sufficient information to identify the protocol.

## 5.11 Confirmation of Review by IRB/IEC

5.11.1 The sponsor should obtain from the investigator/institution:
a.  The name and address of the investigator's/institution's IRB/IEC.
b.  A statement obtained from the IRB/IEC that it is organized and oper-
    ates according to GCP and the applicable laws and regulations.
c.  Documented IRB/IEC approval/favorable opinion and, if requested by
    the sponsor, a current copy of protocol, written informed consent
    form(s) and any other written information to be provided to subjects,
    subject recruiting procedures, and documents related to payments and
    compensation available to the subjects, and any other documents that
    the IRB/IEC may have requested.

5.11.2 If the IRB/IEC conditions its approval/favorable opinion upon change(s) in any aspect of the trial, such as modification(s) of the protocol, written informed consent form and any other written information to be provided to subjects, and/or other procedures, the sponsor should obtain from the investigator/institution a copy of the modification(s) made and the date approval/favorable opinion was given by the IRB/IEC.

5.11.3 The sponsor should obtain from the investigator/institution documentation and dates of any IRB/IEC reapprovals/re-evaluations with favorable opinion, and of any withdrawals or suspensions of approval/favorable opinion.

## 5.12 Information on Investigational Product(s)

5.12.1 When planning trials, the sponsor should ensure that sufficient safety and efficacy data from nonclinical studies and/or clinical trials are available to support human exposure by the route, at the dosages, for the duration, and in the trial population to be studied.

5.12.2 The sponsor should update the Investigator's Brochure as significant new information becomes available (see 7. Investigator's Brochure).

## 5.13 Manufacturing, Packaging, Labeling, and Coding Investigational Product(s)

5.13.1 The sponsor should ensure that the investigational product(s) (including active comparator(s) and placebo, if applicable) is characterized as appropriate to the stage of development of the product(s), is manufactured in accordance with any applicable GMP, and is coded and labeled in a manner that protects the blinding, if applicable. In addition, the labeling should comply with applicable regulatory requirement(s).

5.13.2 The sponsor should determine, for the investigational product(s), acceptable storage temperatures, storage conditions (e.g. protection from light), storage times, reconstitution fluids and procedures, and devices for product infusion, if any. The sponsor should inform all involved parties (e.g. monitors, investigators, pharmacists, storage managers) of these determinations.

5.13.3 The investigational product(s) should be packaged to prevent contamination and unacceptable deterioration during transport and storage.

5.13.4 In blinded trials, the coding system for the investigational product(s) should include a mechanism that permits rapid identification of the product(s) in case of a medical emergency, but does not permit undetectable breaks of the blinding.

5.13.5 If significant formulation changes are made in the investigational or comparator product(s) during the course of clinical development, the results of any additional studies of the formulated product(s) (e.g. stability, dissolution rate, bioavailability) needed to assess whether these changes would significantly alter the pharmacokinetic profile of the product should be available prior to the use of the new formulation in clinical trials.

## 5.14 Supplying and Handling Investigational Product(s)

5.14.1 The sponsor is responsible for supplying the investigator(s)/institution(s) with the investigational product(s).

5.14.2 The sponsor should not supply an investigator/institution with the investigational product(s) until the sponsor obtains all required documentation (e.g. approval/favorable opinion from IRB/IEC and regulatory authority(ies)).

5.14.3 The sponsor should ensure that written procedures include instructions that the investigator/institution should follow for the handling and storage of investigational product(s) for the trial and documentation thereof.

The procedures should address adequate and safe receipt, handling, storage, dispensing, retrieval of unused product from subjects, and return of unused investigational product(s) to the sponsor (or alternative disposition if authorized by the sponsor and in compliance with the applicable regulatory requirement(s)).

5.14.4 The sponsor should:
a.  Ensure timely delivery of investigational product(s) to the investigator(s).
b.  Maintain records that document shipment, receipt, disposition, return, and destruction of the investigational product(s) (see 8. Essential Documents for the Conduct of a Clinical Trial).
c.  Maintain a system for retrieving investigational products and documenting this retrieval (e.g. for deficient product recall, reclaim after trial completion, expired product reclaim).
d.  Maintain a system for the disposition of unused investigational product(s) and for the documentation of this disposition.

5.14.5 The sponsor should:
a.  Take steps to ensure that the investigational product(s) are stable over the period of use.
b.  Maintain sufficient quantities of the investigational product(s) used in the trials to reconfirm specifications, should this become necessary, and maintain records of batch sample analyses and characteristics. To the extent stability permits, samples should be retained either until the analyses of the trial data are complete or as required by the applicable regulatory requirement(s), whichever represents the longer retention period.

## 5.15 Record Access
5.15.1 The sponsor should ensure that it is specified in the protocol or other written agreement that the investigator(s)/institution(s) provide direct access to source data/documents for trial-related monitoring, audits, IRB/IEC review, and regulatory inspection.

5.15.2 The sponsor should verify that each subject has consented, in writing, to direct access to his/her original medical records for trial-related monitoring, audit, IRB/IEC review, and regulatory inspection.

## 5.16 Safety Information
5.16.1 The sponsor is responsible for the ongoing safety evaluation of the investigational product(s).

5.16.2 The sponsor should promptly notify all concerned investigator(s)/institution(s) and the regulatory authority(ies) of findings that could affect adversely the safety of subjects, impact the conduct of the trial, or alter the IRB/IEC's approval/favorable opinion to continue the trial.

## 5.17 Adverse Drug Reaction Reporting

5.17.1 The sponsor should expedite the reporting to all concerned investigator(s)/institutions(s), to the IRB(s)/IEC(s), where required, and to the regulatory authority(ies) of all adverse drug reactions (ADRs) that are both serious and unexpected.

5.17.2 Such expedited reports should comply with the applicable regulatory requirement(s) and with the ICH Guideline for Clinical Safety Data Management: Definitions and Standards for Expedited Reporting.

5.17.3 The sponsor should submit to the regulatory authority(ies) all safety updates and periodic reports, as required by applicable regulatory requirement(s).

## 5.18 Monitoring

5.18.1 Purpose
The purposes of trial monitoring are to verify that:
a.  The rights and well-being of human subjects are protected.
b.  The reported trial data are accurate, complete, and verifiable from source documents.
c.  The conduct of the trial is in compliance with the currently approved protocol/amendment(s), with GCP, and with the applicable regulatory requirement(s).

5.18.2 Selection and Qualifications of Monitors
a.  Monitors should be appointed by the sponsor.
b.  Monitors should be appropriately trained, and should have the scientific and/or clinical knowledge needed to monitor the trial adequately. A monitor's qualifications should be documented.
c.  Monitors should be thoroughly familiar with the investigational product(s), the protocol, written informed consent form and any other written information to be provided to subjects, the sponsor's SOPs, GCP, and the applicable regulatory requirement(s).

5.18.3 *Extent and Nature of Monitoring.* The sponsor should ensure that the trials are adequately monitored. The sponsor should determine the appropriate extent and nature of monitoring. The determination of the extent and nature of monitoring should be based on considerations such as the objective, purpose, design, complexity, blinding, size, and endpoints of the trial. In general there is a need for on-site monitoring, before, during, and after the trial; however in exceptional circumstances the sponsor may determine that central monitoring in conjunction with procedures such as investigators' training and meetings, and extensive written guidance can assure appropriate conduct of the trial in accordance with GCP. Statistically controlled sampling may be an acceptable method for selecting the data to be verified.

5.18.4 *Monitor's Responsibilities.* The monitor(s) in accordance with the sponsor's requirements should ensure that the trial is conducted and documented properly by carrying out the following activities when relevant and necessary to the trial and the trial site:

a. Acting as the main line of communication between the sponsor and the investigator.
b. Verifying that the investigator has adequate qualifications and resources (see 4.1, 4.2, 5.6) and remain adequate throughout the trial period, that facilities, including laboratories, equipment, and staff, are adequate to safely and properly conduct the trial and remain adequate throughout the trial period.
c. Verifying, for the investigational product(s):
   i. That storage times and conditions are acceptable, and that supplies are sufficient throughout the trial.
   ii. That the investigational product(s) are supplied only to subjects who are eligible to receive it and at the protocol specified dose(s).
   iii. That subjects are provided with necessary instruction on properly using, handling, storing, and returning the investigational product(s).
   iv. That the receipt, use, and return of the investigational product(s) at the trial sites are controlled and documented adequately.
   v. That the disposition of unused investigational product(s) at the trial sites complies with applicable regulatory requirement(s) and is in accordance with the sponsor.
d. Verifying that the investigator follows the approved protocol and all approved amendment(s), if any.
e. Verifying that written informed consent was obtained before each subject's participation in the trial.
f. Ensuring that the investigator receives the current Investigator's Brochure, all documents, and all trial supplies needed to conduct the trial properly and to comply with the applicable regulatory requirement(s).
g. Ensuring that the investigator and the investigator's trial staff are adequately informed about the trial.
h. Verifying that the investigator and the investigator's trial staff are performing the specified trial functions, in accordance with the protocol and any other written agreement between the sponsor and the investigator/institution, and have not delegated these functions to unauthorized individuals.
i. Verifying that the investigator is enrolling only eligible subjects.
j. Reporting the subject recruitment rate.
k. Verifying that source documents and other trial records are accurate, complete, kept up-to-date and maintained.

l.   Verifying that the investigator provides all the required reports, notifications, applications, and submissions, and that these documents are accurate, complete, timely, legible, dated, and identify the trial.

m.  Checking the accuracy and completeness of the CRF entries, source documents and other trial-related records against each other. The monitor specifically should verify that:

    i.   The data required by the protocol are reported accurately on the CRFs and are consistent with the source documents.

    ii.  Any dose and/or therapy modifications are well documented for each of the trial subjects.

    iii. Adverse events, concomitant medications and intercurrent illnesses are reported in accordance with the protocol on the CRFs.

    iv.  Visits that the subjects fail to make, tests that are not conducted, and examinations that are not performed are clearly reported as such on the CRFs.

    v.   All withdrawals and dropouts of enrolled subjects from the trial are reported and explained on the CRFs.

n.   Informing the investigator of any CRF entry error, omission, or illegibility. The monitor should ensure that appropriate corrections, additions, or deletions are made, dated, explained (if necessary), and initialed by the investigator or by a member of the investigator's trial staff who is authorized to initial CRF changes for the investigator. This authorization should be documented.

o.   Determining whether all adverse events (AEs) are appropriately reported within the time periods required by GCP, the protocol, the IRB/IEC, the sponsor, and the applicable regulatory requirement(s).

p.   Determining whether the investigator is maintaining the essential documents (see 8. Essential Documents for the Conduct of a Clinical Trial).

q.   Communicating deviations from the protocol, SOPs, GCP, and the applicable regulatory requirements to the investigator and taking appropriate action designed to prevent recurrence of the detected deviations.

5.18.5 *Monitoring Procedures.* The monitor(s) should follow the sponsor's established written SOPs as well as those procedures that are specified by the sponsor for monitoring a specific trial.

5.18.6 *Monitoring Report*

a.   The monitor should submit a written report to the sponsor after each trial-site visit or trial-related communication.

b.   Reports should include the date, site, name of the monitor, and name of the investigator or other individual(s) contacted.

c.   Reports should include a summary of what the monitor reviewed and the monitor's statements concerning the significant findings/facts, deviations and deficiencies, conclusions, actions taken or to be taken and/or actions recommended to secure compliance.

d.   The review and follow-up of the monitoring report with the sponsor should be documented by the sponsor's designated representative.

## 5.19 Audit

If or when sponsors perform audits, as part of implementing quality assurance, they should consider:

5.19.1 *Purpose.* The purpose of a sponsor's audit, which is independent of and separate from routine monitoring or quality control functions, should be to evaluate trial conduct and compliance with the protocol, SOPs, GCP, and the applicable regulatory requirements.

5.19.2 Selection and Qualification of Auditors
a.   The sponsor should appoint individuals, who are independent of the clinical trials/systems, to conduct audits.
b.   The sponsor should ensure that the auditors are qualified by training and experience to conduct audits properly. An auditor's qualifications should be documented.

5.19.3 Auditing Procedures
a.   The sponsor should ensure that the auditing of clinical trials/systems is conducted in accordance with the sponsor's written procedures on what to audit, how to audit, the frequency of audits, and the form and content of audit reports.
b.   The sponsor's audit plan and procedures for a trial audit should be guided by the importance of the trial to submissions to regulatory authorities, the number of subjects in the trial, the type and complexity of the trial, the level of risks to the trial subjects, and any identified problem(s).
c.   The observations and findings of the auditor(s) should be documented.
d.   To preserve the independence and value of the audit function, the regulatory authority(ies) should not routinely request the audit reports. Regulatory authority(ies) may seek access to an audit report on a case by case basis when evidence of serious GCP non-compliance exists, or in the course of legal proceedings.
e.   When required by applicable law or regulation, the sponsor should provide an audit certificate.

## 5.20 Noncompliance

5.20.1 Noncompliance with the protocol, SOPs, GCP, and/or applicable regulatory requirement(s) by an investigator/institution, or by member(s) of the sponsor's staff should lead to prompt action by the sponsor to secure compliance.

5.20.2 If the monitoring and/or auditing identifies serious and/or persistent noncompliance on the part of an investigator/institution, the sponsor should terminate the investigator's/institution's participation in the trial. When an investigator's/institution's participation is terminated because of noncompliance, the sponsor should notify promptly the regulatory authority(ies).

## 5.21 Premature Termination or Suspension of a Trial

If a trial is prematurely terminated or suspended, the sponsor should promptly inform the investigators/institutions, and the regulatory authority(ies) of the termination or suspension and the reason(s) for the termination or suspension. The IRB/IEC should also be informed promptly and provided the reason(s) for the termination or suspension by the sponsor or by the investigator/institution, as specified by the applicable regulatory requirement(s).

## 5.22 Clinical Trial/Study Reports

Whether the trial is completed or prematurely terminated, the sponsor should ensure that the clinical trial reports are prepared and provided to the regulatory agency(ies) as required by the applicable regulatory requirement(s). The sponsor should also ensure that the clinical trial reports in marketing applications meet the standards of the ICH Guideline for Structure and Content of Clinical Study Reports. (NOTE: The ICH Guideline for Structure and Content of Clinical Study Reports specifies that abbreviated study reports may be acceptable in certain cases.)

## 5.23 Multicentre Trials

For multicentre trials, the sponsor should ensure that:

5.23.1 All investigators conduct the trial in strict compliance with the protocol agreed to by the sponsor and, if required, by the regulatory authority(ies), and given approval/favorable opinion by the IRB/IEC.

5.23.2 The CRFs are designed to capture the required data at all multicentre trial sites. For those investigators who are collecting additional data, supplemental CRFs should also be provided that are designed to capture the additional data.

5.23.3 The responsibilities of coordinating investigator(s) and the other participating investigators are documented prior to the start of the trial.

5.23.4 All investigators are given instructions on following the protocol, on complying with a uniform set of standards for the assessment of clinical and laboratory findings, and on completing the CRFs.

5.23.5 Communication between investigators is facilitated.

## 6. Clinical Trial Protocol and Protocol Amendment(s)

The contents of a trial protocol should generally include the following topics. However, site specific information may be provided on separate protocol page(s), or addressed in a separate agreement, and some of the information listed below may be contained in other protocol referenced documents, such as an Investigator's Brochure.

### 6.1 General Information

6.1.1 Protocol title, protocol identifying number, and date. Any amendment(s) should also bear the amendment number(s) and date(s).

6.1.2 Name and address of the sponsor and monitor (if other than the sponsor).

6.1.3 Name and title of the person(s) authorized to sign the protocol and the protocol amendment(s) for the sponsor.

6.1.4 Name, title, address, and telephone number(s) of the sponsor's medical expert (or dentist when appropriate) for the trial.

6.1.5 Name and title of the investigator(s) who is (are) responsible for conducting the trial, and the address and telephone number(s) of the trial site(s).

6.1.6 Name, title, address, and telephone number(s) of the qualified physician (or dentist, if applicable), who is responsible for all trial-site related medical (or dental) decisions (if other than investigator). 6.1.7 Name(s) and address(es) of the clinical laboratory(ies) and other medical and/or technical department(s) and/or institutions involved in the trial.

### 6.2 Background Information

6.2.1 Name and description of the investigational product(s).

6.2.2 A summary of findings from nonclinical studies that potentially have clinical significance and from clinical trials that are relevant to the trial.

6.2.3 Summary of the known and potential risks and benefits, if any, to human subjects.

6.2.4 Description of and justification for the route of administration, dosage, dosage regimen, and treatment period(s).

6.2.5 A statement that the trial will be conducted in compliance with the protocol, GCP and the applicable regulatory requirement(s).

6.2.6 Description of the population to be studied.

6.2.7 References to literature and data that are relevant to the trial, and that provide background for the trial.

## 6.3 Trial Objectives and Purpose
A detailed description of the objectives and the purpose of the trial.

## 6.4 Trial Design
The scientific integrity of the trial and the credibility of the data from the trial depend substantially on the trial design. A description of the trial design, should include:

6.4.1 A specific statement of the primary endpoints and the secondary end-points, if any, to be measured during the trial.

6.4.2 A description of the type/design of trial to be conducted (e.g. double-blind, placebo-controlled, parallel design) and a schematic diagram of trial design, procedures and stages.

6.4.3 A description of the measures taken to minimize/avoid bias, including:
a.   Randomization.
b.   Blinding.

6.4.4 A description of the trial treatment(s) and the dosage and dosage regimen of the investigational product(s). Also include a description of the dosage form, packaging, and labeling of the investigational product(s).

6.4.5 The expected duration of subject participation, and a description of the sequence and duration of all trial periods, including follow-up, if any.

6.4.6 A description of the "stopping rules" or "discontinuation criteria" for individual subjects, parts of trial and entire trial.

6.4.7 Accountability procedures for the investigational product(s), including the placebo(s) and comparator(s), if any.

6.4.8 Maintenance of trial treatment randomization codes and procedures for breaking codes.

6.4.9 The identification of any data to be recorded directly on the CRFs (i.e. no prior written or electronic record of data), and to be considered to be source data.

## 6.5 Selection and Withdrawal of Subjects
6.5.1 Subject inclusion criteria.

6.5.2 Subject exclusion criteria.

6.5.3 Subject withdrawal criteria (i.e. terminating investigational product treatment/trial treatment) and procedures specifying:

a.  When and how to withdraw subjects from the trial/investigational product treatment.
b.  The type and timing of the data to be collected for withdrawn subjects.
c.  Whether and how subjects are to be replaced.
d.  The follow-up for subjects withdrawn from investigational product treatment/trial treatment.

## 6.6 Treatment of Subjects

6.6.1 The treatment(s) to be administered, including the name(s) of all the product(s), the dose(s), the dosing schedule(s), the route/mode(s) of administration, and the treatment period(s), including the follow-up period(s) for subjects for each investigational product treatment/trial treatment group/arm of the trial.

6.6.2 Medication(s)/treatment(s) permitted (including rescue medication) and not permitted before and/or during the trial.

6.6.3 Procedures for monitoring subject compliance.

## 6.7 Assessment of Efficacy

6.7.1 Specification of the efficacy parameters.

6.7.2 Methods and timing for assessing, recording, and analyzing of efficacy parameters.

## 6.8 Assessment of Safety

6.8.1 Specification of safety parameters.

6.8.2 The methods and timing for assessing, recording, and analyzing safety parameters.

6.8.3 Procedures for eliciting reports of and for recording and reporting adverse event and intercurrent illnesses.

6.8.4 The type and duration of the follow-up of subjects after adverse events.

## 6.9 Statistics

6.9.1 A description of the statistical methods to be employed, including timing of any planned interim analysis(ses).

6.9.2 The number of subjects planned to be enrolled. In multicentre trials, the numbers of enrolled subjects projected for each trial site should be specified. Reason for choice of sample size, including reflections on (or calculations of) the power of the trial and clinical justification.

6.9.3 The level of significance to be used.

6.9.4 Criteria for the termination of the trial.

6.9.5 Procedure for accounting for missing, unused, and spurious data.

6.9.6 Procedures for reporting any deviation(s) from the original statistical plan (any deviation(s) from the original statistical plan should be described and justified in protocol and/or in the final report, as appropriate).

6.9.7 The selection of subjects to be included in the analyses (e.g. all randomized subjects, all dosed subjects, all eligible subjects, evaluable subjects).

## 6.10 Direct Access to Source Data/Documents
The sponsor should ensure that it is specified in the protocol or other written agreement that the investigator(s)/institution(s) will permit trial-related monitoring, audits, IRB/IEC review, and regulatory inspection(s), providing direct access to source data/documents.

## 6.11 Quality Control and Quality Assurance

## 6.12 Ethics
Description of ethical considerations relating to the trial.

## 6.13 Data Hand ling and Record Keeping

## 6.14 Financing and Insurance
Financing and insurance if not addressed in a separate agreement.

## 6.15 Publication Policy
Publication policy, if not addressed in a separate agreement.

## 6.16 Supplements
(NOTE: Since the protocol and the clinical trial/study report are closely related, further relevant information can be found in the ICH Guideline for Structure and Content of Clinical Study Reports.).

# 7. Investigator's Brochure

## 7.1 Introduction
The Investigator's Brochure (IB) is a compilation of the clinical and nonclinical data on the investigational product(s) that are relevant to the study of the product(s) in human subjects. Its purpose is to provide the investigators and others involved in the trial with the information to facilitate their understanding of the rationale for, and their compliance with, many key features of the protocol, such as the dose, dose frequency/interval, methods of adminis-

tration: and safety monitoring procedures. The IB also provides insight to support the clinical management of the study subjects during the course of the clinical trial. The information should be presented in a concise, simple, objective, balanced, and non-promotional form that enables a clinician, or potential investigator, to understand it and make his/her own unbiased risk-benefit assessment of the appropriateness of the proposed trial. For this reason, a medically qualified person should generally participate in the editing of an IB, but the contents of the IB should be approved by the disciplines that generated the described data.

This guideline delineates the minimum information that should be included in an IB and provides suggestions for its layout. It is expected that the type and extent of information available will vary with the stage of development of the investigational product. If the investigational product is marketed and its pharmacology is widely understood by medical practitioners, an extensive IB may not be necessary. Where permitted by regulatory authorities, a basic product information brochure, package leaflet, or labeling may be an appropriate alternative, provided that it includes current, comprehensive, and detailed information on all aspects of the investigational product that might be of importance to the investigator. If a marketed product is being studied for a new use (i.e., a new indication), an IB specific to that new use should be prepared. The IB should be reviewed at least annually and revised as necessary in compliance with a sponsor's written procedures. More frequent revision may be appropriate depending on the stage of development and the generation of relevant new information. However, in accordance with Good Clinical Practice, relevant new information may be so important that it should be communicated to the investigators, and possibly to the Institutional Review Boards (IRBs)/Independent Ethics Committees (IECs) and/or regulatory authorities before it is included in a revised IB.

Generally, the sponsor is responsible for ensuring that an up-to-date IB is made available to the investigator(s) and the investigators are responsible for providing the up-to-date IB to the responsible IRBs/IECs. In the case of an investigator sponsored trial, the sponsor-investigator should determine whether a brochure is available from the commercial manufacturer. If the investigational product is provided by the sponsor-investigator, then he or she should provide the necessary information to the trial personnel. In cases where preparation of a formal IB is impractical, the sponsor-investigator should provide, as a substitute, an expanded background information section in the trial protocol that contains the minimum current information described in this guideline.

## 7.2 General Considerations
The IB should include:

7.2.1 *Title Page.* This should provide the sponsor's name, the identity of each investigational product (i.e., research number, chemical or approved generic name, and trade name(s) where legally permissible and desired by the sponsor), and the release date. It is also suggested that an edition number, and a reference to the number and date of the edition it supersedes, be provided. An example is given in Appendix 1.

7.2.2 *Confidentiality Statement.* The sponsor may wish to include a statement instructing the investigator/recipients to treat the IB as a confidential document for the sole information and use of the investigator's team and the IRB/IEC.

### 7.3 Contents of the Investigator's Brochure
The IB should contain the following sections, each with literature references where appropriate:

7.3.1 *Table of Contents.* An example of the Table of Contents is given in Appendix 2

7.3.2 *Summary.* A brief summary (preferably not exceeding two pages) should be given, highlighting the significant physical, chemical, pharmaceutical, pharmacological, toxicological, pharmacokinetic, metabolic, and clinical information available that is relevant to the stage of clinical development of the investigational product.

7.3.3 *Introduction.* A brief introductory statement should be provided that contains the chemical name (and generic and trade name(s) when approved) of the investigational product(s), all active ingredients, the investigational product (s ) pharmacological class and its expected position within this class (e.g. advantages), the rationale for performing research with the investigational product(s), and the anticipated prophylactic, therapeutic, or diagnostic indication(s). Finally, the introductory statement should provide the general approach to be followed in evaluating the investigational product.

7.3.4 *Physical, Chemical, and Pharmaceutical Properties and Formulation.* A description should be provided of the investigational product substance(s) (including the chemical and/or structural formula(e)), and a brief summary should be given of the relevant physical, chemical, and pharmaceutical properties. To permit appropriate safety measures to be taken in the course of the trial, a description of the formulation(s) to be used, including excipients, should be provided and justified if clinically relevant. Instructions for the storage and handling of the dosage form(s) should also be given. Any structural similarities to other known compounds should be mentioned.

7.3.5 *Nonclinical Studies.* Introduction: The results of all relevant nonclinical pharmacology, toxicology, pharmacokinetic, and investigational product metabolism studies should be provided in summary form. This summary should address the methodology used, the results, and a discussion of the relevance of the findings to the investigated therapeutic and the possible unfavorable and unintended effects in humans.

The information provided may include the following, as appropriate, if known/available:

- Species tested
- Number and sex of animals in each group
- Unit dose (e.g., milligram/kilogram (mg/kg))
- Dose interval
- Route of administration
- Duration of dosing
- Information on systemic distribution
- Duration of post-exposure follow-up
- Results, including the following aspects:
- Nature and frequency of pharmacological or toxic effects
- Severity or intensity of pharmacological or toxic effects
- Time to onset of effects
- Reversibility of effects
- Duration of effects
- Dose response

Tabular format/listings should be used whenever possible to enhance the clarity of the presentation. The following sections should discuss the most important findings from the studies, including the dose response of observed effects, the relevance to humans, and any aspects to be studied in humans. If applicable, the effective and nontoxic dose findings in the same animal species should be compared (i.e., the therapeutic index should be discussed). The relevance of this information to the proposed human dosing should be addressed. Whenever possible, comparisons should be made in terms of blood/tissue levels rather than on a mg/kg basis.

a. *Nonclinical Pharmacology.* A summary of the pharmacological aspects of the investigational product and, where appropriate, its significant metabolites studied in animals, should be included. Such a summary should incorporate studies that assess potential therapeutic activity (e.g. efficacy models, receptor binding, and specificity) as well as those that assess safety (e.g., special studies to assess pharmacological actions other than the intended therapeutic effect(s)).

b. *Pharmacokinetics and Product Metabolism in Animals.* A summary of the pharmacokinetics and biological transformation and disposition of the investigational product in all species studied should be given. The discussion of the findings should address the absorption and the local and systemic bioavailability of the investigational product and its metabolites, and their relationship to the pharmacological and toxicological findings in animal species.

c. *Toxicology.* A summary of the toxicological effects found in relevant studies conducted in different animal species should be described under the following headings where appropriate:

- Single dose
- Repeated dose
- Carcinogenicity
- Special studies (e.g. irritancy and sensitization)
- Reproductive toxicity
- Genotoxicity (mutagenicity)

7.3.6 *Effects in Humans.* Introduction: A thorough discussion of the known effects of the investigational product(s) in humans should be provided, including information on pharmacokinetics, metabolism, pharmacodynamics, dose response, safety, efficacy, and other pharmacological activities. Where possible, a summary of each completed clinical trial should be provided. Information should also be provided regarding results of any use of the investigational product(s) other than from in clinical trials, such as from experience during marketing.

a. *Pharmacokinetics and Product Metabolism in Humans.* A summary of information on the pharmacokinetics of the investigational product(s) should be presented, including the following, if available:
  - Pharmacokinetics (including metabolism, as appropriate, and absorption, plasma protein binding, distribution, and elimination).
  - Bioavailability of the investigational product (absolute, where possible, and/or relative) using a reference dosage form.
  - Population subgroups (e.g., gender, age, and impaired organ function).
  - Interactions (e.g., product-product interactions and effects of food).
  - Other pharmacokinetic data (e.g., results of population studies performed within clinical trial(s).

b. *Safety and Efficacy.* A summary of information should be provided about the investigational product's/products' (including metabolites, where appropriate) safety, pharmacodynamics, efficacy, and dose response that were obtained from preceding trials in humans (healthy volunteers and/or patients). The implications of this information should be discussed. In cases where a number of clinical trials have been completed, the use of summaries of safety and efficacy across multiple trials by indications in subgroups may provide a clear presentation of the data. Tabular summaries of adverse drug reactions for all the clinical trials (including those for all the studied indications) would be useful. Important differences in adverse drug reaction patterns/incidences across indications or subgroups should be discussed. The IB should provide a description of the possible risks and adverse drug reactions to be anticipated on the basis of prior experiences with the product under investigation and with related products. A description should also be provided of the precautions or special monitoring to be done as part of the investigational use of the product(s).

c. *Marketing Experience.* The IB should identify countries where the investigational product has been marketed or approved. Any significant information arising from the marketed use should be summarized (e.g., formulations, dosages, routes of administration, and adverse product reactions). The IB should also identify all the countries where the investigational product did not receive approval/registration for marketing or was withdrawn from marketing/registration.

*7.3.7 Summary of Data and Guidance for the Investigator.* This section should provide an overall discussion of the nonclinical and clinical data, and should summarize the information from various sources on different aspects of the investigational product(s), wherever possible. In this way, the investigator can be provided with the most informative interpretation of the available data and with an assessment of the implications of the information for future clinical trials. Where appropriate, the published reports on related products should be discussed. This could help the investigator to anticipate adverse drug reactions or other problems in clinical trials.

The overall aim of this section is to provide the investigator with a clear understanding of the possible risks and adverse reactions, and of the specific tests, observations, and precautions that may be needed for a clinical trial. This understanding should be based on the available physical, chemical, pharmaceutical, pharmacological, toxicological, and clinical information on the investigational product(s). Guidance should also be provided to the clinical investigator on the recognition and treatment of possible overdose and adverse drug reactions that is based on previous human experience and on the pharmacology of the investigational product.

## 7.4 APPENDIX 1:
Title Page (Example)

SPONSOR'S NAME
Product:
Research Number:
Name(s): Chemical, Generic (if approved)
Trade Name(s) (if legally permissible and desired by the sponsor)
INVESTIGATOR'S BROCHURE
Edition Number:
Release Date:
Replaces Previous Edition Number:
Date:

## 7.5 APPENDIX 2:
Table of Contents of Investigator's Brochure (Example)

Confidentiality Statement (optional)
Signature Page (optional)
1 Table of Contents
2 Summary
3 Introduction
4 Physical, Chemical, and Pharmaceutical Properties and Formulation
5 Nonclinical Studies
5.1 Nonclinical Pharmacology
5.2 Pharmacokinetics and Product Metabolism in Animals
5.3 Toxicology
6 Effects in Humans
6.1 Pharmacokinetics and Product Metabolism in Humans
6.2 Safety and Efficacy
6.3 Marketing Experience
7 Summary of Data and Guidance for the Investigator
NB: References on (These references should be found at the end of each chapter)
1 Publications
2 Reports
Appendices (if any).

## 8. Essential Documents for the Conduct of a Clinical Trial

### 8.1 Introduction

Essential Documents are those documents which individually and collectively permit evaluation of the conduct of a trial and the quality of the data produced. These documents serve to demonstrate the compliance of the investigator, sponsor and monitor with the standards of Good Clinical Practice and with all applicable regulatory requirements. Essential Documents also serve a number of other important purposes. Filing essential documents at the investigator/institution and sponsor sites in a timely manner can greatly assist in the successful management of a trial by the investigator, sponsor and monitor. These documents are also the ones which are usually audited by the sponsor's independent audit function and inspected by the regulatory authority (ies) as part of the process to confirm the validity of the trial conduct and the integrity of data collected. The minimum list of essential documents which has been developed follows. The various documents are grouped in three sections according to the stage of the trial during which they will normally be generated: 1) before the clinical phase of the trial commences, 2) during the clinical conduct of the trial, and 3) after completion or termination of the trial. A description is given of the purpose of each document, and whether it should be filed in either the investigator/institution or sponsor files, or both. It is acceptable to combine some of the documents, provided the individual elements are readily identifiable. Trial master files should be established at the beginning of the trial, both at the investigator/institution's site and at the sponsor's office. A final close-out of a trial can only be done when the monitor has reviewed both investigator/institution and sponsor files and confirmed that all necessary documents are in the appropriate files.

Any or all of the documents addressed in this guideline may be subject to, and should be available for, audit by the sponsor's auditor and inspection by the regulatory authority(ies).

## 8.2 Before the clinical phase of the trial commences

During this planning stage the following documents should be generated and should be on file before the trial formally starts

| Title of Document/Purpose | Located in the files of | |
|---|:---:|:---:|
| | **Invest/ Site** | **Sponsor** |
| 8.2.1 **Investigator's Brochure** To document that relevant and current scientific information about the investigational product has been provided to the investigator | X | X |
| 8.2.2 **Signed Protocol, Amendments, If Any, & Sample CRF** To document investigator and sponsor agreement to the protocol/amendment(s) and crf | X | X |
| 8.2.3 **Info. Given to Trial Subject** | X | X |
|   – *Informed Consent Form* Including all applicable translations) to document the informed consent. | X | X |
|   – *Any Other Written Information* To document that subjects will be given appropriate written information (content and wording) to support their ability to give fully informed consent. | X | X |
|   – *Advertisement For Subject Recruitment* (if used) to document that recruitment measures are appropriate and not coercive. | X | |
| 8.2.4 **Financial Aspects of the Trial** To document the financial agreement between the investigator/institution and the sponsor for the trial | X | X |

\* if applicable/required, \*\* third party if applicable, \*\*\* if destroyed at the site

| | Title of Document/Purpose | Located in the files of | |
|---|---|:---:|:---:|
| | | Invest/ Site | Sponsor |
| 8.2.5 | **Insurance Statement** (where required) to document that compensation to subject(s) for trial-related injury will be available | X | X |
| 8.2.6 | **Signed Agreement Between Involved Parties** To document agreements. E.g.: Investigator/ institution & sponsor – investigator/institution & cro – sponsor & cro –investigator/institution & authority(ies)* | X | X |
| 8.2.7 | **Dated, Documented Approval/Favorable Opinion of IRB/IEC of the Following:** – *Protocol and Any Amendments* – *CRF (If Applicable)* – *Informed Consent Form(s)* – *Any Other Written Information to be Provided to the Subject(s)* – *Advertisement For Subject Recruitment (If Used)* – *Subject Compensation (If Any)* – *Any Other Documents Given Approval/Favorable Opinion* To document that the trial has been subject to IRB/IEC review and given approval/favorable opinion. To identify the version number and date of the document(s) | X | X |
| 8.2.8 | **IRB/Independent Ethics Committee Composition** To document that the irb/iec is constituted in Agreement with GCP | X | X* |
| 8.2.9 | **Regulatory Authority(ies) Authorization/Approval/ Notification of Protocol** (Where Required) To document appropriate authorisation/approval/ notification by the regulatory authority(ies) has been obtained prior to initiation of the trial in compliance with the applicable regulatory requirement(s) | X* | X* |

* if applicable/required, ** third party if applicable, *** if destroyed at the site

|  | Title of Document/Purpose | Located in the files of | |
|---|---|---|---|
|  |  | Invest/ Site | Sponsor |
| 8.2.10 | **Curriculum Vitae and/or Other Relevant Documents Evidencing Qualifications of Investigator(s) and Sub-Investigator(s)** To document qualifications and eligibility to conduct trial and/or provide medical supervision of subjects | X | X |
| 8.2.11 | **Normal Value(s)/Range(s) For Medical/ Laboratory/Technical Procedure(s) and/or Test(s) Included in the Protocol** To document normal values and/or ranges of thetests | X | X |
| 8.2.12 | **Medical/Laboratory/Technical ProceduresTests** – *Certification or* – *Accreditation or* – *Established Quality Control and/or External Quality Assessment or* – *Other Validation\** To document competence of facility to perform required test(s) , and support reliability of results | X* | X |
| 8.2.13 | **Sample of Label(s) Attached to Investigational Product Container(s)** To document compliance with applicable labeling regulations and appropriateness of instructions provided to the subjects |  | X |
| 8.2.14 | **Instructions For Handling of Investigational Product(s) and Trial-Related Materials (If Not Included in Protocol or Investigator's Brochure)** To document instructions needed to ensure proper storage, packaging, dispensing and disposition of investigational products and trial- related materials | X | X |

* if applicable/required, ** third party if applicable, *** if destroyed at the site

| | Title of Document/Purpose | Located in the files of | |
|---|---|---|---|
| | | Invest/ Site | Sponsor |
| 8.2.15 | **Shipping Records For Investigational Product(s) and Trial-Related Materials** To document shipment dates, batch numbers and method of shipment of investigational product(s) and trial-related materials. Allows tracking of product batch, review of shipping conditions, and accountability | X | X |
| 8.2.16 | **Certificate(s) of Analysis of Investigational Product(s) Shipped** To document identity, purity, and strength of investigational product(s) to be used in the trial | | X |
| 8.2.17 | **Decoding Procedures For Blinded Trials** To document how, in case of an emergency, identity of blinded investigational product can be revealed without breaking the blind for the remaining subjects' treatment | X | X** |
| 8.2.18 | **Master Randomization List** To document method for randomization of trial subjects | | X** |
| 8.2.19 | **Pre-Trial Monitoring Report** To document that the site is suitable for the trial (may be combined with 8.2.20) | | X |
| 8.2.20 | **Trial Initiation Monitoring Report** To document that trial procedures were reviewed with the investigator and the investigator's trial staff ( may be combined with 8.2.19) | X | X |

## 8.3 during the clinical conduct of the trial

In addition to having on file the above documents, the following should be added to the files during the trial as evidence that all new relevant information is documented as it becomes available.

\* if applicable/required, \*\* third party if applicable, \*\*\* if destroyed at the site

| | Title of Document/Purpose | Located in the files of | |
|---|---|:---:|:---:|
| | | **Invest/ Site** | **Sponsor** |
| 8.3.1 | **Investigator's Brochure Updates** <br> To document that investigator is informed in a timely manner of relevant information as it becomes available | X | X |
| 8.3.2 | **Any Revision to:** <br> – *Protocol/Amendment(s) and CRF* <br> – *Informed Consent Form* <br> – *Any Other Written Information Provided to Subjects* <br> – *Advertisement For Subject Recruitment (If Used)* <br> To document revisions of these trial related documents that take effect during trial | X | X |
| 8.3.3 | **Dated, Documented Approval/Favorable Opinion of IRB/IEC of the Following:** <br> – *Protocol Amendment(s)* <br> – *Revision(s) of:* <br>   – *Informed Consent Form* <br>   – *Any Other Written Information to be Provided to the Subject* <br>   – *Advertisement For Subject Recruitment* <br> – *Any Other Documents Given Approval/Favorable Opinion* <br> – *Continuing Review of Trial\** <br> To document that the amendment(s) and/or revision(s) have been subject to irb/iec review and were given approval/favourable opinion. To identify the version number and date of the document(s). | X | X |
| 8.3.4 | **Regulatory Authority(ies) Authorizations/Approvals/ Notifications Where Required For:** <br> – *Protocol Amendment(s) and Other Documents* <br> To document compliance with applicable regulatory requirements. | X\* | X |

\* if applicable/required, \*\* third party if applicable, \*\*\* if destroyed at the site

| | | Located in the files of | |
|---|---|---|---|
| | Title of Document/Purpose | Invest/ Site | Sponsor |
| 8.3.5 | **CVs For New Investigator(s) and/or Sub-Investigator(s)** (see 8.2.10) | X | X |
| 8.3.6 | **Updates to Normal Value(s)/Range(s) For Medical/Laboratory/Technical Procedure(s)/ Test(s) Included in the Protocol** To document normal values and ranges that are revised during the trial (see 8.2.11). | X | X |
| 8.3.7 | **Updates of Medical/Laboratory/Technical Procedures/Tests** – *Certification or* – *Accreditation or* – *Established Quality Control and/or External Quality Assessment or* – *Other Validation (Where Required)* To document that tests remain adequate throughout the trial period (see 8.2.12). | X* | X |
| 8.3.8 | **Documentation of Investigational Product(s) and Trial-Related Materials Shipment** (see 8.2.15.) | X | X |
| 8.3.9 | **Certificate(s) of Analysis For New Batches of Investigational Products** (see 8.2.16) | | X |
| 8.3.10 | **Monitoring Visit Reports** To document site visits by, and findings of, the monitor | | X |

* if applicable/required, ** third party if applicable, *** if destroyed at the site

|  | Title of Document/Purpose | Located in the files of |  |
|---|---|---|---|
|  |  | Invest/ Site | Sponsor |
| 8.3.11 | **Relevant Communications Other Than Site Visits** | X | X |
|  | – *Letters* |  |  |
|  | – *Meeting Notes* |  |  |
|  | – *Notes of Telephone Calls* |  |  |
|  | To document any agreements or significant discussions regarding trial administration, protocol violations, trial conduct, adverse event(ae) reporting. |  |  |
| 8.3.12 | **Signed Informed Consent Forms** | X |  |
|  | To document that consent is obtained in accordance with gcp and protocol and dated prior to participation of each subject in trial. Also to document direct access permission (see 8.2.3). |  |  |
| 8.3.13 | **Source Documents** | X |  |
|  | To document the existence of the subject and substantiate integrity of trial data collected. To include original documents related to the trial, to medical treatment, and history of subject |  |  |
| 8.3.14 | **Signed, Dated and Completed Case Report Forms (CRF)** | X copy | X orig. |
|  | To document that the investigator or authorized member of the investigator's staff confirms the observations recorded |  |  |
| 8.3.15 | **Documentation of CRF Corrections** | X copy | X orig. |
|  | To document all changes/additions or corrections made to crf after initial data were recorded |  |  |
| 8.3.16 | **Notification By Originating Investigator to Sponsor of Serious Adverse Events and Related Reports** | X | X |
|  | Notification by originating investigator to sponsor of serious adverse events and related reports in accordance with 4.11 |  |  |

* if applicable/required, ** third party if applicable, *** if destroyed at the site

| | Title of Document/Purpose | Located in the files of | |
|---|---|---|---|
| | | Invest/ Site | Sponsor |
| 8.3.17 | **Notification By Sponsor and/or Investigator, If Needed, to Regulatory Authority(ies) and IRB(s)/IEC(s) of Unexpected Serious Adverse Drug Reactions and of Other Safety Information** Notification by sponsor and/or investigator, where applicable, to regulatory authorities and irb(s)/iec(s) of unexpected serious adverse drug reactions in accordance with 5.17 and 4.11.1 and of other safety information in accordance with 5.16.2 and 4.11.2. | X* | X |
| 8.3.18 | **Notification By Sponsor to Investigators of Safety Information** Notification by sponsor to investigators of safety information in accordance with 5.16.2. | X | X |
| 8.3.19 | **Interim or Annual Reports to IRB/IEC and Authority(ies)** Interim or annual reports provided to irb/iec in accordance with 4.10 and to authority(ies) in accordance with 5.17.3. | X | X* |
| 8.3.20 | **Subject Screening Log** To document identification of subjects who entered pre-trial screening. | X | X* |
| 8.3.21 | **Subject Identification Code List** To document that investigator/institution keeps a confidential list of names of all subjects allocated to trial numbers on enrolling in the trial. Allows investigator/institution to reveal identity of any subject. | X | |
| 8.3.22 | **Subject Enrolment Log** To document chronological enrolment of subjects by trial number. | X | |
| 8.3.23 | **Investigational Products Accountability atthe Site** To document that investigational product(s) have been used according to the protocol. | X | X |

* if applicable/required, ** third party if applicable, *** if destroyed at the site

| | Title of Document/Purpose | Located in the files of Invest/ Site | Sponsor |
|---|---|---|---|
| 8.3.24 | **Signature Sheet** To document signatures and initials of all persons authorised to make entries and/or corrections on CRFs. | X | X |
| 8.3.25 | **Record of Retained Body Fluids/Tissue Samples (If Any)** To document location and identification of retained samples if assays need to be repeated. | X | X |

## 8.4 After completion or termination of the trial

After completion or termination of the trial, all of the documents identified in sections 8.2 and 8.3 should be in the file together with the following

| | Title of Document/Purpose | Located in the files of Invest/ Site | Sponsor |
|---|---|---|---|
| 8.4.1 | **Investigational Product(s) Accountability at the Site** To document that the investigational product(s) have been used according to the protocol. To documents the final accounting of investigational product(s) received at the site, dispensed to subjects, returned by the subjects, and returned to sponsor. | X | X |
| 8.4.2 | **Documentation of Investigational Product Destruction** To document destruction of unused investigational products by sponsor or at site. | X*** | X |
| 8.4.3 | **Completed Subject Identification Code List** To permit identification of all subjects enrolled in the trial in case follow-up is required. List should be kept in a confidential manner and for agreed upon time. | X | |
| 8.4.4 | **Audit Certificate (if available)** to document that audit was performed. | | X |

* if applicable/required, ** third party if applicable, *** if destroyed at the site

| Title of Document/Purpose | Located in the files of | |
| --- | --- | --- |
| | Invest/ Site | Sponsor |
| **8.4.5 Final Trial Close-Out Monitoring Report** To document that all activities required for trial close-out are completed, and copies of essential documents are held in the appropriate files. | | X |
| **8.4.6 Treatment Allocation and Decoding Documentation** Returned to sponsor to document any decoding that may have occurred. | | X |
| **8.4.7 Final Report By Investigator to IRB/IEC Where Required, and Where Applicable, to the Regulatory Authority(ies)** To document completion of the trial. | X | |
| **8.4.8 Clinical Study Report** To document results and interpretation of trial. | X* | X |

* if applicable/required, ** third party if applicable, *** if destroyed at the site

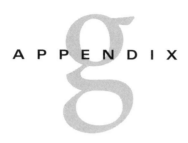

# A P P E N D I X g

# Code of Federal Regulations

## 21 CFR—Food and Drugs
### Chapter 1: Food and Drug Administration, Department of Health and Human Services

### Part 50—Protection of Human Subjects

50.51    Clinical investigations not involving greater than minimal risk.

50.52    Clinical investigations involving greater than minimal risk but presenting the prospect of direct benefit to individual subjects.

50.53    Clinical investigations involving greater than minimal risk and no prospect of direct benefit to individual subjects, but likely to yield generalizable knowledge about the subjects' disorder or condition.

50.54    Clinical investigations not otherwise approvable that present an opportunity to understand, prevent, or alleviate a serious problem affecting the health or welfare of children.

50.55    Requirements for permission by parents or guardians and for assent by children.

50.56    Wards.

Authority: 21 U.S.C 321, 343, 346, 346a, 348, 350a, 350b, 352, 353, 355, 360, 360c-360f, 360h-360j, 371, 379e, 381; 42 U.S.C. 216, 241, 262, 263b-263n.

Source: 45 FR 36390, May 30, 1980, unless otherwise noted.

## Subpart A—General Provisions

### §50.1 Scope.

(a) This part applies to all clinical investigations regulated by the Food and Drug Administration under sections 505(i) and 520(g) of the Federal Food, Drug, and Cosmetic Act, as well as clinical investigations that support applications for research or marketing permits for products regulated by the Food and Drug Administration, including foods, including dietary supplements, that bear a nutrient content claim or a health claim, infant formulas, food and color additives, drugs for human use, medical devices for human use, biological products for human use, and electronic products. Additional specific obligations and commitments of, and standards of conduct for, persons who sponsor or monitor clinical investigations involving particular test articles may also be found in other parts (e.g., parts 312 and 812). Compliance with these parts is intended to protect the rights and safety of subjects involved in investigations filed with the Food and Drug Administration pursuant to sections 403, 406, 409, 412, 413, 502, 503, 505, 510, 513-516, 518-520, 721, and 801 of the Federal Food, Drug, and Cosmetic Act and sections 351 and 354-360F of the Public Health Service Act.

(b) References in this part to regulatory sections of the Code of Federal Regulations are to chapter I of title 21, unless otherwise noted.
[45 FR 36390, May 30, 1980; 46 FR 8979, Jan. 27, 1981, as amended at 63 FR 26697, May 13, 1998; 64 FR 399, Jan. 5, 1999; 66 FR 20597, Apr. 24, 2001]

**§50.3 Definitions.**

As used in this part:

(a) *Act* means the Federal Food, Drug, and Cosmetic Act, as amended (secs. 201—902, 52 Stat. 1040 *et seq.* as amended (21 U.S.C. 321—392)).

(b) *Application for research or marketing permit* includes:

(1) A color additive petition, described in part 71.

(2) A food additive petition, described in parts 171 and 571.

(3) Data and information about a substance submitted as part of the procedures for establishing that the substance is generally recognized as safe for use that results or may reasonably be expected to result, directly or indirectly, in its becoming a component or otherwise affecting the characteristics of any food, described in §§170.30 and 570.30.

(4) Data and information about a food additive submitted as part of the procedures for food additives permitted to be used on an interim basis pending additional study, described in §180.1.

(5) Data and information about a substance submitted as part of the procedures for establishing a tolerance for unavoidable contaminants in food and food-packaging materials, described in section 406 of the act.

(6) An investigational new drug application, described in part 312 of this chapter.

(7) A new drug application, described in part 314.
(8) Data and information about the bioavailability or bioequivalence of drugs for human use submitted as part of the procedures for issuing, amending, or repealing a bioequivalence requirement, described in part 320.

(9) Data and information about an over-the-counter drug for human use submitted as part of the procedures for classifying these drugs as generally recognized as safe and effective and not misbranded, described in part 330.

(10) Data and information about a prescription drug for human use submitted as part of the procedures for classifying these drugs as generally recognized as safe and effective and not misbranded, described in this chapter.

(11) [Reserved]

(12) An application for a biologics license, described in part 601 of this chapter.

(13) Data and information about a biological product submitted as part of the procedures for determining that licensed biological products are safe and effective and not misbranded, described in part 601.

(14) Data and information about an in vitro diagnostic product submitted as part of the procedures for establishing, amending, or repealing a standard for these products, described in part 809.

(15) An *Application for an Investigational Device Exemption*, described in part 812.

(16) Data and information about a medical device submitted as part of the procedures for classifying these devices, described in section 513.

(17) Data and information about a medical device submitted as part of the procedures for establishing, amending, or repealing a standard for these devices, described in section 514.

(18) An application for premarket approval of a medical device, described in section 515.

(19) A product development protocol for a medical device, described in section 515.

(20) Data and information about an electronic product submitted as part of the procedures for establishing, amending, or repealing a standard for these products, described in section 358 of the Public Health Service Act.

(21) Data and information about an electronic product submitted as part of the procedures for obtaining a variance from any electronic product performance standard, as described in §1010.4.

(22) Data and information about an electronic product submitted as part of the procedures for granting, amending, or extending an exemption from a radiation safety performance standard, as described in §1010.5.

(23) Data and information about a clinical study of an infant formula when submitted as part of an infant formula notification under section 412(c) of the Federal Food, Drug, and Cosmetic Act.

(24) Data and information submitted in a petition for a nutrient content claim, described in §101.69 of this chapter, or for a health claim, described in §101.70 of this chapter.

(25) Data and information from investigations involving children submitted in a new dietary ingredient notification, described in §190.6 of this chapter.

(c) *Clinical investigation* means any experiment that involves a test article and one or more human subjects and that either is subject to requirements for prior submission to the Food and Drug Administration under section 505(i) or 520(g) of the act, or is not subject to requirements for prior submission to the Food and Drug Administration under these sections of the act, but the results of which are intended to be submitted later to, or held for inspection by, the Food and Drug Administration as part of an application for a research or marketing permit. The term does not include experiments that are subject to the provisions of part 58 of this chapter, regarding nonclinical laboratory studies.

(d) *Investigator* means an individual who actually conducts a clinical investigation, i.e., under whose immediate direction the test article is administered or dispensed to, or used involving, a subject, or, in the event of an investigation conducted by a team of individuals, is the responsible leader of that team.

(e) *Sponsor* means a person who initiates a clinical investigation, but who does not actually conduct the investigation, i.e., the test article is administered or dispensed to or used involving, a subject under the immediate direction of another individual. A person other than an individual (e.g., corporation or agency) that uses one or more of its own employees to conduct a clinical investigation it has initiated is considered to be a sponsor (not a sponsor-investigator), and the employees are considered to be investigators.

(f) *Sponsor-investigator* means an individual who both initiates and actually conducts, alone or with others, a clinical investigation, i.e., under whose immediate direction the test article is administered or dispensed to, or used involving, a subject. The term does not include any person other than an individual, e.g., corporation or agency.

(g) *Human subject* means an individual who is or becomes a participant in research, either as a recipient of the test article or as a control. A subject may be either a healthy human or a patient.

(h) *Institution* means any public or private entity or agency (including Federal, State, and other agencies). The word facility as used in section 520(g) of the act is deemed to be synonymous with the term *institution* for purposes of this part.

(i) *Institutional review board (IRB)* means any board, committee, or other group formally designated by an institution to review biomedical research involving humans as subjects, to approve the initiation of and conduct periodic review of such research. The term has the same meaning as the phrase *institutional review committee* as used in section 520(g) of the act.

(j) *Test article* means any drug (including a biological product for human use), medical device for human use, human food additive, color additive, electronic product, or any other article subject to regulation under the act or under sections 351 and 354-360F of the Public Health Service Act (42 U.S.C. 262 and 263b-263n).

(k) *Minimal risk* means that the probability and magnitude of harm or discomfort anticipated in the research are not greater in and of themselves than those ordinarily encountered in daily life or during the performance of routine physical or psychological examinations or tests.

(l) *Legally authorized representative* means an individual or judicial or other body authorized under applicable law to consent on behalf of a prospective subject to the subject's particpation in the procedure(s) involved in the research.

(m) *Family member* means any one of the following legally competent persons: Spouse; parents; children (including adopted children); brothers, sisters, and spouses of brothers and sisters; and any individual related by blood or affinity whose close association with the subject is the equivalent of a family relationship.

(n) *Assent* means a child's affirmative agreement to participate in a clinical investigation. Mere failure to object may not, absent affirmative agreement, be construed as assent.

(o) *Children* means persons who have not attained the legal age for consent to treatments or procedures involved in clinical investigations, under the applicable law of the jurisdiction in which the clinical investigation will be conducted.

(p) *Parent* means a child's biological or adoptive parent.

(q) *Ward* means a child who is placed in the legal custody of the State or other agency, institution, or entity, consistent with applicable Federal, State, or local law.

(r) *Permission* means the agreement of parent(s) or guardian to the participation of their child or ward in a clinical investigation. Permission must be obtained in compliance with subpart B of this part and must include the elements of informed consent described in §50.25.

(s) *Guardian* means an individual who is authorized under applicable State or local law to consent on behalf of a child to general medical care when general medical care includes participation in research. For purposes of subpart D of this part, a guardian also means an individual who is authorized to consent on behalf of a child to participate in research.

[45 FR 36390, May 30, 1980, as amended at 46 FR 8950, Jan. 27, 1981; 54 FR 9038, Mar. 3, 1989; 56 FR 28028, June 18, 1991; 61 FR 51528, Oct. 2, 1996; 62 FR 39440, July 23, 1997; 64 FR 399, Jan. 5, 1999; 64 FR 56448, Oct. 20, 1999; 66 FR 20597, Apr. 24, 2001]

## Subpart B—Informed Consent of Human Subjects

Source: 46 FR 8951, Jan. 27, 1981, unless otherwise noted.

**§50.20 General requirements for informed consent.**

Except as provided in §§50.23 and 50.24, no investigator may involve a human being as a subject in research covered by these regulations unless the investigator has obtained the legally effective informed consent of the subject or the subject's legally authorized representative. An investigator shall seek such consent only under circumstances that provide the prospective subject or the representative sufficient opportunity to consider whether or not to participate and that minimize the possibility of coercion or undue influence. The information that is given to the subject or the representative shall be in language understandable to the subject or the representative. No informed consent, whether oral or written, may include any exculpatory language through which the subject or the representative is made to waive or appear to waive any of the subject's legal rights, or releases or appears to release the investigator, the sponsor, the institution, or its agents from liability for negligence.

[46 FR 8951, Jan. 27, 1981, as amended at 64 FR 10942, Mar. 8, 1999]

**§50.23 Exception from general requirements.**

(a) The obtaining of informed consent shall be deemed feasible unless, before use of the test article (except as provided in paragraph (b) of this section), both the investigator and a physician who is not otherwise participating in the clinical investigation certify in writing all of the following:

(1) The human subject is confronted by a life-threatening situation necessitating the use of the test article.
(2) Informed consent cannot be obtained from the subject because of an inability to communicate with, or obtain legally effective consent from, the subject.

(3) Time is not sufficient to obtain consent from the subject's legal representative.

(4) There is available no alternative method of approved or generally recognized therapy that provides an equal or greater likelihood of saving the life of the subject.

(b) If immediate use of the test article is, in the investigator's opinion, required to preserve the life of the subject, and time is not sufficient to obtain the independent determination required in paragraph (a) of this section in advance of using the test article, the determinations of the clinical investigator shall be made and, within 5 working days after the use of the article, be reviewed and evaluated in writing by a physician who is not participating in the clinical investigation.

(c) The documentation required in paragraph (a) or (b) of this section shall be submitted to the IRB within 5 working days after the use of the test article.

(d)(1) Under 10 U.S.C. 1107(f) the President may waive the prior consent requirement for the administration of an investigational new drug to a member of the armed forces in connection with the member's participation in a particular military operation. The statute specifies that only the President may waive informed consent in this connection and the President may grant such a waiver only if the President determines in writing that obtaining consent: Is not feasible; is contrary to the best interests of the military member; or is not in the interests of national security. The statute further provides that in making a determination to waive prior informed consent on the ground that it is not feasible or the ground that it is contrary to the best interests of the military members involved, the President shall apply the standards and criteria that are set forth in the relevant FDA regulations for a waiver of the prior informed consent requirements of section 505(i)(4) of the Federal Food, Drug, and Cosmetic Act (21 U.S.C. 355(i)(4)). Before such a determination may be made that obtaining informed consent from military personnel prior to the use of an investigational drug (including an antibiotic or biological product) in a specific protocol under an investigational new drug application (IND) sponsored by the Department of Defense (DOD) and limited to specific military personnel involved in a particular military operation is not feasible or is contrary to the best interests of the military members involved the Secretary of Defense must first request such a determination from the President, and certify and document to the President that the following standards and criteria contained in paragraphs (d)(1) through (d)(4) of this section have been met.

(i) The extent and strength of evidence of the safety and effectiveness of the investigational new drug in relation to the medical risk that could be encountered during the military operation supports the drug's administration under an IND.

(ii) The military operation presents a substantial risk that military personnel may be subject to a chemical, biological, nuclear, or other exposure likely to produce death or serious or life-threatening injury or illness.

(iii) There is no available satisfactory alternative therapeutic or preventive treatment in relation to the intended use of the investigational new drug.

(iv) Conditioning use of the investigational new drug on the voluntary participation of each member could significantly risk the safety and health of any individual member who would decline its use, the safety of other military personnel, and the accomplishment of the military mission.

(v) A duly constituted institutional review board (IRB) established and operated in accordance with the requirements of paragraphs (d)(2) and (d)(3) of this section, responsible for review of the study, has reviewed and approved the investigational new drug protocol and the administration of the investigational new drug without informed consent. DOD's request is to include the documentation required by §56.115(a)(2) of this chapter.

(vi) DOD has explained:

(A) The context in which the investigational drug will be administered, e.g., the setting or whether it will be self-administered or it will be administered by a health professional;
(B) The nature of the disease or condition for which the preventive or therapeutic treatment is intended; and

(C) To the extent there are existing data or information available, information on conditions that could alter the effects of the investigational drug.

(vii) DOD's recordkeeping system is capable of tracking and will be used to track the proposed treatment from supplier to the individual recipient.

(viii) Each member involved in the military operation will be given, prior to the administration of the investigational new drug, a specific written information sheet (including information required by 10 U.S.C. 1107(d)) concerning the investigational new drug, the risks and benefits of its use, potential side effects, and other pertinent information about the appropriate use of the product.

(ix) Medical records of members involved in the military operation will accurately document the receipt by members of the notification required by paragraph (d)(1)(viii) of this section.

(x) Medical records of members involved in the military operation will accurately document the receipt by members of any investigational new drugs in accordance with FDA regulations including part 312 of this chapter.

(xi) DOD will provide adequate followup to assess whether there are beneficial or adverse health consequences that result from the use of the investigational product.

(xii) DOD is pursuing drug development, including a time line, and marketing approval with due diligence.

(xiii) FDA has concluded that the investigational new drug protocol may proceed subject to a decision by the President on the informed consent waiver request.

(xiv) DOD will provide training to the appropriate medical personnel and potential recipients on the specific investigational new drug to be administered prior to its use.

(xv) DOD has stated and justified the time period for which the waiver is needed, not to exceed one year, unless separately renewed under these standards and criteria.

(xvi) DOD shall have a continuing obligation to report to the FDA and to the President any changed circumstances relating to these standards and criteria (including the time period referred to in paragraph (d)(1)(xv) of this section) or that otherwise might affect the determination to use an investigational new drug without informed consent.

(xvii) DOD is to provide public notice as soon as practicable and consistent with classification requirements through notice in the FEDERAL REGISTER describing each waiver of informed consent determination, a summary of the most updated scientific information on the products used, and other pertinent information.

(xviii) Use of the investigational drug without informed consent otherwise conforms with applicable law.

(2) The duly constituted institutional review board, described in paragraph (d)(1)(v) of this section, must include at least 3 nonaffiliated members who shall not be employees or officers of the Federal Government (other than for purposes of membership on the IRB) and shall be required to obtain any necessary security clearances. This IRB shall review the proposed IND protocol at a convened meeting at which a majority of the members are present including at least one member whose primary concerns are in nonscientific areas and, if feasible, including a majority of the nonaffiliated members. The

information required by §56.115(a)(2) of this chapter is to be provided to the Secretary of Defense for further review.

(3) The duly constituted institutional review board, described in paragraph (d)(1)(v) of this section, must review and approve:

(i) The required information sheet;

(ii) The adequacy of the plan to disseminate information, including distribution of the information sheet to potential recipients, on the investigational product (e.g., in forms other than written);

(iii) The adequacy of the information and plans for its dissemination to health care providers, including potential side effects, contraindications, potential interactions, and other pertinent considerations; and

(iv) An informed consent form as required by part 50 of this chapter, in those circumstances in which DOD determines that informed consent may be obtained from some or all personnel involved.

(4) DOD is to submit to FDA summaries of institutional review board meetings at which the proposed protocol has been reviewed.

(5) Nothing in these criteria or standards is intended to preempt or limit FDA's and DOD's authority or obligations under applicable statutes and regulations.

[46 FR 8951, Jan. 27, 1981, as amended at 55 FR 52817, Dec. 21, 1990; 64 FR 399, Jan. 5, 1999; 64 FR 54188, Oct. 5, 1999]

## §50.24 Exception from informed consent requirements for emergency research.

(a) The IRB responsible for the review, approval, and continuing review of the clinical investigation described in this section may approve that investigation without requiring that informed consent of all research subjects be obtained if the IRB (with the concurrence of a licensed physician who is a member of or consultant to the IRB and who is not otherwise participating in the clinical investigation) finds and documents each of the following:
(1) The human subjects are in a life-threatening situation, available treatments are unproven or unsatisfactory, and the collection of valid scientific evidence, which may include evidence obtained through randomized placebo-controlled investigations, is necessary to determine the safety and effectiveness of particular interventions.

(2) Obtaining informed consent is not feasible because:

(i) The subjects will not be able to give their informed consent as a result of their medical condition;

(ii) The intervention under investigation must be administered before consent from the subjects' legally authorized representatives is feasible; and

(iii) There is no reasonable way to identify prospectively the individuals likely to become eligible for participation in the clinical investigation.

(3) Participation in the research holds out the prospect of direct benefit to the subjects because:

(i) Subjects are facing a life-threatening situation that necessitates intervention;

(ii) Appropriate animal and other preclinical studies have been conducted, and the information derived from those studies and related evidence support the potential for the intervention to provide a direct benefit to the individual subjects; and

(iii) Risks associated with the investigation are reasonable in relation to what is known about the medical condition of the potential class of subjects, the risks and benefits of standard therapy, if any, and what is known about the risks and benefits of the proposed intervention or activity.

(4) The clinical investigation could not practicably be carried out without the waiver.

(5) The proposed investigational plan defines the length of the potential therapeutic window based on scientific evidence, and the investigator has committed to attempting to contact a legally authorized representative for each subject within that window of time and, if feasible, to asking the legally authorized representative contacted for consent within that window rather than proceeding without consent. The investigator will summarize efforts made to contact legally authorized representatives and make this information available to the IRB at the time of continuing review.

(6) The IRB has reviewed and approved informed consent procedures and an informed consent document consistent with §50.25. These procedures and the informed consent document are to be used with subjects or their legally authorized representatives in situations where use of such procedures and documents is feasible. The IRB has reviewed and approved procedures and information to be used when providing an opportunity for a family member to object to a subject's participation in the clinical investigation consistent with paragraph (a)(7)(v) of this section.

(7) Additional protections of the rights and welfare of the subjects will be provided, including, at least:

(i) Consultation (including, where appropriate, consultation carried out by the IRB) with representatives of the communities in which the clinical investigation will be conducted and from which the subjects will be drawn;

(ii) Public disclosure to the communities in which the clinical investigation will be conducted and from which the subjects will be drawn, prior to initiation of the clinical investigation, of plans for the investigation and its risks and expected benefits;

(iii) Public disclosure of sufficient information following completion of the clinical investigation to apprise the community and researchers of the study, including the demographic characteristics of the research population, and its results;

(iv) Establishment of an independent data monitoring committee to exercise oversight of the clinical investigation; and

(v) If obtaining informed consent is not feasible and a legally authorized representative is not reasonably available, the investigator has committed, if feasible, to attempting to contact within the therapeutic window the subject's family member who is not a legally authorized representative, and asking whether he or she objects to the subject's participation in the clinical investigation. The investigator will summarize efforts made to contact family members and make this information available to the IRB at the time of continuing review.

(b) The IRB is responsible for ensuring that procedures are in place to inform, at the earliest feasible opportunity, each subject, or if the subject remains incapacitated, a legally authorized representative of the subject, or if such a representative is not reasonably available, a family member, of the subject's inclusion in the clinical investigation, the details of the investigation and other information contained in the informed consent document. The IRB shall also ensure that there is a procedure to inform the subject, or if the subject remains incapacitated, a legally authorized representative of the subject, or if such a representative is not reasonably available, a family member, that he or she may discontinue the subject's participation at any time without penalty or loss of benefits to which the subject is otherwise entitled. If a legally authorized representative or family member is told about the clinical investigation and the subject's condition improves, the subject is also to be informed as soon as feasible. If a subject is entered into a clinical investigation with waived consent and the subject dies before a legally authorized representative or family member can be contacted, information about the clinical investigation is to be provided to the subject's legally authorized representative or family member, if feasible.

(c) The IRB determinations required by paragraph (a) of this section and the documentation required by paragraph (e) of this section are to be retained by the IRB for at least 3 years after completion of the clinical investigation, and the records shall be accessible for inspection and copying by FDA in accordance with §56.115(b) of this chapter.

(d) Protocols involving an exception to the informed consent requirement under this section must be performed under a separate investigational new drug application (IND) or investigational device exemption (IDE) that clearly identifies such protocols as protocols that may include subjects who are unable to consent. The submission of those protocols in a separate IND/IDE is required even if an IND for the same drug product or an IDE for the same device already exists. Applications for investigations under this section may not be submitted as amendments under §§312.30 or 812.35 of this chapter.

(e) If an IRB determines that it cannot approve a clinical investigation because the investigation does not meet the criteria in the exception provided under paragraph (a) of this section or because of other relevant ethical concerns, the IRB must document its findings and provide these findings promptly in writing to the clinical investigator and to the sponsor of the clinical investigation. The sponsor of the clinical investigation must promptly disclose this information to FDA and to the sponsor's clinical investigators who are participating or are asked to participate in this or a substantially equivalent clinical investigation of the sponsor, and to other IRB's that have been, or are, asked to review this or a substantially equivalent investigation by that sponsor.

[61 FR 51528, Oct. 2, 1996]

**§50.25 Elements of informed consent.**

(a) *Basic elements of informed consent.* In seeking informed consent, the following information shall be provided to each subject:

(1) A statement that the study involves research, an explanation of the purposes of the research and the expected duration of the subject's participation, a description of the procedures to be followed, and identification of any procedures which are experimental.

(2) A description of any reasonably foreseeable risks or discomforts to the subject.

(3) A description of any benefits to the subject or to others which may reasonably be expected from the research.

(4) A disclosure of appropriate alternative procedures or courses of treatment, if any, that might be advantageous to the subject.

(5) A statement describing the extent, if any, to which confidentiality of records identifying the subject will be maintained and that notes the possibility that the Food and Drug Administration may inspect the records.

(6) For research involving more than minimal risk, an explanation as to whether any compensation and an explanation as to whether any medical treatments are available if injury occurs and, if so, what they consist of, or where further information may be obtained.

(7) An explanation of whom to contact for answers to pertinent questions about the research and research subjects' rights, and whom to contact in the event of a research-related injury to the subject.

(8) A statement that participation is voluntary, that refusal to participate will involve no penalty or loss of benefits to which the subject is otherwise entitled, and that the subject may discontinue participation at any time without penalty or loss of benefits to which the subject is otherwise entitled.

(b) *Additional elements of informed consent.* When appropriate, one or more of the following elements of information shall also be provided to each subject:
(1) A statement that the particular treatment or procedure may involve risks to the subject (or to the embryo or fetus, if the subject is or may become pregnant) which are currently unforeseeable.

(2) Anticipated circumstances under which the subject's participation may be terminated by the investigator without regard to the subject's consent.

(3) Any additional costs to the subject that may result from participation in the research.

(4) The consequences of a subject's decision to withdraw from the research and procedures for orderly termination of participation by the subject.

(5) A statement that significant new findings developed during the course of the research which may relate to the subject's willingness to continue participation will be provided to the subject.

(6) The approximate number of subjects involved in the study.

(c) The informed consent requirements in these regulations are not intended to preempt any applicable Federal, State, or local laws which require additional information to be disclosed for informed consent to be legally effective.

(d) Nothing in these regulations is intended to limit the authority of a physician to provide emergency medical care to the extent the physician is permitted to do so under applicable Federal, State, or local law.

## §50.27 Documentation of informed consent.

(a) Except as provided in §56.109(c), informed consent shall be documented by the use of a written consent form approved by the IRB and signed and dated by the subject or the subject's legally authorized representative at the time of consent. A copy shall be given to the person signing the form.

(b) Except as provided in §56.109(c), the consent form may be either of the following:

(1) A written consent document that embodies the elements of informed consent required by §50.25. This form may be read to the subject or the subject's legally authorized representative, but, in any event, the investigator shall give either the subject or the representative adequate opportunity to read it before it is signed.

(2) A *short form* written consent document stating that the elements of informed consent required by §50.25 have been presented orally to the subject or the subject's legally authorized representative. When this method is used, there shall be a witness to the oral presentation. Also, the IRB shall approve a written summary of what is to be said to the subject or the representative. Only the short form itself is to be signed by the subject or the representative. However, the witness shall sign both the short form and a copy of the summary, and the person actually obtaining the consent shall sign a copy of the summary. A copy of the summary shall be given to the subject or the representative in addition to a copy of the short form.

[46 FR 8951, Jan. 27, 1981, as amended at 61 FR 57280, Nov. 5, 1996]

## Subpart C [Reserved]

## Subpart D—Additional Safeguards for Children in Clinical Investigations
Source: 66 FR 20598, Apr. 24, 2001, unless otherwise noted.

§50.50 IRB duties.

In addition to other responsibilities assigned to IRBs under this part and part 56 of this chapter, each IRB must review clinical investigations involving children as subjects covered by this subpart D and approve only those clinical investigations that satisfy the criteria described in §50.51, §50.52, or §50.53 and the conditions of all other applicable sections of this subpart D.

**§50.51 Clinical investigations not involving greater than minimal risk.**

Any clinical investigation within the scope described in §§50.1 and 56.101 of this chapter in which no greater than minimal risk to children is presented may involve children as subjects only if the IRB finds and documents that adequate provisions are made for soliciting the assent of the children and the permission of their parents or guardians as set forth in §50.55.

**§50.52 Clinical investigations involving greater than minimal risk but presenting the prospect of direct benefit to individual subjects.**

Any clinical investigation within the scope described in §§50.1 and 56.101 of this chapter in which more than minimal risk to children is presented by an intervention or procedure that holds out the prospect of direct benefit for the individual subject, or by a monitoring procedure that is likely to contribute to the subject's well-being, may involve children as subjects only if the IRB finds and documents that:

(a) The risk is justified by the anticipated benefit to the subjects;
(b) The relation of the anticipated benefit to the risk is at least as favorable to the subjects as that presented by available alternative approaches; and

(c) Adequate provisions are made for soliciting the assent of the children and permission of their parents or guardians as set forth in §50.55.

**§50.53 Clinical investigations involving greater than minimal risk and no prospect of direct benefit to individual subjects, but likely to yield generalizable knowledge about the subjects' disorder or condition.**

Any clinical investigation within the scope described in §§50.1 and56.101 of this chapter in which more than minimal risk to children is presented by an intervention or procedure that does not hold out the prospect of direct benefit for the individual subject, or by a monitoring procedure that is not likely to contribute to the well-being of the subject, may involve children as subjects only if the IRB finds and documents that:

(a) The risk represents a minor increase over minimal risk;

(b) The intervention or procedure presents experiences to subjects that are reasonably commensurate with those inherent in their actual or expected medical, dental, psychological, social, or educational situations;

(c) The intervention or procedure is likely to yield generalizable knowledge about the subjects' disorder or condition that is of vital importance for the understanding or amelioration of the subjects' disorder or condition; and

(d) Adequate provisions are made for soliciting the assent of the children and permission of their parents or guardians as set forth in §50.55.

**§50.54 Clinical investigations not otherwise approvable that present an opportunity to understand, prevent, or alleviate a serious problem affecting the health or welfare of children.**

If an IRB does not believe that a clinical investigation within the scope described in §§50.1 and 56.101 of this chapter and involving children as subjects meets the requirements of §50.51, §50.52, or §50.53, the clinical investigation may proceed only if:

(a) The IRB finds and documents that the clinical investigation presents a reasonable opportunity to further the understanding, prevention, or alleviation of a serious problem affecting the health or welfare of children; and

(b) The Commissioner of Food and Drugs, after consultation with a panel of experts in pertinent disciplines (for example: science, medicine, education, ethics, law) and following opportunity for public review and comment, determines either:

(1) That the clinical investigation in fact satisfies the conditions of §50.51, §50.52, or §50.53, as applicable, or

(2) That the following conditions are met:

(i) The clinical investigation presents a reasonable opportunity to further the understanding, prevention, or alleviation of a serious problem affecting the health or welfare of children;

(ii) The clinical investigation will be conducted in accordance with sound ethical principles; and

(iii) Adequate provisions are made for soliciting the assent of children and the permission of their parents or guardians as set forth in §50.55.

**§50.55 Requirements for permission by parents or guardians and for assent by children.**

(a) In addition to the determinations required under other applicable sections of this subpart D, the IRB must determine that adequate provisions are made for soliciting the assent of the children when in the judgment of the IRB the children are capable of providing assent.

(b) In determining whether children are capable of providing assent, the IRB must take into account the ages, maturity, and psychological state of the children involved. This judgment may be made for all children to be involved in clinical investigations under a particular protocol, or for each child, as the IRB deems appropriate.

(c) The assent of the children is not a necessary condition for proceeding with the clinical investigation if the IRB determines:

(1) That the capability of some or all of the children is so limited that they cannot reasonably be consulted, or

(2) That the intervention or procedure involved in the clinical investigation holds out a prospect of direct benefit that is important to the health or well-being of the children and is available only in the context of the clinical investigation.

(d) Even where the IRB determines that the subjects are capable of assenting, the IRB may still waive the assent requirement if it finds and documents that:

(1) The clinical investigation involves no more than minimal risk to the subjects;

(2) The waiver will not adversely affect the rights and welfare of the subjects;

(3) The clinical investigation could not practicably be carried out without the waiver; and

(4) Whenever appropriate, the subjects will be provided with additional pertinent information after participation.

(e) In addition to the determinations required under other applicable sections of this subpart D, the IRB must determine that the permission of each child's parents or guardian is granted.

(1) Where parental permission is to be obtained, the IRB may find that the permission of one parent is sufficient, if consistent with State law, for clinical investigations to be conducted under §50.51 or §50.52.

(2) Where clinical investigations are covered by §50.53 or §50.54 and permission is to be obtained from parents, both parents must give their permission

unless one parent is deceased, unknown, incompetent, or not reasonably available, or when only one parent has legal responsibility for the care and custody of the child if consistent with State law.

(f) Permission by parents or guardians must be documented in accordance with and to the extent required by §50.27.

(g) When the IRB determines that assent is required, it must also determine whether and how assent must be documented.

## §50.56 Wards.

(a) Children who are wards of the State or any other agency, institution, or entity can be included in clinical investigations approved under §50.53 or §50.54 only if such clinical investigations are:

(1) Related to their status as wards; or

(2) Conducted in schools, camps, hospitals, institutions, or similar settings in which the majority of children involved as subjects are not wards.

(b) If the clinical investigation is approved under paragraph (a) of this section, the IRB must require appointment of an advocate for each child who is a ward.

(1) The advocate will serve in addition to any other individual acting on behalf of the child as guardian or in loco parentis.

(2) One individual may serve as advocate for more than one child.

(3) The advocate must be an individual who has the background and experience to act in, and agrees to act in, the best interest of the child for the duration of the child's participation in the clinical investigation.

(4) The advocate must not be associated in any way (except in the role as advocate or member of the IRB) with the clinical investigation, the investigator(s), or the guardian organization.

# PART 54—FINANCIAL DISCLOSURE BY CLINICAL INVESTIGATORS

Authority: 21 U.S.C. 321, 331, 351, 352, 353, 355, 360, 360c-360j, 371, 372, 373, 374, 375, 376, 379; 42 U.S.C. 262.

Source: 63 FR 5250, Feb. 2, 1998, unless otherwise noted.

## §54.1 Purpose.

(a) The Food and Drug Administration (FDA) evaluates clinical studies submitted in marketing applications, required by law, for new human drugs and biological products and marketing applications and reclassification petitions for medical devices.

(b) The agency reviews data generated in these clinical studies to determine whether the applications are approvable under the statutory requirements. FDA may consider clinical studies inadequate and the data inadequate if, among other things, appropriate steps have not been taken in the design, conduct, reporting, and analysis of the studies to minimize bias. One potential source of bias in clinical studies is a financial interest of the clinical investigator in the outcome of the study because of the way payment is arranged (e.g., a royalty) or because the investigator has a proprietary interest in the product (e.g., a patent) or because the investigator has an equity interest in the sponsor of the covered study. This section and conforming regulations require an applicant whose submission relies in part on clinical data to disclose certain financial arrangements between sponsor(s) of the covered studies and the clinical investigators and certain interests of the clinical investigators in the product under study or in the sponsor of the covered studies. FDA will use this information, in conjunction with information about the design and purpose of the study, as well as information obtained through on-site inspections, in the agency's assessment of the reliability of the data.

## §54.2 Definitions.

For the purposes of this part:

(a) *Compensation affected by the outcome of clinical studies* means compensation that could be higher for a favorable outcome than for an unfavorable outcome, such as compensation that is explicitly greater for a favorable result or compensation to the investigator in the form of an equity interest in the sponsor of a covered study or in the form of compensation tied to sales of the product, such as a royalty interest.

(b) *Significant equity interest in the sponsor of a covered study* means any ownership interest, stock options, or other financial interest whose value cannot be readily determined through reference to public prices (generally, interests in a nonpublicly traded corporation), or any equity interest in a publicly traded corporation that exceeds $50,000 during the time the clinical investigator is carrying out the study and for 1 year following completion of the study.

(c) *Proprietary interest in the tested product* means property or other financial interest in the product including, but not limited to, a patent, trademark, copyright or licensing agreement.

(d) *Clinical investigator* means only a listed or identified investigator or subinvestigator who is directly involved in the treatment or evaluation of research subjects. The term also includes the spouse and each dependent child of the investigator.

(e) *Covered clinical study* means any study of a drug or device in humans submitted in a marketing application or reclassification petition subject to this part that the applicant or FDA relies on to establish that the product is effective (including studies that show equivalence to an effective product) or any study in which a single investigator makes a significant contribution to the demonstration of safety. This would, in general, not include phase l tolerance studies or pharmacokinetic studies, most clinical pharmacology studies (unless they are critical to an efficacy determination), large open safety studies conducted at multiple sites, treatment protocols, and parallel track protocols. An applicant may consult with FDA as to which clinical studies constitute "covered clinical studies" for purposes of complying with financial disclosure requirements.

(f) *Significant payments of other sorts* means payments made by the sponsor of a covered study to the investigator or the institution to support activities of the investigator that have a monetary value of more than $25,000, exclusive of the costs of conducting the clinical study or other clinical studies, (e.g., a grant to fund ongoing research, compensation in the form of equipment or retainers for ongoing consultation or honoraria) during the time the clinical investigator is carrying out the study and for 1 year following the completion of the study.

(g) *Applicant* means the party who submits a marketing application to FDA for approval of a drug, device, or biologic product. The applicant is responsible for submitting the appropriate certification and disclosure statements required in this part.

(h) *Sponsor of the covered clinical study* means the party supporting a particular study at the time it was carried out.

[63 FR 5250, Feb. 2, 1998, as amended at 63 FR 72181, Dec. 31, 1998]

## §54.3 Scope.

The requirements in this part apply to any applicant who submits a marketing application for a human drug, biological product, or device and who submits covered clinical studies. The applicant is responsible for making the appropriate certification or disclosure statement where the applicant either contracted with one or more clinical investigators to conduct the studies or submitted studies conducted by others not under contract to the applicant.

## §54.4 Certification and disclosure requirements.

For purposes of this part, an applicant must submit a list of all clinical investigators who conducted covered clinical studies to determine whether the applicant's product meets FDA's marketing requirements, identifying those clinical investigators who are full-time or part-time employees of the sponsor of each covered study. The applicant must also completely and accurately disclose or certify information concerning the financial interests of a clinical investigator who is not a full-time or part-time employee of the sponsor for each covered clinical study. Clinical investigators subject to investigational new drug or investigational device exemption regulations must provide the sponsor of the study with sufficient accurate information needed to allow subsequent disclosure or certification. The applicant is required to submit for each clinical investigator who participates in a covered study, either a certification that none of the financial arrangements described in §54.2 exist, or disclose the nature of those arrangements to the agency. Where the applicant acts with due diligence to obtain the information required in this section but is unable to do so, the applicant shall certify that despite the applicant's due diligence in attempting to obtain the information, the applicant was unable to obtain the information and shall include the reason.

(a) The applicant (of an application submitted under sections 505, 506, 510(k), 513, or 515 of the Federal Food, Drug, and Cosmetic Act, or section 351 of the Public Health Service Act) that relies in whole or in part on clinical studies shall submit, for each clinical investigator who participated in a covered clinical study, either a certification described in paragraph (a)(1) of this section or a disclosure statement described in paragraph (a)(3) of this section.

(1) Certification: The applicant covered by this section shall submit for all clinical investigators (as defined in §54.2(d)), to whom the certification applies, a completed Form FDA 3454 attesting to the absence of financial interests and arrangements described in paragraph (a)(3) of this section. The form shall be dated and signed by the chief financial officer or other responsible corporate official or representative.

(2) If the certification covers less than all covered clinical data in the application, the applicant shall include in the certification a list of the studies covered by this certification.

(3) Disclosure Statement: For any clinical investigator defined in §54.2(d) for whom the applicant does not submit the certification described in paragraph (a)(1) of this section, the applicant shall submit a completed Form FDA 3455 disclosing completely and accurately the following:

(i) Any financial arrangement entered into between the sponsor of the covered study and the clinical investigator involved in the conduct of a covered clinical trial, whereby the value of the compensation to the clinical investigator for conducting the study could be influenced by the outcome of the study;

(ii) Any significant payments of other sorts from the sponsor of the covered study, such as a grant to fund ongoing research, compensation in the form of equipment, retainer for ongoing consultation, or honoraria;

(iii) Any proprietary interest in the tested product held by any clinical investigator involved in a study;

(iv) Any significant equity interest in the sponsor of the covered study held by any clinical investigator involved in any clinical study; and

(v) Any steps taken to minimize the potential for bias resulting from any of the disclosed arrangements, interests, or payments.

(b) The clinical investigator shall provide to the sponsor of the covered study sufficient accurate financial information to allow the sponsor to submit complete and accurate certification or disclosure statements as required in paragraph (a) of this section. The investigator shall promptly update this information if any relevant changes occur in the course of the investigation or for 1 year following completion of the study.

(c) *Refusal to file application.* FDA may refuse to file any marketing application described in paragraph (a) of this section that does not contain the information required by this section or a certification by the applicant that the applicant has acted with due diligence to obtain the information but was unable to do so and stating the reason.

[63 FR 5250, Feb. 2, 1998; 63 FR 35134, June 29, 1998, as amended at 64 FR 399, Jan. 5, 1999]

## §54.5 Agency evaluation of financial interests.

(a) *Evaluation of disclosure statement.* FDA will evaluate the information disclosed under §54.4(a)(2) about each covered clinical study in an application to determine the impact of any disclosed financial interests on the reliability of the study. FDA may consider both the size and nature of a disclosed financial interest (including the potential increase in the value of the interest if the product is approved) and steps that have been taken to minimize the potential for bias.

(b) *Effect of study design.* In assessing the potential of an investigator's financial interests to bias a study, FDA will take into account the design and purpose of the study. Study designs that utilize such approaches as multiple investigators (most of whom do not have a disclosable interest), blinding, objective endpoints, or measurement of endpoints by someone other than the investigator may adequately protect against any bias created by a disclosable financial interest.

(c) *Agency actions to ensure reliability of data.* If FDA determines that the financial interests of any clinical investigator raise a serious question about the integrity of the data, FDA will take any action it deems necessary to ensure the reliability of the data including:

(1) Initiating agency audits of the data derived from the clinical investigator in question;

(2) Requesting that the applicant submit further analyses of data, e.g., to evaluate the effect of the clinical investigator's data on overall study outcome;

(3) Requesting that the applicant conduct additional independent studies to confirm the results of the questioned study; and

(4) Refusing to treat the covered clinical study as providing data that can be the basis for an agency action.

## §54.6 Recordkeeping and record retention.

(a) *Financial records of clinical investigators to be retained.* An applicant who has submitted a marketing application containing covered clinical studies shall keep on file certain information pertaining to the financial interests of clinical investigators who conducted studies on which the application relies and who are not full or part-time employees of the applicant, as follows:

(1) Complete records showing any financial interest or arrangement as described in §54.4(a)(3)(i) paid to such clinical investigators by the sponsor of the covered study.

(2) Complete records showing significant payments of other sorts, as described in §54.4(a)(3)(ii), made by the sponsor of the covered clinical study to the clinical investigator.

(3) Complete records showing any financial interests held by clinical investigators as set forth in §54.4(a)(3)(iii) and (a)(3)(iv).

(b) *Requirements for maintenance of clinical investigators' financial records.*

(1) For any application submitted for a covered product, an applicant shall retain records as described in paragraph (a) of this section for 2 years after the date of approval of the application.

(2) The person maintaining these records shall, upon request from any properly authorized officer or employee of FDA, at reasonable times, permit such officer or employee to have access to and copy and verify these records.

# Part 56—Institutional Review Boards

## Subpart A—General Provisions

## Subpart B—Organization and Personnel

## Subpart C—IRB Functions and Operations

## Subpart D—Records and Reports

## Subpart E—Administrative Actions for Noncompliance

Authority: 21 U.S.C. 321, 343, 346, 346a, 348, 350a, 350b, 351, 352, 353, 355, 360, 360c-360f, 360h-360j, 371, 379e, 381; 42 U.S.C. 216, 241, 262, 263b-263n.

Source: 46 FR 8975, Jan. 27, 1981, unless otherwise noted.

## Subpart A—General Provisions

### §56.101 Scope.

(a) This part contains the general standards for the composition, operation, and responsibility of an Institutional Review Board (IRB) that reviews clinical investigations regulated by the Food and Drug Administration under sections 505(i) and 520(g) of the act, as well as clinical investigations that support applications for research or marketing permits for products regulated by the Food and Drug Administration, including foods, including dietary supplements, that bear a nutrient content claim or a health claim, infant formulas, food and color additives, drugs for human use, medical devices for human use, biological products for human use, and electronic products. Compliance with this part is intended to protect the rights and welfare of human subjects involved in such investigations.

(b) References in this part to regulatory sections of the Code of Federal Regulations are to chapter I of title 21, unless otherwise noted.

[46 FR 8975, Jan. 27, 1981, as amended at 64 FR 399, Jan. 5, 1999; 66 FR 20599, Apr. 24, 2001]

**§56.102 Definitions.**

As used in this part:

(a) *Act* means the Federal Food, Drug, and Cosmetic Act, as amended (secs. 201-902, 52 Stat. 1040 *et seq.*, as amended (21 U.S.C. 321-392)).

(b) *Application for research or marketing permit* includes:

(1) A color additive petition, described in part 71.

(2) Data and information regarding a substance submitted as part of the procedures for establishing that a substance is generally recognized as safe for a use which results or may reasonably be expected to result, directly or indirectly, in its becoming a component or otherwise affecting the characteristics of any food, described in §170.35.
(3) A food additive petition, described in part 171.

(4) Data and information regarding a food additive submitted as part of the procedures regarding food additives permitted to be used on an interim basis pending additional study, described in §180.1.

(5) Data and information regarding a substance submitted as part of the procedures for establishing a tolerance for unavoidable contaminants in food and food-packaging materials, described in section 406 of the act.

(6) An investigational new drug application, described in part 312 of this chapter.

(7) A new drug application, described in part 314.

(8) Data and information regarding the bioavailability or bioequivalence of drugs for human use submitted as part of the procedures for issuing, amending, or repealing a bioequivalence requirement, described in part 320.

(9) Data and information regarding an over-the-counter drug for human use submitted as part of the procedures for classifying such drugs as generally recognized as safe and effective and not misbranded, described in part 330.

(10) An application for a biologics license, described in part 601 of this chapter.

(11) Data and information regarding a biological product submitted as part of the procedures for determining that licensed biological products are safe and effective and not misbranded, as described in part 601 of this chapter.

(12) An *Application for an Investigational Device Exemption*, described in parts 812 and 813.

(13) Data and information regarding a medical device for human use submitted as part of the procedures for classifying such devices, described in part 860.

(14) Data and information regarding a medical device for human use submitted as part of the procedures for establishing, amending, or repealing a standard for such device, described in part 861.

(15) An application for premarket approval of a medical device for human use, described in section 515 of the act.

(16) A product development protocol for a medical device for human use, described in section 515 of the act.

(17) Data and information regarding an electronic product submitted as part of the procedures for establishing, amending, or repealing a standard for such products, described in section 358 of the Public Health Service Act.

(18) Data and information regarding an electronic product submitted as part of the procedures for obtaining a variance from any electronic product performance standard, as described in §1010.4.

(19) Data and information regarding an electronic product submitted as part of the procedures for granting, amending, or extending an exemption from a radiation safety performance standard, as described in §1010.5.

(20) Data and information regarding an electronic product submitted as part of the procedures for obtaining an exemption from notification of a radiation safety defect or failure of compliance with a radiation safety performance standard, described in subpart D of part 1003.

(21) Data and information about a clinical study of an infant formula when submitted as part of an infant formula notification under section 412(c) of the Federal Food, Drug, and Cosmetic Act.

(22) Data and information submitted in a petition for a nutrient content claim, described in §101.69 of this chapter, and for a health claim, described in §101.70 of this chapter.

(23) Data and information from investigations involving children submitted in a new dietary ingredient notification, described in §190.6 of this chapter.

(c) *Clinical investigation* means any experiment that involves a test article and one or more human subjects, and that either must meet the requirements for prior submission to the Food and Drug Administration under section 505(i) or 520(g) of the act, or need not meet the requirements for prior submission to the Food and Drug Administration under these sections of the act, but the results of which are intended to be later submitted to, or held for inspection by, the Food and Drug Administration as part of an application for a research or marketing permit. The term does not include experiments that must meet the provisions of part 58, regarding nonclinical laboratory studies. The terms *research, clinical research, clinical study, study,* and *clinical investigation* are deemed to be synonymous for purposes of this part.

(d) *Emergency use* means the use of a test article on a human subject in a life-threatening situation in which no standard acceptable treatment is available, and in which there is not sufficient time to obtain IRB approval.

(e) *Human subject* means an individual who is or becomes a participant in research, either as a recipient of the test article or as a control. A subject may be either a healthy individual or a patient.

(f) *Institution* means any public or private entity or agency (including Federal, State, and other agencies). The term facility as used in section 520(g) of the act is deemed to be synonymous with the term *institution* for purposes of this part.

(g) *Institutional Review Board* (IRB) means any board, committee, or other group formally designated by an institution to review, to approve the initiation of, and to conduct periodic review of, biomedical research involving human subjects. The primary purpose of such review is to assure the protection of the rights and welfare of the human subjects. The term has the same meaning as the phrase *institutional review committee* as used in section 520(g) of the act.

(h) *Investigator* means an individual who actually conducts a clinical investigation (i.e., under whose immediate direction the test article is administered or dispensed to, or used involving, a subject) or, in the event of an investigation conducted by a team of individuals, is the responsible leader of that team.

(i) *Minimal risk* means that the probability and magnitude of harm or discomfort anticipated in the research are not greater in and of themselves than those ordinarily encountered in daily life or during the performance of routine physical or psychological examinations or tests.

(j) *Sponsor* means a person or other entity that initiates a clinical investigation, but that does not actually conduct the investigation, i.e., the test article is administered or dispensed to, or used involving, a subject under the immediate direction of another individual. A person other than an individual (e.g., a corporation or agency) that uses one or more of its own employees to conduct an investigation that it has initiated is considered to be a sponsor (not a sponsor-investigator), and the employees are considered to be investigators.

(k) *Sponsor-investigator* means an individual who both initiates and actually conducts, alone or with others, a clinical investigation, i.e., under whose immediate direction the test article is administered or dispensed to, or used involving, a subject. The term does not include any person other than an individual, e.g., it does not include a corporation or agency. The obligations of a sponsor-investigator under this part include both those of a sponsor and those of an investigator.

(l) *Test article* means any drug for human use, biological product for human use, medical device for human use, human food additive, color additive, electronic product, or any other article subject to regulation under the act or under sections 351 or 354-360F of the Public Health Service Act.

(m) IRB *approval* means the determination of the IRB that the clinical investigation has been reviewed and may be conducted at an institution within the constraints set forth by the IRB and by other institutional and Federal requirements.

[46 FR 8975, Jan. 27, 1981, as amended at 54 FR 9038, Mar. 3, 1989; 56 FR 28028, June 18, 1991; 64 FR 399, Jan. 5, 1999; 64 FR 56448, Oct. 20, 1999; 65 FR 52302, Aug. 29, 2000; 66 FR 20599, Apr. 24, 2001]

**§56.103 Circumstances in which IRB review is required.**

(a) Except as provided in §§56.104 and 56.105, any clinical investigation which must meet the requirements for prior submission (as required in parts 312, 812, and 813) to the Food and Drug Administration shall not be initiated unless that investigation has been reviewed and approved by, and remains subject to continuing review by, an IRB meeting the requirements of this part.

(b) Except as provided in §§56.104 and 56.105, the Food and Drug Administration may decide not to consider in support of an application for a research or marketing permit any data or information that has been derived from a clinical investigation that has not been approved by, and that was not subject to initial and continuing review by, an IRB meeting the requirements of this part. The determination that a clinical investigation may not be considered in support of an application for a research or marketing permit does not, however, relieve the applicant for such a permit of any obligation under any other applicable regulations to submit the results of the investigation to the Food and Drug Administration.

(c) Compliance with these regulations will in no way render inapplicable pertinent Federal, State, or local laws or regulations.

[46 FR 8975, Jan. 27, 1981; 46 FR 14340, Feb. 27, 1981]

**§56.104 Exemptions from IRB requirement.**

The following categories of clinical investigations are exempt from the requirements of this part for IRB review:
(a) Any investigation which commenced before July 27, 1981 and was subject to requirements for IRB review under FDA regulations before that date, provided that the investigation remains subject to review of an IRB which meets the FDA requirements in effect before July 27, 1981.

(b) Any investigation commenced before July 27, 1981 and was not otherwise subject to requirements for IRB review under Food and Drug Administration regulations before that date.

(c) Emergency use of a test article, provided that such emergency use is reported to the IRB within 5 working days. Any subsequent use of the test article at the institution is subject to IRB review.

(d) Taste and food quality evaluations and consumer acceptance studies, if wholesome foods without additives are consumed or if a food is consumed that contains a food ingredient at or below the level and for a use found to be safe, or agricultural, chemical, or environmental contaminant at or below the level found to be safe, by the Food and Drug Administration or approved by the Environmental Protection Agency or the Food Safety and Inspection Service of the U.S. Department of Agriculture.

[46 FR 8975, Jan. 27, 1981, as amended at 56 FR 28028, June 18, 1991]

## §56.105 Waiver of IRB requirement.

On the application of a sponsor or sponsor-investigator, the Food and Drug Administration may waive any of the requirements contained in these regulations, including the requirements for IRB review, for specific research activities or for classes of research activities, otherwise covered by these regulations.

## Subpart B—Organization and Personnel

### §56.107 IRB membership.

(a) Each IRB shall have at least five members, with varying backgrounds to promote complete and adequate review of research activities commonly conducted by the institution. The IRB shall be sufficiently qualified through the experience and expertise of its members, and the diversity of the members, including consideration of race, gender, cultural backgrounds, and sensitivity to such issues as community attitudes, to promote respect for its advice and counsel in safeguarding the rights and welfare of human subjects. In addition to possessing the professional competence necessary to review the specific research activities, the IRB shall be able to ascertain the acceptability of proposed research in terms of institutional commitments and regulations, applicable law, and standards or professional conduct and practice. The IRB shall therefore include persons knowledgeable in these areas. If an IRB regularly reviews research that involves a vulnerable catgory of subjects, such as children, prisoners, pregnant women, or handicapped or mentally disabled persons, consideration shall be given to the inclusion of one or more individuals who are knowledgeable about and experienced in working with those subjects.

(b) Every nondiscriminatory effort will be made to ensure that no IRB consists entirely of men or entirely of women, including the instituton's consideration of qualified persons of both sexes, so long as no selection is made to the IRB on the basis of gender. No IRB may consist entirely of members of one profession.

(c) Each IRB shall include at least one member whose primary concerns are in the scientific area and at least one member whose primary concerns are in nonscientific areas.

(d) Each IRB shall include at least one member who is not otherwise affiliated with the institution and who is not part of the immediate family of a person who is affiliated with the institution.

(e) No IRB may have a member participate in the IRB's initial or continuing review of any project in which the member has a conflicting interest, except to provide information requested by the IRB.

(f) An IRB may, in its discretion, invite individuals with competence in special areas to assist in the review of complex issues which require expertise beyond or in addition to that available on the IRB. These individuals may not vote with the IRB.

[46 FR 8975, Jan 27, 1981, as amended at 56 FR 28028, June 18, 1991; 56 FR 29756, June 28, 1991]

### Subpart C—IRB Functions and Operations

§56.108 IRB functions and operations.

In order to fulfill the requirements of these regulations, each IRB shall:

(a) Follow written procedures: (1) For conducting its initial and continuing review of research and for reporting its findings and actions to the investigator and the institution; (2) for determining which projects require review more often than annually and which projects need verification from sources other than the investigator that no material changes have occurred since previous IRB review; (3) for ensuring prompt reporting to the IRB of changes in research activity; and (4) for ensuring that changes in approved research, during the period for which IRB approval has already been given, may not be initiated without IRB review and approval except where necessary to eliminate apparent immediate hazards to the human subjects.

(b) Follow written procedures for ensuring prompt reporting to the IRB, appropriate institutional officials, and the Food and Drug Administration of: (1) Any unanticipated problems involving risks to human subjects or others; (2) any instance of serious or continuing noncompliance with these regulations or the requirements or determinations of the IRB; or (3) any suspension or termination of IRB approval.

(c) Except when an expedited review procedure is used (see §56.110), review proposed research at convened meetings at which a majority of the members of the IRB are present, including at least one member whose primary concerns are in nonscientific areas. In order for the research to be approved, it shall receive the approval of a majority of those members present at the meeting.

[46 FR 8975, Jan. 27, 1981, as amended at 56 FR 28028, June 18, 1991; 67 FR 9585, Mar. 4, 2002]

## §56.109 IRB review of research.

(a) An IRB shall review and have authority to approve, require modifications in (to secure approval), or disapprove all research activities covered by these regulations.

(b) An IRB shall require that information given to subjects as part of informed consent is in accordance with §50.25. The IRB may require that information, in addition to that specifically mentioned in §50.25, be given to the subjects when in the IRB's judgment the information would meaningfully add to the protection of the rights and welfare of subjects.

(c) An IRB shall require documentation of informed consent in accordance with §50.27 of this chapter, except as follows:

(1) The IRB may, for some or all subjects, waive the requirement that the subject, or the subject's legally authorized representative, sign a written consent form if it finds that the research presents no more than minimal risk of harm to subjects and involves no procedures for which written consent is normally required outside the research context; or

(2) The IRB may, for some or all subjects, find that the requirements in §50.24 of this chapter for an exception from informed consent for emergency research are met.

(d) In cases where the documentation requirement is waived under paragraph (c)(1) of this section, the IRB may require the investigator to provide subjects with a written statement regarding the research.

(e) An IRB shall notify investigators and the institution in writing of its decision to approve or disapprove the proposed research activity, or of modifications required to secure IRB approval of the research activity. If the IRB decides to disapprove a research activity, it shall include in its written notification a statement of the reasons for its decision and give the investigator an opportunity to respond in person or in writing. For investigations involving an exception to informed consent under §50.24 of this chapter, an IRB shall promptly notify in writing the investigator and the sponsor of the research when an IRB determines that it cannot approve the research because it does not meet the criteria in the exception provided under §50.24(a) of this chapter or because of other relevant ethical concerns. The written notification shall include a statement of the reasons for the IRB's determination.

(f) An IRB shall conduct continuing review of research covered by these regulations at intervals appropriate to the degree of risk, but not less than once per year, and shall have authority to observe or have a third party observe the consent process and the research.

(g) An IRB shall provide in writing to the sponsor of research involving an exception to informed consent under §50.24 of this chapter a copy of information that has been publicly disclosed under §50.24(a)(7)(ii) and (a)(7)(iii) of this chapter. The IRB shall provide this information to the sponsor promptly so that the sponsor is aware that such disclosure has occurred. Upon receipt, the sponsor shall provide copies of the information disclosed to FDA.

(h) When some or all of the subjects in a study are children, an IRB must determine that the research study is in compliance with part 50, subpart D of this chapter, at the time of its initial review of the research. When some or all of the subjects in a study that is ongoing on April 30, 2001 are children, an IRB must conduct a review of the research to determine compliance with part 50, subpart D of this chapter, either at the time of continuing review or, at the discretion of the IRB, at an earlier date.

[46 FR 8975, Jan. 27, 1981, as amended at 61 FR 51529, Oct. 2, 1996; 66 FR 20599, Apr. 24, 2001]

**§56.110 Expedited review procedures for certain kinds of research involving no more than minimal risk, and for minor changes in approved research.**

(a) The Food and Drug Administration has established, and published in the FEDERAL REGISTER, a list of categories of research that may be reviewed by the IRB through an expedited review procedure. The list will be amended, as appropriate, through periodic republication in the FEDERAL REGISTER.

(b) An IRB may use the expedited review procedure to review either or both of the following: (1) Some or all of the research appearing on the list and found by the reviewer(s) to involve no more than minimal risk, (2) minor changes in previously approved research during the period (of 1 year or less) for which approval is authorized. Under an expedited review procedure, the review may be carried out by the IRB chairperson or by one or more experienced reviewers designated by the IRB chairperson from among the members of the IRB. In reviewing the research, the reviewers may exercise all of the authorities of the IRB except that the reviewers may not disapprove the research. A research activity may be disapproved only after review in accordance with the nonexpedited review procedure set forth in §56.108(c).

(c) Each IRB which uses an expedited review procedure shall adopt a method for keeping all members advised of research proposals which have been approved under the procedure.

(d) The Food and Drug Administration may restrict, suspend, or terminate an institution's or IRB's use of the expedited review procedure when necessary to protect the rights or welfare of subjects.

[46 FR 8975, Jan. 27, 1981, as amended at 56 FR 28029, June 18, 1991]

### §56.111 Criteria for IRB approval of research.

(a) In order to approve research covered by these regulations the IRB shall determine that all of the following requirements are satisfied:

(1) Risks to subjects are minimized: (i) By using procedures which are consistent with sound research design and which do not unnecessarily expose subjects to risk, and (ii) whenever appropriate, by using procedures already being performed on the subjects for diagnostic or treatment purposes.

(2) Risks to subjects are reasonable in relation to anticipated benefits, if any, to subjects, and the importance of the knowledge that may be expected to result. In evaluating risks and benefits, the IRB should consider only those risks and benefits that may result from the research (as distinguished from risks and benefits of therapies that subjects would receive even if not participating in the research). The IRB should not consider possible long-range effects of applying knowledge gained in the research (for example, the possible effects of the research on public policy) as among those research risks that fall within the purview of its responsibility.

(3) Selection of subjects is equitable. In making this assessment the IRB should take into account the purposes of the research and the setting in which the research will be conducted and should be particularly cognizant of the special problems of research involving vulnerable populations, such as children, prisoners, pregnant women, handicapped, or mentally disabled persons, or economically or educationally disadvantaged persons.

(4) Informed consent will be sought from each prospective subject or the subject's legally authorized representative, in accordance with and to the extent required by part 50.

(5) Informed consent will be appropriately documented, in accordance with and to the extent required by §50.27.

(6) Where appropriate, the research plan makes adequate provision for monitoring the data collected to ensure the safety of subjects.

(7) Where appropriate, there are adequate provisions to protect the privacy of subjects and to maintain the confidentiality of data.

(b) When some or all of the subjects, such as children, prisoners, pregnant women, handicapped, or mentally disabled persons, or economically or educationally disadvantaged persons, are likely to be vulnerable to coercion or undue influence additional safeguards have been included in the study to protect the rights and welfare of these subjects.

(c) In order to approve research in which some or all of the subjects are children, an IRB must determine that all research is in compliance with part 50, subpart D of this chapter.

[46 FR 8975, Jan. 27, 1981, as amended at 56 FR 28029, June 18, 1991; 66 FR 20599, Apr. 24, 2001]

### §56.112 Review by institution.

Research covered by these regulations that has been approved by an IRB may be subject to further appropriate review and approval or disapproval by officials of the institution. However, those officials may not approve the research if it has not been approved by an IRB.

### §56.113 Suspension or termination of IRB approval of research.

An IRB shall have authority to suspend or terminate approval of research that is not being conducted in accordance with the IRB's requirements or that has been associated with unexpected serious harm to subjects. Any suspension or termination of approval shall include a statement of the reasons for the IRB's action and shall be reported promptly to the investigator, appropriate institutional officials, and the Food and Drug Administration.

### §56.114 Cooperative research.

In complying with these regulations, institutions involved in multi-institutional studies may use joint review, reliance upon the review of another qualified IRB, or similar arrangements aimed at avoidance of duplication of effort.

## Subpart D—Records and Reports

### §56.115 IRB records.

(a) An institution, or where appropriate an IRB, shall prepare and maintain adequate documentation of IRB activities, including the following:

(1) Copies of all research proposals reviewed, scientific evaluations, if any, that accompany the proposals, approved sample consent documents, progress reports submitted by investigators, and reports of injuries to subjects.

(2) Minutes of IRB meetings which shall be in sufficient detail to show attendance at the meetings; actions taken by the IRB; the vote on these actions including the number of members voting for, against, and abstaining; the basis for requiring changes in or disapproving research; and a written summary of the discussion of controverted issues and their resolution.

(3) Records of continuing review activities.

(4) Copies of all correspondence between the IRB and the investigators.

(5) A list of IRB members identified by name; earned degrees; representative capacity; indications of experience such as board certifications, licenses, etc., sufficient to describe each member's chief anticipated contributions to IRB deliberations; and any employment or other relationship between each member and the institution; for example: full-time employee, part-time employee, a member of governing panel or board, stockholder, paid or unpaid consultant.

(6) Written procedures for the IRB as required by §56.108 (a) and (b).

(7) Statements of significant new findings provided to subjects, as required by §50.25.
(b) The records required by this regulation shall be retained for at least 3 years after completion of the research, and the records shall be accessible for inspection and copying by authorized representatives of the Food and Drug Administration at reasonable times and in a reasonable manner.

(c) The Food and Drug Administration may refuse to consider a clinical investigation in support of an application for a research or marketing permit if the institution or the IRB that reviewed the investigation refuses to allow an inspection under this section.

[46 FR 8975, Jan. 27, 1981, as amended at 56 FR 28029, June 18, 1991; 67 FR 9585, Mar. 4, 2002]

## Subpart E—Administrative Actions for Noncompliance

**§56.120 Lesser administrative actions.**

(a) If apparent noncompliance with these regulations in the operation of an IRB is observed by an FDA investigator during an inspection, the inspector will present an oral or written summary of observations to an appropriate representative of the IRB. The Food and Drug Administration may subsequently send a letter describing the noncompliance to the IRB and to the parent institution. The agency will require that the IRB or the parent institution respond to this letter within a time period specified by FDA and describe the corrective actions that will be taken by the IRB, the institution, or both to achieve compliance with these regulations.

(b) On the basis of the IRB's or the institution's response, FDA may schedule a reinspection to confirm the adequacy of corrective actions. In addition, until the IRB or the parent institution takes appropriate corrective action, the agency may:

(1) Withhold approval of new studies subject to the requirements of this part that are conducted at the institution or reviewed by the IRB;

(2) Direct that no new subjects be added to ongoing studies subject to this part;

(3) Terminate ongoing studies subject to this part when doing so would not endanger the subjects; or

(4) When the apparent noncompliance creates a significant threat to the rights and welfare of human subjects, notify relevant State and Federal regulatory agencies and other parties with a direct interest in the agency's action of the deficiencies in the operation of the IRB.

(c) The parent institution is presumed to be responsible for the operation of an IRB, and the Food and Drug Administration will ordinarily direct any administrative action under this subpart against the institution. However, depending on the evidence of responsibility for deficiencies, determined during the investigation, the Food and Drug Administration may restrict its administrative actions to the IRB or to a component of the parent institution determined to be responsible for formal designation of the IRB.

## §56.121 Disqualification of an IRB or an institution.

(a) Whenever the IRB or the institution has failed to take adequate steps to correct the noncompliance stated in the letter sent by the agency under §56.120(a), and the Commissioner of Food and Drugs determines that this noncompliance may justify the disqualification of the IRB or of the parent institution, the Commissioner will institute proceedings in accordance with the requirements for a regulatory hearing set forth in part 16.

(b) The Commissioner may disqualify an IRB or the parent institution if the Commissioner determines that:

(1) The IRB has refused or repeatedly failed to comply with any of the regulations set forth in this part, and

(2) The noncompliance adversely affects the rights or welfare of the human subjects in a clinical investigation.

(c) If the Commissioner determines that disqualification is appropriate, the Commissioner will issue an order that explains the basis for the determination and that prescribes any actions to be taken with regard to ongoing clinical research conducted under the review of the IRB. The Food and Drug Administration will send notice of the disqualification to the IRB and the parent institution. Other parties with a direct interest, such as sponsors and clinical investigators, may also be sent a notice of the disqualification. In addition, the agency may elect to publish a notice of its action in the FEDERAL REGISTER.

(d) The Food and Drug Administration will not approve an application for a research permit for a clinical investigation that is to be under the review of a disqualified IRB or that is to be conducted at a disqualified institution, and it may refuse to consider in support of a marketing permit the data from a clinical investigation that was reviewed by a disqualified IRB as conducted at a disqualified institution, unless the IRB or the parent institution is reinstated as provided in §56.123.

### §56.122 Public disclosure of information regarding revocation.

A determination that the Food and Drug Administration has disqualified an institution and the administrative record regarding that determination are disclosable to the public under part 20.

### §56.123 Reinstatement of an IRB or an institution.

An IRB or an institution may be reinstated if the Commissioner determines, upon an evaluation of a written submission from the IRB or institution that explains the corrective action that the institution or IRB plans to take, that the IRB or institution has provided adequate assurance that it will operate in compliance with the standards set forth in this part. Notification of reinstatement shall be provided to all persons notified under §56.121(c).

### §56.124 Actions alternative or additional to disqualification.

Disqualification of an IRB or of an institution is independent of, and neither in lieu of nor a precondition to, other proceedings or actions authorized by the act. The Food and Drug Administration may, at any time, through the Department of Justice institute any appropriate judicial proceedings (civil or criminal) and any other appropriate regulatory action, in addition to or in lieu of, and before, at the time of, or after, disqualification. The agency may also refer pertinent matters to another Federal, State, or local government agency for any action that that agency determines to be appropriate.

# Part 312—Investigational New Drug Application

Authority: 21 U.S.C. 321, 331, 351, 352, 353, 355, 371; 42 U.S.C. 262.
Source: 52 FR 8831, Mar. 19, 1987, unless otherwise noted.

**Subpart A—General Provisions**

§312.1 Scope.

(a) This part contains procedures and requirements governing the use of investigational new drugs, including procedures and requirements for the submission to, and review by, the Food and Drug Administration of investigational new drug applications (IND's). An investigational new drug for which an IND is in effect in accordance with this part is exempt from the premarketing approval requirements that are otherwise applicable and may be shipped lawfully for the purpose of conducting clinical investigations of that drug.

(b) References in this part to regulations in the Code of Federal Regulations are to chapter I of title 21, unless otherwise noted.

## §312.2 Applicability.

(a) *Applicability*. Except as provided in this section, this part applies to all clinical investigations of products that are subject to section 505 of the Federal Food, Drug, and Cosmetic Act or to the licensing provisions of the Public Health Service Act (58 Stat. 632, as amended (42 U.S.C. 201 *et seq.*)).

(b) *Exemptions*. (1) The clinical investigation of a drug product that is lawfully marketed in the United States is exempt from the requirements of this part if all the following apply:

(i) The investigation is not intended to be reported to FDA as a well-controlled study in support of a new indication for use nor intended to be used to support any other significant change in the labeling for the drug;

(ii) If the drug that is undergoing investigation is lawfully marketed as a prescription drug product, the investigation is not intended to support a significant change in the advertising for the product;

(iii) The investigation does not involve a route of administration or dosage level or use in a patient population or other factor that significantly increases the risks (or decreases the acceptability of the risks) associated with the use of the drug product;

(iv) The investigation is conducted in compliance with the requirements for institutional review set forth in part 56 and with the requirements for informed consent set forth in part 50; and
(v) The investigation is conducted in compliance with the requirements of §312.7.

(2)(i) A clinical investigation involving an in vitro diagnostic biological product listed in paragraph (b)(2)(ii) of this section is exempt from the requirements of this part if (a) it is intended to be used in a diagnostic procedure that confirms the diagnosis made by another, medically established, diagnostic product or procedure and (b) it is shipped in compliance with §312.160.

(ii) In accordance with paragraph (b)(2)(i) of this section, the following products are exempt from the requirements of this part: *(a)* blood grouping serum; *(b)* reagent red blood cells; and *(c)* anti-human globulin.

(3) A drug intended solely for tests in vitro or in laboratory research animals is exempt from the requirements of this part if shipped in accordance with §312.160.

(4) FDA will not accept an application for an investigation that is exempt under the provisions of paragraph (b)(1) of this section.

(5) A clinical investigation involving use of a placebo is exempt from the requirements of this part if the investigation does not otherwise require submission of an IND.

(6) A clinical investigation involving an exception from informed consent under §50.24 of this chapter is not exempt from the requirements of this part.

(c) *Bioavailability studies.* The applicability of this part to in vivo bioavailability studies in humans is subject to the provisions of §320.31.

(d) *Unlabeled indication.* This part does not apply to the use in the practice of medicine for an unlabeled indication of a new drug product approved under part 314 or of a licensed biological product.

(e) *Guidance.* FDA may, on its own initiative, issue guidance on the applicability of this part to particular investigational uses of drugs. On request, FDA will advise on the applicability of this part to a planned clinical investigation.

[52 FR 8831, Mar. 19, 1987, as amended at 61 FR 51529, Oct. 2, 1996; 64 FR 401, Jan. 5, 1999]

### §312.3 Definitions and interpretations.

(a) The definitions and interpretations of terms contained in section 201 of the Act apply to those terms when used in this part:

(b) The following definitions of terms also apply to this part:

*Act* means the Federal Food, Drug, and Cosmetic Act (secs. 201-902, 52 Stat. 1040 *et seq.*, as amended (21 U.S.C. 301-392)).

*Clinical investigation* means any experiment in which a drug is administered or dispensed to, or used involving, one or more human subjects. For the purposes of this part, an experiment is any use of a drug except for the use of a marketed drug in the course of medical practice.

*Contract research organization* means a person that assumes, as an independent contractor with the sponsor, one or more of the obligations of a sponsor, e.g., design of a protocol, selection or monitoring of investigations, evaluation of reports, and preparation of materials to be submitted to the Food and Drug Administration.

FDA means the Food and Drug Administration.

IND means an investigational new drug application. For purposes of this part, "IND" is synonymous with "Notice of Claimed Investigational Exemption for a New Drug."

*Investigational new drug* means a new drug or biological drug that is used in a clinical investigation. The term also includes a biological product that is used in vitro for diagnostic purposes. The terms "investigational drug" and "investigational new drug" are deemed to be synonymous for purposes of this part.

*Investigator* means an individual who actually conducts a clinical investigation (i.e., under whose immediate direction the drug is administered or dispensed to a subject). In the event an investigation is conducted by a team of individuals, the investigator is the responsible leader of the team. "Subinvestigator" includes any other individual member of that team.

*Marketing application* means an application for a new drug submitted under section 505(b) of the act or a biologics license application for a biological product submitted under the Public Health Service Act.

*Sponsor* means a person who takes responsibility for and initiates a clinical investigation. The sponsor may be an individual or pharmaceutical company, governmental agency, academic institution, private organization, or other organization. The sponsor does not actually conduct the investigation unless the sponsor is a sponsor-investigator. A person other than an individual that uses one or more of its own employees to conduct an investigation that it has initiated is a sponsor, not a sponsor-investigator, and the employees are investigators.

*Sponsor-Investigator* means an individual who both initiates and conducts an investigation, and under whose immediate direction the investigational drug is administered or dispensed. The term does not include any person other than an individual. The requirements applicable to a sponsor-investigator under this part include both those applicable to an investigator and a sponsor.

*Subject* means a human who participates in an investigation, either as a recipient of the investigational new drug or as a control. A subject may be a healthy human or a patient with a disease.

[52 FR 8831, Mar. 19, 1987, as amended at 64 FR 401, Jan. 5, 1999; 64 FR 56449, Oct. 20, 1999]

### §312.6 Labeling of an investigational new drug.

(a) The immediate package of an investigational new drug intended for human use shall bear a label with the statement "Caution: New Drug— Limited by Federal (or United States) law to investigational use."

(b) The label or labeling of an investigational new drug shall not bear any statement that is false or misleading in any particular and shall not represent that the investigational new drug is safe or effective for the purposes for which it is being investigated.

### §312.7 Promotion and charging for investigational drugs.

(a) *Promotion of an investigational new drug.* A sponsor or investigator, or any person acting on behalf of a sponsor or investigator, shall not represent in a promotional context that an investigational new drug is safe or effective for the purposes for which it is under investigation or otherwise promote the drug. This provision is not intended to restrict the full exchange of scientific information concerning the drug, including dissemination of scientific findings in scientific or lay media. Rather, its intent is to restrict promotional claims of safety or effectiveness of the drug for a use for which it is under investigation and to preclude commercialization of the drug before it is approved for commercial distribution.

(b) *Commercial distribution of an investigational new drug.* A sponsor or investigator shall not commercially distribute or test market an investigational new drug.

(c) *Prolonging an investigation.* A sponsor shall not unduly prolong an investigation after finding that the results of the investigation appear to establish sufficient data to support a marketing application.

(d) *Charging for and commercialization of investigational drugs*—(1) *Clinical trials under an* IND. Charging for an investigational drug in a clinical trial under an IND is not permitted without the prior written approval of FDA. In requesting such approval, the sponsor shall provide a full written explanation of why charging is necessary in order for the sponsor to undertake or continue the clinical trial, e.g., why distribution of the drug to test subjects should not be considered part of the normal cost of doing business.

(2) *Treatment protocol or treatment* IND. A sponsor or investigator may charge for an investigational drug for a treatment use under a treatment protocol or treatment IND provided: (i) There is adequate enrollment in the ongoing clinical investigations under the authorized IND; (ii) charging does not constitute commercial marketing of a new drug for which a marketing application has not been approved; (iii) the drug is not being commercially promoted or advertised; and (iv) the sponsor of the drug is actively pursuing marketing approval with due diligence. FDA must be notified in writing in advance of commencing any such charges, in an information amendment submitted under §312.31. Authorization for charging goes into effect automatically 30 days after receipt by FDA of the information amendment, unless the sponsor is notified to the contrary.

(3) *Noncommercialization of investigational drug.* Under this section, the sponsor may not commercialize an investigational drug by charging a price larger than that necessary to recover costs of manufacture, research, development, and handling of the investigational drug.

(4) *Withdrawal of authorization.* Authorization to charge for an investigational drug under this section may be withdrawn by FDA if the agency finds that the conditions underlying the authorization are no longer satisfied.

[52 FR 8831, Mar. 19, 1987, as amended at 52 FR 19476, May 22, 1987; 67 FR 9585, Mar. 4, 2002]

**§312.10 Waivers.**

(a) A sponsor may request FDA to waive applicable requirement under this part. A waiver request may be submitted either in an IND or in an information amendment to an IND. In an emergency, a request may be made by telephone or other rapid communication means. A waiver request is required to contain at least one of the following:

(1) An explanation why the sponsor's compliance with the requirement is unnecessary or cannot be achieved;

(2) A description of an alternative submission or course of action that satisfies the purpose of the requirement; or

(3) Other information justifying a waiver.

(b) FDA may grant a waiver if it finds that the sponsor's noncompliance would not pose a significant and unreasonable risk to human subjects of the investigation and that one of the following is met:

(1) The sponsor's compliance with the requirement is unnecessary for the agency to evaluate the application, or compliance cannot be achieved;

(2) The sponsor's proposed alternative satisfies the requirement; or

(3) The applicant's submission otherwise justifies a waiver.

[52 FR 8831, Mar. 19, 1987, as amended at 52 FR 23031, June 17, 1987; 67 FR 9585, Mar. 4, 2002]

### Subpart B—Investigational New Drug Application (IND)

§312.20 Requirement for an IND.

(a) A sponsor shall submit an IND to FDA if the sponsor intends to conduct a clinical investigation with an investigational new drug that is subject to §312.2(a).

(b) A sponsor shall not begin a clinical investigation subject to §312.2(a) until the investigation is subject to an IND which is in effect in accordance with §312.40.

(c) A sponsor shall submit a separate IND for any clinical investigation involving an exception from informed consent under §50.24 of this chapter. Such a clinical investigation is not permitted to proceed without the prior written authorization from FDA. FDA shall provide a written determination 30 days after FDA receives the IND or earlier.

[52 FR 8831, Mar. 19, 1987, as amended at 61 FR 51529, Oct. 2, 1996; 62 FR 32479, June 16, 1997]

§312.21 Phases of an investigation.

An IND may be submitted for one or more phases of an investigation. The clinical investigation of a previously untested drug is generally divided into three phases. Although in general the phases are conducted sequentially, they may overlap. These three phases of an investigation are a follows:

(a) *Phase 1.* (1) Phase 1 includes the initial introduction of an investigational new drug into humans. Phase 1 studies are typically closely monitored and may be conducted in patients or normal volunteer subjects. These studies are designed to determine the metabolism and pharmacologic actions of the drug in humans, the side effects associated with increasing doses, and, if possible, to gain early evidence on effectiveness. During Phase 1, sufficient information about the drug's pharmacokinetics and pharmacological effects should be obtained to permit the design of well-controlled, scientifically valid, Phase 2 studies. The total number of subjects and patients included in Phase 1 studies varies with the drug, but is generally in the range of 20 to 80.

(2) Phase 1 studies also include studies of drug metabolism, structure-activity relationships, and mechanism of action in humans, as well as studies in which investigational drugs are used as research tools to explore biological phenomena or disease processes.

(b) *Phase 2.* Phase 2 includes the controlled clinical studies conducted to evaluate the effectiveness of the drug for a particular indication or indications in patients with the disease or condition under study and to determine the common short-term side effects and risks associated with the drug. Phase 2 studies are typically well controlled, closely monitored, and conducted in a relatively small number of patients, usually involving no more than several hundred subjects.

(c) *Phase 3.* Phase 3 studies are expanded controlled and uncontrolled trials. They are performed after preliminary evidence suggesting effectiveness of the drug has been obtained, and are intended to gather the additional information about effectiveness and safety that is needed to evaluate the overall benefit-risk relationship of the drug and to provide an adequate basis for physician labeling. Phase 3 studies usually include from several hundred to several thousand subjects.

## §312.22 General principles of the IND submission.

(a) FDA's primary objectives in reviewing an IND are, in all phases of the investigation, to assure the safety and rights of subjects, and, in Phase 2 and 3, to help assure that the quality of the scientific evaluation of drugs is adequate to permit an evaluation of the drug's effectiveness and safety. Therefore, although FDA's review of Phase 1 submissions will focus on assessing the safety of Phase 1 investigations, FDA's review of Phases 2 and 3 submissions will also include an assessment of the scientific quality of the clinical investigations and the likelihood that the investigations will yield data capable of meeting statutory standards for marketing approval.

(b) The amount of information on a particular drug that must be submitted in an IND to assure the accomplishment of the objectives described in paragraph (a) of this section depends upon such factors as the novelty of the drug, the extent to which it has been studied previously, the known or suspected risks, and the developmental phase of the drug.

(c) The central focus of the initial IND submission should be on the general investigational plan and the protocols for specific human studies. Subsequent amendments to the IND that contain new or revised protocols should build logically on previous submissions and should be supported by additional information, including the results of animal toxicology studies or other human studies as appropriate. Annual reports to the IND should serve as the focus for reporting the status of studies being conducted under the IND and should update the general investigational plan for the coming year.

(d) The IND format set forth in §312.23 should be followed routinely by sponsors in the interest of fostering an efficient review of applications. Sponsors are expected to exercise considerable discretion, however, regarding the content of information submitted in each section, depending upon the kind of drug being studied and the nature of the available information. Section 312.23 outlines the information needed for a commercially sponsored IND for a new molecular entity. A sponsor-investigator who uses, as a research tool, an investigational new drug that is already subject to a manufacturer's IND or marketing application should follow the same general format, but ordinarily may, if authorized by the manufacturer, refer to the manufacturer's IND or marketing application in providing the technical information supporting the proposed clinical investigation. A sponsor-investigator who uses an investigational drug not subject to a manufacturer's IND or marketing application is ordinarily required to submit all technical information supporting the IND, unless such information may be referenced from the scientific literature.

## §312.23 IND content and format.

(a) A sponsor who intends to conduct a clinical investigation subject to this part shall submit an "Investigational New Drug Application" (IND) including, in the following order:

(1) *Cover sheet (Form FDA-1571).* A cover sheet for the application containing the following:

(i) The name, address, and telephone number of the sponsor, the date of the application, and the name of the investigational new drug.

(ii) Identification of the phase or phases of the clinical investigation to be conducted.

(iii) A commitment not to begin clinical investigations until an IND covering the investigations is in effect.

(iv) A commitment that an Institutional Review Board (IRB) that complies with the requirements set forth in part 56 will be responsible for the initial and continuing review and approval of each of the studies in the proposed clinical investigation and that the investigator will report to the IRB proposed changes in the research activity in accordance with the requirements of part 56.

(v) A commitment to conduct the investigation in accordance with all other applicable regulatory requirements.

(vi) The name and title of the person responsible for monitoring the conduct and progress of the clinical investigations.

(vii) The name(s) and title(s) of the person(s) responsible under §312.32 for review and evaluation of information relevant to the safety of the drug.

(viii) If a sponsor has transferred any obligations for the conduct of any clinical study to a contract research organization, a statement containing the name and address of the contract research organization, identification of the clinical study, and a listing of the obligations transferred. If all obligations governing the conduct of the study have been transferred, a general statement of this transfer—in lieu of a listing of the specific obligations transferred—may be submitted.

(ix) The signature of the sponsor or the sponsor's authorized representative. If the person signing the application does not reside or have a place of business within the United States, the IND is required to contain the name and address of, and be countersigned by, an attorney, agent, or other authorized official who resides or maintains a place of business within the United States.

(2) *A table of contents.*

(3) *Introductory statement and general investigational plan.* (i) A brief introductory statement giving the name of the drug and all active ingredients, the drug's pharmacological class, the structural formula of the drug (if known), the formulation of the dosage form(s) to be used, the route of administration, and the broad objectives and planned duration of the proposed clinical investigation(s).

(ii) A brief summary of previous human experience with the drug, with reference to other IND's if pertinent, and to investigational or marketing experience in other countries that may be relevant to the safety of the proposed clinical investigation(s).

(iii) If the drug has been withdrawn from investigation or marketing in any country for any reason related to safety or effectiveness, identification of the country(ies) where the drug was withdrawn and the reasons for the withdrawal.

(iv) A brief description of the overall plan for investigating the drug product for the following year. The plan should include the following: (a) The rationale for the drug or the research study; (b) the indication(s) to be studied; (c) the general approach to be followed in evaluating the drug; (d ) the kinds of clinical trials to be conducted in the first year following the submission (if plans are not developed for the entire year, the sponsor should so indicate); (e) the estimated number of patients to be given the drug in those studies; and (f) any risks of particular severity or seriousness anticipated on the basis of the toxicological data in animals or prior studies in humans with the drug or related drugs.

(4) [Reserved]

(5) *Investigator's brochure.* If required under §312.55, a copy of the investigator's brochure, containing the following information:

(i) A brief description of the drug substance and the formulation, including the structural formula, if known.

(ii) A summary of the pharmacological and toxicological effects of the drug in animals and, to the extent known, in humans.

(iii) A summary of the pharmacokinetics and biological disposition of the drug in animals and, if known, in humans.

(iv) A summary of information relating to safety and effectiveness in humans obtained from prior clinical studies. (Reprints of published articles on such studies may be appended when useful.)

(v) A description of possible risks and side effects to be anticipated on the basis of prior experience with the drug under investigation or with related drugs, and of precautions or special monitoring to be done as part of the investigational use of the drug.

(6) *Protocols.* (i) A protocol for each planned study. (Protocols for studies not submitted initially in the IND should be submitted in accordance with §312.30(a).) In general, protocols for Phase 1 studies may be less detailed and more flexible than protocols for Phase 2 and 3 studies. Phase 1 protocols should be directed primarily at providing an outline of the investigation— an estimate of the number of patients to be involved, a description of safety exclusions, and a description of the dosing plan including duration, dose, or method to be used in determining dose—and should specify in detail only those elements of the study that are critical to safety, such as necessary monitoring of vital signs and blood chemistries. Modifications of the experimental design of Phase 1 studies that do not affect critical safety assessments are required to be reported to FDA only in the annual report.

(ii) In Phases 2 and 3, detailed protocols describing all aspects of the study should be submitted. A protocol for a Phase 2 or 3 investigation should be designed in such a way that, if the sponsor anticipates that some deviation from the study design may become necessary as the investigation progresses, alternatives or contingencies to provide for such deviation are built into the protocols at the outset. For example, a protocol for a controlled short-term study might include a plan for an early crossover of nonresponders to an alternative therapy.

(iii) A protocol is required to contain the following, with the specific elements and detail of the protocol reflecting the above distinctions depending on the phase of study:

(a) A statement of the objectives and purpose of the study.

(b ) The name and address and a statement of the qualifications (curriculum vitae or other statement of qualifications) of each investigator, and the name of each subinvestigator (e.g., research fellow, resident) working under the supervision of the investigator; the name and address of the research facilities to be used; and the name and address of each reviewing Institutional Review Board.

(c) The criteria for patient selection and for exclusion of patients and an estimate of the number of patients to be studied.

(d ) A description of the design of the study, including the kind of control group to be used, if any, and a description of methods to be used to minimize bias on the part of subjects, investigators, and analysts.

(e ) The method for determining the dose(s) to be administered, the planned maximum dosage, and the duration of individual patient exposure to the drug.

(f) A description of the observations and measurements to be made to fulfill the objectives of the study.

(g ) A description of clinical procedures, laboratory tests, or other measures to be taken to monitor the effects of the drug in human subjects and to minimize risk.

(7) *Chemistry, manufacturing, and control information.* (i) As appropriate for the particular investigations covered by the IND, a section describing the composition, manufacture, and control of the drug substance and the drug product. Although in each phase of the investigation sufficient information is required to be submitted to assure the proper identification, quality, purity, and strength of the investigational drug, the amount of information needed to make that assurance will vary with the phase of the investigation, the proposed duration of the investigation, the dosage form, and the amount of information otherwise available. FDA recognizes that modifications to the method of preparation of the new drug substance and dosage

form and changes in the dosage form itself are likely as the investigation progresses. Therefore, the emphasis in an initial Phase 1 submission should generally be placed on the identification and control of the raw materials and the new drug substance. Final specifications for the drug substance and drug product are not expected until the end of the investigational process.

(ii) It should be emphasized that the amount of information to be submitted depends upon the scope of the proposed clinical investigation. For example, although stability data are required in all phases of the IND to demonstrate that the new drug substance and drug product are within acceptable chemical and physical limits for the planned duration of the proposed clinical investigation, if very short-term tests are proposed, the supporting stability data can be correspondingly limited.

(iii) As drug development proceeds and as the scale or production is changed from the pilot-scale production appropriate for the limited initial clinical investigations to the larger-scale production needed for expanded clinical trials, the sponsor should submit information amendments to supplement the initial information submitted on the chemistry, manufacturing, and control processes with information appropriate to the expanded scope of the investigation.

(iv) Reflecting the distinctions described in this paragraph (a)(7), and based on the phase(s) to be studied, the submission is required to contain the following:

(a) *Drug substance.* A description of the drug substance, including its physical, chemical, or biological characteristics; the name and address of its manufacturer; the general method of preparation of the drug substance; the acceptable limits and analytical methods used to assure the identity, strength, quality, and purity of the drug substance; and information sufficient to support stability of the drug substance during the toxicological studies and the planned clinical studies. Reference to the current edition of the United States Pharmacopeia—National Formulary may satisfy relevant requirements in this paragraph.

(b) *Drug product.* A list of all components, which may include reasonable alternatives for inactive compounds, used in the manufacture of the investigational drug product, including both those components intended to appear in the drug product and those which may not appear but which are used in the manufacturing process, and, where applicable, the quantitative composition of the investigational drug product, including any reasonable variations that may be expected during the investigational stage; the name and address of the drug product manufacturer; a brief general description of the manufacturing and packaging procedure as appropriate for the product; the acceptable limits and analytical methods used to assure the identity, strength, quality, and purity of the drug product; and information sufficient to assure the product's stability during the planned clinical studies. Reference to the current edition of the United States Pharmacopeia—National Formulary may satisfy certain requirements in this paragraph.

(c) A brief general description of the composition, manufacture, and control of any placebo used in a controlled clinical trial.

(d) *Labeling.* A copy of all labels and labeling to be provided to each investigator.

(e) *Environmental analysis requirements.* A claim for categorical exclusion under §25.30 or 25.31 or an environmental assessment under §25.40.

(8) *Pharmacology and toxicology information.* Adequate information about pharmacological and toxicological studies of the drug involving laboratory animals or in vitro, on the basis of which the sponsor has concluded that it is reasonably safe to conduct the proposed clinical investigations. The kind, duration, and scope of animal and other tests required varies with the duration and nature of the proposed clinical investigations. Guidance documents are available from FDA that describe ways in which these requirements may be met. Such information is required to include the identification and qualifications of the individuals who evaluated the results of such studies and concluded that it is reasonably safe to begin the proposed investigations and a statement of where the investigations were conducted and where the records are available for inspection. As drug development proceeds, the sponsor is required to submit informational amendments, as appropriate, with additional information pertinent to safety.

(i) *Pharmacology and drug disposition.* A section describing the pharmacological effects and mechanism(s) of action of the drug in animals, and information on the absorption, distribution, metabolism, and excretion of the drug, if known.

(ii) *Toxicology.* (a ) An integrated summary of the toxicological effects of the drug in animals and in vitro. Depending on the nature of the drug and the phase of the investigation, the description is to include the results of acute, subacute, and chronic toxicity tests; tests of the drug's effects on reproduction and the developing fetus; any special toxicity test related to the drug's particular mode of administration or conditions of use (e.g., inhalation, dermal, or ocular toxicology); and any in vitro studies intended to evaluate drug toxicity.

(b ) For each toxicology study that is intended primarily to support the safety of the proposed clinical investigation, a full tabulation of data suitable for detailed review.

(iii) For each nonclinical laboratory study subject to the good laboratory practice regulations under part 58, a statement that the study was conducted in compliance with the good laboratory practice regulations in part 58, or, if the study was not conducted in compliance with those regulations, a brief statement of the reason for the noncompliance.

(9) *Previous human experience with the investigational drug.* A summary of previous human experience known to the applicant, if any, with the investigational drug. The information is required to include the following:

(i) If the investigational drug has been investigated or marketed previously, either in the United States or other countries, detailed information about such experience that is relevant to the safety of the proposed investigation or to the investigation's rationale. If the durg has been the subject of controlled trials, detailed information on such trials that is relevant to an assessment of the drug's effectiveness for the proposed investigational use(s) should also be provided. Any published material that is relevant to the safety of the proposed investigation or to an assessment of the drug's effectiveness for its proposed investigational use should be provided in full. Published material that is less directly relevant may be supplied by a bibliography.

(ii) If the drug is a combination of drugs previously investigated or marketed, the information required under paragraph (a)(9)(i) of this section should be provided for each active drug component. However, if any component in such combination is subject to an approved marketing application or is otherwise lawfully marketed in the United States, the sponsor is not required to submit published material concerning that active drug component unless such material relates directly to the proposed investigational use (including publications relevant to component-component interaction).

(iii) If the drug has been marketed outside the United States, a list of the countries in which the drug has been marketed and a list of the countries in which the drug has been withdrawn from marketing for reasons potentially related to safety or effectiveness.

(10) *Additional information.* In certain applications, as described below, information on special topics may be needed. Such information shall be submitted in this section as follows:

(i) *Drug dependence and abuse potential.* If the drug is a psychotropic substance or otherwise has abuse potential, a section describing relevant clinical studies and experience and studies in test animals.

(ii) *Radioactive drugs.* If the drug is a radioactive drug, sufficient data from animal or human studies to allow a reasonable calculation of radiation-absorbed dose to the whole body and critical organs upon administration to a human subject. Phase 1 studies of radioactive drugs must include studies which will obtain sufficient data for dosimetry calculations.

(iii) *Pediatric studies.* Plans for assessing pediatric safety and effectiveness.

(iv) *Other information.* A brief statement of any other information that would aid evaluation of the proposed clinical investigations with respect to their safety or their design and potential as controlled clinical trials to support marketing of the drug.

(11) *Relevant information.* If requested by FDA, any other relevant information needed for review of the application.

(b) *Information previously submitted.* The sponsor ordinarily is not required to resubmit information previously submitted, but may incorporate the information by reference. A reference to information submitted previously must identify the file by name, reference number, volume, and page number where the information can be found. A reference to information submitted to the agency by a person other than the sponsor is required to contain a written statement that authorizes the reference and that is signed by the person who submitted the information.

(c) *Material in a foreign language.* The sponsor shall submit an accurate and complete English translation of each part of the IND that is not in English. The sponsor shall also submit a copy of each original literature publication for which an English translation is submitted.

(d) *Number of copies.* The sponsor shall submit an original and two copies of all submissions to the IND file, including the original submission and all amendments and reports.

(e) *Numbering of IND submissions.* Each submission relating to an IND is required to be numbered serially using a single, three-digit serial number. The initial IND is required to be numbered 000; each subsequent submission (e.g., amendment, report, or correspondence) is required to be numbered chronologically in sequence.

(f) *Identification of exception from informed consent.* If the investigation involves an exception from informed consent under §50.24 of this chapter, the sponsor shall prominently identify on the cover sheet that the investigation is subject to the requirements in §50.24 of this chapter.

[52 FR 8831, Mar. 19, 1987, as amended at 52 FR 23031, June 17, 1987; 53 FR 1918, Jan. 25, 1988; 61 FR 51529, Oct. 2, 1996; 62 FR 40599, July 29, 1997; 63 FR 66669, Dec. 2, 1998; 65 FR 56479, Sept. 19, 2000; 67 FR 9585, Mar. 4, 2002]

## §312.30 Protocol amendments.

Once an IND is in effect, a sponsor shall amend it as needed to ensure that the clinical investigations are conducted according to protocols included in the application. This section sets forth the provisions under which new protocols may be submitted and changes in previously submitted protocols may be made. Whenever a sponsor intends to conduct a clinical investigation with an exception from informed consent for emergency research as set forth in §50.24 of this chapter, the sponsor shall submit a separate IND for such investigation.

(a) *New protocol.* Whenever a sponsor intends to conduct a study that is not covered by a protocol already contained in the IND, the sponsor shall submit to FDA a protocol amendment containing the protocol for the study. Such study may begin provided two conditions are met: (1) The sponsor has submitted the protocol to FDA for its review; and (2) the protocol has been approved by the Institutional Review Board (IRB) with responsibility for review and approval of the study in accordance with the requirements of part 56. The sponsor may comply with these two conditions in either order.

(b) *Changes in a protocol.* (1) A sponsor shall submit a protocol amendment describing any change in a Phase 1 protocol that significantly affects the safety of subjects or any change in a Phase 2 or 3 protocol that significantly affects the safety of subjects, the scope of the investigation, or the scientific quality of the study. Examples of changes requiring an amendment under this paragraph include:

(i) Any increase in drug dosage or duration of exposure of individual subjects to the drug beyond that in the current protocol, or any significant increase in the number of subjects under study.

(ii) Any significant change in the design of a protocol (such as the addition or dropping of a control group).

(iii) The addition of a new test or procedure that is intended to improve monitoring for, or reduce the risk of, a side effect or adverse event; or the dropping of a test intended to monitor safety.

(2)(i) A protocol change under paragraph (b)(1) of this section may be made provided two conditions are met:

(a) The sponsor has submitted the change to FDA for its review; and

(b) The change has been approved by the IRB with responsibility for review and approval of the study. The sponsor may comply with these two conditions in either order.

(ii) Notwithstanding paragraph (b)(2)(i) of this section, a protocol change intended to eliminate an apparent immediate hazard to subjects may be implemented immediately provided FDA is subsequently notified by protocol amendment and the reviewing IRB is notified in accordance with §56.104(c).

(c) *New investigator.* A sponsor shall submit a protocol amendment when a new investigator is added to carry out a previously submitted protocol, except that a protocol amendment is not required when a licensed practitioner is added in the case of a treatment protocol under §312.34. Once the investigator is added to the study, the investigational drug may be shipped to the investigator and the investigator may begin participating in the study. The sponsor shall notify FDA of the new investigator within 30 days of the investigator being added.

(d) *Content and format.* A protocol amendment is required to be prominently identified as such (i.e., "Protocol Amendment: New Protocol", "Protocol Amendment: Change in Protocol", or "Protocol Amendment: New Investigator"), and to contain the following:

(1)(i) In the case of a new protocol, a copy of the new protocol and a brief description of the most clinically significant differences between it and previous protocols.

(ii) In the case of a change in protocol, a brief description of the change and reference (date and number) to the submission that contained the protocol. (iii) In the case of a new investigator, the investigator's name, the qualifications to conduct the investigation, reference to the previously submitted protocol, and all additional information about the investigator's study as is required under §312.23(a)(6)(iii)(b).

(2) Reference, if necessary, to specific technical information in the IND or in a concurrently submitted information amendment to the IND that the sponsor relies on to support any clinically significant change in the new or amended protocol. If the reference is made to supporting information already in the IND, the sponsor shall identify by name, reference number, volume, and page number the location of the information.

(3) If the sponsor desires FDA to comment on the submission, a request for such comment and the specific questions FDA's response should address.

(e) *When submitted.* A sponsor shall submit a protocol amendment for a new protocol or a change in protocol before its implementation. Protocol amendments to add a new investigator or to provide additional information about investigators may be grouped and submitted at 30-day intervals. When several submissions of new protocols or protocol changes are anticipated during a short period, the sponsor is encouraged, to the extent feasible, to include these all in a single submission.

[52 FR 8831, Mar. 19, 1987, as amended at 52 FR 23031, June 17, 1987; 53 FR 1918, Jan. 25, 1988; 61 FR 51530, Oct. 2, 1996; 67 FR 9585, Mar. 4, 2002]

### §312.31 Information amendments.

(a) *Requirement for information amendment.* A sponsor shall report in an information amendment essential information on the IND that is not within the scope of a protocol amendment, IND safety reports, or annual report. Examples of information requiring an information amendment include:

(1) New toxicology, chemistry, or other technical information; or

(2) A report regarding the discontinuance of a clinical investigation.

(b) *Content and format of an information amendment.* An information amendment is required to bear prominent identification of its contents (e.g., "Information Amendment: Chemistry, Manufacturing, and Control", "Information Amendment: Pharmacology-Toxicology", "Information Amendment: Clinical"), and to contain the following:

(1) A statement of the nature and purpose of the amendment.

(2) An organized submission of the data in a format appropriate for scientific review.

(3) If the sponsor desires FDA to comment on an information amendment, a request for such comment.

(c) *When submitted.* Information amendments to the IND should be submitted as necessary but, to the extent feasible, not more than every 30 days.

[52 FR 8831, Mar. 19, 1987, as amended at 52 FR 23031, June 17, 1987; 53 FR 1918, Jan. 25, 1988; 67 FR 9585, Mar. 4, 2002]

### §312.32 IND safety reports.

(a) *Definitions.* The following definitions of terms apply to this section:-

Associated with the use of the drug. There is a reasonable possibility that the experience may have been caused by the drug.

*Disability.* A substantial disruption of a person's ability to conduct normal life functions.

*Life-threatening adverse drug experience.* Any adverse drug experience that places the patient or subject, in the view of the investigator, at immediate risk of death from the reaction as it occurred, i.e., it does not include a reaction that, had it occurred in a more severe form, might have caused death.

*Serious adverse drug experience:* Any adverse drug experience occurring at any dose that results in any of the following outcomes: Death, a life-threatening adverse drug experience, inpatient hospitalization or prolongation of existing hospitalization, a persistent or significant disability/incapacity, or a congenital anomaly/birth defect. Important medical events that may not result in death, be life-threatening, or require hospitalization may be considered a serious adverse drug experience when, based upon appropriate medical judgment, they may jeopardize the patient or subject and may require medical or surgical intervention to prevent one of the outcomes listed in this definition. Examples of such medical events include allergic bronchospasm requiring intensive treatment in an emergency room or at home, blood dyscrasias or convulsions that do not result in inpatient hospitalization, or the development of drug dependency or drug abuse.

*Unexpected adverse drug experience:* Any adverse drug experience, the specificity or severity of which is not consistent with the current investigator brochure; or, if an investigator brochure is not required or available, the specificity or severity of which is not consistent with the risk information described in the general investigational plan or elsewhere in the current application, as amended. For example, under this definition, hepatic necrosis would be unexpected (by virtue of greater severity) if the investigator brochure only referred to elevated hepatic enzymes or hepatitis. Similarly, cerebral thromboembolism and cerebral vasculitis would be unexpected (by virtue of greater specificity) if the investigator brochure only listed cerebral vascular accidents. "Unexpected," as used in this definition, refers to an adverse drug experience that has not been previously observed (e.g., included in the investigator brochure) rather than from the perspective of such experience not being anticipated from the pharmacological properties of the pharmaceutical product.

(b) *Review of safety information.* The sponsor shall promptly review all information relevant to the safety of the drug obtained or otherwise received by the sponsor from any source, foreign or domestic, including information derived from any clinical or epidemiological investigations, animal investigations, commercial marketing experience, reports in the scientific literature, and unpublished scientific papers, as well as reports from foreign regulatory authorities that have not already been previously reported to the agency by the sponsor.

(c) IND *safety reports.* (1) *Written reports*—(i) The sponsor shall notify FDA and all participating investigators in a written IND safety report of:

(A) Any adverse experience associated with the use of the drug that is both serious and unexpected; or

(B) Any finding from tests in laboratory animals that suggests a significant risk for human subjects including reports of mutagenicity, teratogenicity, or carcinogenicity. Each notification shall be made as soon as possible and in no event later than 15 calendar days after the sponsor's initial receipt of the information. Each written notification may be submitted on FDA Form 3500A or in a narrative format (foreign events may be submitted either on an FDA Form 3500A or, if preferred, on a CIOMS I form; reports from animal or epidemiological studies shall be submitted in a narrative format) and shall bear prominent identification of its contents, i.e., "IND Safety Report." Each written notification to FDA shall be transmitted to the FDA new drug review division in the Center for Drug Evaluation and Research or the product review division in the Center for Biologics Evaluation and Research that has responsibility for review of the IND. If FDA determines that additional data are needed, the agency may require further data to be submitted.

(ii) In each written IND safety report, the sponsor shall identify all safety reports previously filed with the IND concerning a similar adverse experience, and shall analyze the significance of the adverse experience in light of the previouos, similar reports.

(2) *Telephone and facsimile transmission safety reports.* The sponsor shall also notify FDA by telephone or by facsimile transmission of any unexpected fatal or life-threatening experience associated with the use of the drug as soon as possible but in no event later than 7 calendar days after the sponsor's initial receipt of the information. Each telephone call or facsimile transmission to FDA shall be transmitted to the FDA new drug review division in the Center for Drug Evaluation and Research or the product review division in the Center for Biologics Evaluation and Research that has responsibility for review of the IND.

(3) *Reporting format or frequency.* FDA may request a sponsor to submit IND safety reports in a format or at a frequency different than that required under this paragraph. The sponsor may also propose and adopt a different reporting format or frequency if the change is agreed to in advance by the director of the new drug review division in the Center for Drug Evaluation and Research or the director of the products review division in the Center for Biologics Evaluation and Research which is responsible for review of the IND.

(4) A sponsor of a clinical study of a marketed drug is not required to make a safety report for any adverse experience associated with use of the drug that is not from the clinical study itself.

(d) *Followup.* (1) The sponsor shall promptly investigate all safety information received by it.

(2) Followup information to a safety report shall be submitted as soon as the relevant information is available.

(3) If the results of a sponsor's investigation show that an adverse drug experience not initially determined to be reportable under paragraph (c) of this section is so reportable, the sponsor shall report such experience in a written safety report as soon as possible, but in no event later than 15 calendar days after the determination is made.

(4) Results of a sponsor's investigation of other safety information shall be submitted, as appropriate, in an information amendment or annual report.

(e) *Disclaimer.* A safety report or other information submitted by a sponsor under this part (and any release by FDA of that report or information) does not necessarily reflect a conclusion by the sponsor or FDA that the report or information constitutes an admission that the drug caused or contributed to an adverse experience. A sponsor need not admit, and may deny, that the report or information submitted by the sponsor constitutes an admission that the drug caused or contributed to an adverse experience.

[52 FR 8831, Mar. 19, 1987, as amended at 52 FR 23031, June 17, 1987; 55 FR 11579, Mar. 29, 1990; 62 FR 52250, Oct. 7, 1997; 67 FR 9585, Mar. 4, 2002]

## §312.33 Annual reports.

A sponsor shall within 60 days of the anniversary date that the IND went into effect, submit a brief report of the progress of the investigation that includes:

(a) *Individual study information.* A brief summary of the status of each study in progress and each study completed during the previous year. The summary is required to include the following information for each study:

(1) The title of the study (with any appropriate study identifiers such as protocol number), its purpose, a brief statement identifying the patient population, and a statement as to whether the study is completed.

(2) The total number of subjects initially planned for inclusion in the study; the number entered into the study to date, tabulated by age group, gender, and race; the number whose participation in the study was completed as planned; and the number who dropped out of the study for any reason.

(3) If the study has been completed, or if interim results are known, a brief description of any available study results.

(b) *Summary information.* Information obtained during the previous year's clinical and nonclinical investigations, including:

(1) A narrative or tabular summary showing the most frequent and most serious adverse experiences by body system.

(2) A summary of all IND safety reports submitted during the past year.

(3) A list of subjects who died during participation in the investigation, with the cause of death for each subject.

(4) A list of subjects who dropped out during the course of the investigation in association with any adverse experience, whether or not thought to be drug related.

(5) A brief description of what, if anything, was obtained that is pertinent to an understanding of the drug's actions, including, for example, information about dose response, information from controlled trails, and information about bioavailability.

(6) A list of the preclinical studies (including animal studies) completed or in progress during the past year and a summary of the major preclinical findings.

(7) A summary of any significant manufacturing or microbiological changes made during the past year.

(c) A description of the general investigational plan for the coming year to replace that submitted 1 year earlier. The general investigational plan shall contain the information required under §312.23(a)(3)(iv).

(d) If the investigator brochure has been revised, a description of the revision and a copy of the new brochure.

(e) A description of any significant Phase 1 protocol modifications made during the previous year and not previously reported to the IND in a protocol amendment.

(f) A brief summary of significant foreign marketing developments with the drug during the past year, such as approval of marketing in any country or withdrawal or suspension from marketing in any country.

(g) If desired by the sponsor, a log of any outstanding business with respect to the IND for which the sponsor requests or expects a reply, comment, or meeting.

[52 FR 8831, Mar. 19, 1987, as amended at 52 FR 23031, June 17, 1987; 63 FR 6862, Feb. 11, 1998; 67 FR 9585, Mar. 4, 2002]

## §312.34 Treatment use of an investigational new drug.

(a) *General.* A drug that is not approved for marketing may be under clinical investigation for a serious or immediately life-threatening disease condition in patients for whom no comparable or satisfactory alternative drug or other therapy is available. During the clinical investigation of the drug, it may be appropriate to use the drug in the treatment of patients not in the clinical trials, in accordance with a treatment protocol or treatment IND. The purpose of this section is to facilitate the availability of promising new drugs to desperately ill patients as early in the drug development process as possible, before general marketing begins, and to obtain additional data on the drug's safety and effectiveness. In the case of a serious disease, a drug ordinarily may be made available for treatment use under this section during Phase 3 investigations or after all clinical trials have been completed; however, in appropriate circumstances, a drug may be made available for treatment use during Phase 2. In the case of an immediately life-threatening disease, a drug may be made available for treatment use under this section earlier than Phase 3, but ordinarily not earlier than Phase 2. For purposes of this section, the "treatment use" of a drug includes the use of a drug for diagnostic purposes. If a protocol for an investigational drug meets the criteria of this section, the protocol is to be submitted as a treatment protocol under the provisions of this section.

(b) *Criteria.* (1) FDA shall permit an investigational drug to be used for a treatment use under a treatment protocol or treatment IND if:

(i) The drug is intended to treat a serious or immediately life-threatening disease;

(ii) There is no comparable or satisfactory alternative drug or other therapy available to treat that stage of the disease in the intended patient population;

(iii) The drug is under investigation in a controlled clinical trial under an IND in effect for the trial, or all clinical trials have been completed; and

(iv) The sponsor of the controlled clinical trial is actively pursuing marketing approval of the investigational drug with due diligence.

(2) *Serious disease.* For a drug intended to treat a serious disease, the Commissioner may deny a request for treatment use under a treatment protocol or treatment IND if there is insufficient evidence of safety and effectiveness to support such use.

(3) *Immediately life-threatening disease.* (i) For a drug intended to treat an immediately life-threatening disease, the Commissioner may deny a request for treatment use of an investigational drug under a treatment protocol or treatment IND if the available scientific evidence, taken as a whole, fails to provide a reasonable basis for concluding that the drug:

(A) May be effective for its intended use in its intended patient population; or

(B) Would not expose the patients to whom the drug is to be administered to an unreasonable and significant additional risk of illness or injury.

(ii) For the purpose of this section, an "immediately life-threatening" disease means a stage of a disease in which there is a reasonable likelihood that death will occur within a matter of months or in which premature death is likely without early treatment.

(c) *Safeguards.* Treatment use of an investigational drug is conditioned on the sponsor and investigators complying with the safeguards of the IND process, including the regulations governing informed consent (21 CFR part 50) and institutional review boards (21 CFR part 56) and the applicable provisions of part 312, including distribution of the drug through qualified experts, maintenance of adequate manufacturing facilities, and submission of IND safety reports.

(d) *Clinical hold.* FDA may place on clinical hold a proposed or ongoing treatment protocol or treatment IND in accordance with §312.42.

[52 FR 19476, May 22, 1987, as amended at 57 FR 13248, Apr. 15, 1992]

### §312.35 Submissions for treatment use.

(a) *Treatment protocol submitted by* IND *sponsor.* Any sponsor of a clinical investigation of a drug who intends to sponsor a treatment use for the drug shall submit to FDA a treatment protocol under §312.34 if the sponsor believes the criteria of §312.34 are satisfied. If a protocol is not submitted under §312.34, but FDA believes that the protocol should have been submitted under this section, FDA may deem the protocol to be submitted under §312.34. A treatment use under a treatment protocol may begin 30 days after FDA receives the protocol or on earlier notification by FDA that the treatment use described in the protocol may begin.

(1) A treatment protocol is required to contain the following:

(i) The intended use of the drug.

(ii) An explanation of the rationale for use of the drug, including, as appropriate, either a list of what available regimens ordinarily should be tried before using the investigational drug or an explanation of why the use of the investigational drug is preferable to the use of available marketed treatments.

(iii) A brief description of the criteria for patient selection.

(iv) The method of administration of the drug and the dosages.

(v) A description of clinical procedures, laboratory tests, or other measures to monitor the effects of the drug and to minimize risk.

(2) A treatment protocol is to be supported by the following:

(i) Informational brochure for supplying to each treating physician.

(ii) The technical information that is relevant to safety and effectiveness of the drug for the intended treatment purpose. Information contained in the sponsor's IND may be incorporated by reference.

(iii) A commitment by the sponsor to assure compliance of all participating investigators with the informed consent requirements of 21 CFR part 50.

(3) A licensed practioner who receives an investigational drug for treatment use under a treatment protocol is an "investigator" under the protocol and is responsible for meeting all applicable investigator responsibilities under this part and 21 CFR parts 50 and 56.

(b) *Treatment* IND *submitted by licensed practitioner.* (1) If a licensed medical practitioner wants to obtain an investigational drug subject to a controlled clinical trial for a treatment use, the practitioner should first attempt to obtain the drug from the sponsor of the controlled trial under a treatment protocol. If the sponsor of the controlled clinical investigation of the drug will not establish a treatment protocol for the drug under paragraph (a) of this section, the licensed medical practitioner may seek to obtain the drug from the sponsor and submit a treatment IND to FDA requesting authorization to use the investigational drug for treatment use. A treatment use under a treatment IND may begin 30 days after FDA receives the IND or on earlier notification by FDA that the treatment use under the IND may begin. A treatment IND is required to contain the following:

(i) A cover sheet (Form FDA 1571) meeting §312.23(g)(1).

(ii) Information (when not provided by the sponsor) on the drug's chemistry, manufacturing, and controls, and prior clinical and nonclinical experience with the drug submitted in accordance with §312.23. A sponsor of a clinical investigation subject to an IND who supplies an investigational drug to a licensed medical practitioner for purposes of a separate treatment clinical investigation shall be deemed to authorize the incorporation-by-reference of the technical information contained in the sponsor's IND into the medical practitioner's treatment IND.

(iii) A statement of the steps taken by the practitioner to obtain the drug under a treatment protocol from the drug sponsor.

(iv) A treatment protocol containing the same information listed in paragraph (a)(1) of this section.

(v) A statement of the practitioner's qualifications to use the investigational drug for the intended treatment use.

(vi) The practitioner's statement of familiarity with information on the drug's safety and effectiveness derived from previous clinical and nonclinical experience with the drug.

(vii) Agreement to report to FDA safety information in accordance with §312.32.

(2) A licensed practitioner who submits a treatment IND under this section is the sponsor-investigator for such IND and is responsible for meeting all applicable sponsor and investigator responsibilities under this part and 21 CFR parts 50 and 56.

[52 FR 19477, May 22, 1987, as amended at 57 FR 13249, Apr. 15, 1992; 67 FR 9585, Mar. 4, 2002]

## §312.36 Emergency use of an investigational new drug (IND).

Need for an investigational drug may arise in an emergency situation that does not allow time for submission of an IND in accordance with 312.23 or 312.34. In such a case, FDA may authorize shipment of the drug for a specified use in advance of submission of an IND. A request for such authorization may be transmitted to FDA by telephone or other rapid communication means. For investigational biological drugs regulated by the Center for Biologics Evaluation and Research, the request should be directed to the Office of Communication, Training and Manufacturers Assistance (HFM-40), Center for Biologics Evaluation and Research, 301-827-2000. For all other investigational drugs, the request for authorization should be directed to the Division of Drug Information (HFD-240), Center for Drug Evaluation and Research, 301-827-4570. After normal working hours, eastern standard time, the request should be directed to the FDA Office of Emergency Operations (HFA-615), 301-443-1240. Except in extraordinary circumstances, such authorization will be conditioned on the sponsor making an appropriate IND submission as soon as practicable after receiving the authorization.

[69 FR 17927, Apr. 6, 2004]

§312.38 Withdrawal of an IND.

(a) At any time a sponsor may withdraw an effective IND without prejudice.

(b) If an IND is withdrawn, FDA shall be so notified, all clinical investigations conducted under the IND shall be ended, all current investigators notified, and all stocks of the drug returned to the sponsor or otherwise disposed of at the request of the sponsor in accordance with §312.59.

(c) If an IND is withdrawn because of a safety reason, the sponsor shall promptly so inform FDA, all participating investigators, and all reviewing Institutional Review Boards, together with the reasons for such withdrawal. [52 FR 8831, Mar. 19, 1987, as amended at 52 FR 23031, June 17, 1987; 67 FR 9586, Mar. 4, 2002]

## Subpart C—Administrative Actions

§312.40 General requirements for use of an investigational new drug in a clinical investigation.

(a) An investigational new drug may be used in a clinical investigation if the following conditions are met:

(1) The sponsor of the investigation submits an IND for the drug to FDA; the IND is in effect under paragraph (b) of this section; and the sponsor complies with all applicable requirements in this part and parts 50 and 56 with respect to the conduct of the clinical investigations; and

(2) Each participating investigator conducts his or her investigation in compliance with the requirements of this part and parts 50 and 56.
(b) An IND goes into effect:

(1) Thirty days after FDA receives the IND, unless FDA notifies the sponsor that the investigations described in the IND are subject to a clinical hold under §312.42; or

(2) On earlier notification by FDA that the clinical investigations in the IND may begin. FDA will notify the sponsor in writing of the date it receives the IND.

(c) A sponsor may ship an investigational new drug to investigators named in the IND:

(1) Thirty days after FDA receives the IND; or

(2) On earlier FDA authorization to ship the drug.

(d) An investigator may not administer an investigational new drug to human subjects until the IND goes into effect under paragraph (b) of this section.

## §312.41 Comment and advice on an IND.

(a) FDA may at any time during the course of the investigation communicate with the sponsor orally or in writing about deficiencies in the IND or about FDA's need for more data or information.

(b) On the sponsor's request, FDA will provide advice on specific matters relating to an IND. Examples of such advice may include advice on the adequacy of technical data to support an investigational plan, on the design of a clinical trial, and on whether proposed investigations are likely to produce the data and information that is needed to meet requirements for a marketing application.

(c) Unless the communication is accompanied by a clinical hold order under §312.42, FDA communications with a sponsor under this section are solely advisory and do not require any modification in the planned or ongoing clinical investigations or response to the agency.

[52 FR 8831, Mar. 19, 1987, as amended at 52 FR 23031, June 17, 1987; 67 FR 9586, Mar. 4, 2002]

## §312.42 Clinical holds and requests for modification.

(a) *General.* A clinical hold is an order issued by FDA to the sponsor to delay a proposed clinical investigation or to suspend an ongoing investigation. The clinical hold order may apply to one or more of the investigations covered by an IND. When a proposed study is placed on clinical hold, subjects may not be given the investigational drug. When an ongoing study is placed on clinical hold, no new subjects may be recruited to the study and placed on the investigational drug; patients already in the study should be taken off therapy involving the investigational drug unless specifically permitted by FDA in the interest of patient safety.

(b) *Grounds for imposition of clinical hold*—(1) *Clinical hold of a Phase 1 study under an* IND. FDA may place a proposed or ongoing Phase 1 investigation on clinical hold if it finds that:

(i) Human subjects are or would be exposed to an unreasonable and significant risk of illness or injury;

(ii) The clinical investigators named in the IND are not qualified by reason of their scientific training and experience to conduct the investigation described in the IND;

(iii) The investigator brochure is misleading, erroneous, or materially incomplete; or

(iv) The IND does not contain sufficient information required under §312.23 to assess the risks to subjects of the proposed studies.

(v) The IND is for the study of an investigational drug intended to treat a life-threatening disease or condition that affects both genders, and men or women with reproductive potential who have the disease or condition being studied are excluded from eligibility because of a risk or potential risk from use of the investigational drug of reproductive toxicity (i.e., affecting reproductive organs) or developmental toxicity (i.e., affecting potential offspring). The phrase "women with reproductive potential" does not include pregnant women. For purposes of this paragraph, "life-threatening illnesses or diseases" are defined as "diseases or conditions where the likelihood of death is high unless the course of the disease is interrupted." The clinical hold would not apply under this paragraph to clinical studies conducted:

(A) Under special circumstances, such as studies pertinent only to one gender (e.g., studies evaluating the excretion of a drug in semen or the effects on menstrual function);

(B) Only in men or women, as long as a study that does not exclude members of the other gender with reproductive potential is being conducted concurrently, has been conducted, or will take place within a reasonable time agreed upon by the agency; or

(C) Only in subjects who do not suffer from the disease or condition for which the drug is being studied.

(2) *Clinical hold of a Phase 2 or 3 study under an* IND. FDA may place a proposed or ongoing Phase 2 or 3 investigation on clinical hold if it finds that:

(i) Any of the conditions in paragraphs (b)(1)(i) through (b)(1)(v) of this section apply; or
(ii) The plan or protocol for the investigation is clearly deficient in design to meet its stated objectives.

(3) Clinical hold of a treatment IND or treatment protocol.

(i) *Proposed use.* FDA may place a proposed treatment IND or treatment protocol on clinical hold if it is determined that:

(A) The pertinent criteria in §312.34(b) for permitting the treatment use to begin are not satisfied; or

(B) The treatment protocol or treatment IND does not contain the information required under §312.35 (a) or (b) to make the specified determination under §312.34(b).

(ii) *Ongoing use.* FDA may place an ongoing treatment protocol or treatment IND on clinical hold if it is determined that:

(A) There becomes available a comparable or satisfactory alternative drug or other therapy to treat that stage of the disease in the intended patient population for which the investigational drug is being used;

(B) The investigational drug is not under investigation in a controlled clinical trial under an IND in effect for the trial and not all controlled clinical trials necessary to support a marketing application have been completed, or a clinical study under the IND has been placed on clinical hold:

(C) The sponsor of the controlled clinical trial is not pursuing marketing approval with due diligence;

(D) If the treatment IND or treatment protocol is intended for a serious disease, there is insufficient evidence of safety and effectiveness to support such use; or

(E) If the treatment protocol or treatment IND was based on an immediately life-threatening disease, the available scientific evidence, taken as a whole, fails to provide a reasonable basis for concluding that the drug:
(1) May be effective for its intended use in its intended population; or

(2 ) Would not expose the patients to whom the drug is to be administered to an unreasonable and significant additional risk of illness or injury.

(iii) FDA may place a proposed or ongoing treatment IND or treatment protocol on clinical hold if it finds that any of the conditions in paragraph (b)(4)(i) through (b)(4)(viii) of this section apply.

(4) *Clinical hold of any study that is not designed to be adequate and well-controlled.* FDA may place a proposed or ongoing investigation that is not designed to be adequate and well-controlled on clinical hold if it finds that:

(i) Any of the conditions in paragraph (b)(1) or (b)(2) of this section apply; or

(ii) There is reasonable evidence the investigation that is not designed to be adequate and well-controlled is impeding enrollment in, or otherwise interfering with the conduct or completion of, a study that is designed to be an adequate and well-controlled investigation of the same or another investigational drug; or

(iii) Insufficient quantities of the investigational drug exist to adequately conduct both the investigation that is not designed to be adequate and well-controlled and the investigations that are designed to be adequate and well-controlled; or

(iv) The drug has been studied in one or more adequate and well-controlled investigations that strongly suggest lack of effectiveness; or

(v) Another drug under investigation or approved for the same indication and available to the same patient population has demonstrated a better potential benefit/risk balance; or

(vi) The drug has received marketing approval for the same indication in the same patient population; or

(vii) The sponsor of the study that is designed to be an adequate and well-controlled investigation is not actively pursuing marketing approval of the investigational drug with due diligence; or

(viii) The Commissioner determines that it would not be in the public interest for the study to be conducted or continued. FDA ordinarily intends that clinical holds under paragraphs (b)(4)(ii), (b)(4)(iii) and (b)(4)(v) of this section would only apply to additional enrollment in nonconcurrently controlled trials rather than eliminating continued access to individuals already receiving the investigational drug.

(5) *Clinical hold of any investigation involving an exception from informed consent under §50.24 of this chapter.* FDA may place a proposed or ongoing investigation involving an exception from informed consent under §50.24 of this chapter on clinical hold if it is determined that:

(i) Any of the conditions in paragraphs (b)(1) or (b)(2) of this section apply; or

(ii) The pertinent criteria in §50.24 of this chapter for such an investigation to begin or continue are not submitted or not satisfied.

(6) Clinical hold of any investigation involving an exception from informed consent under §50.23(d) of this chapter. FDA may place a proposed or ongo-

ing investigation involving an exception from informed consent under §50.23(d) of this chapter on clinical hold if it is determined that:

(i) Any of the conditions in paragraphs (b)(1) or (b)(2) of this section apply; or

(ii) A determination by the President to waive the prior consent requirement for the administration of an investigational new drug has not been made.

(c) *Discussion of deficiency.* Whenever FDA concludes that a deficiency exists in a clinical investigation that may be grounds for the imposition of clinical hold FDA will, unless patients are exposed to immediate and serious risk, attempt to discuss and satisfactorily resolve the matter with the sponsor before issuing the clinical hold order.

(d) *Imposition of clinical hold.* The clinical hold order may be made by telephone or other means of rapid communication or in writing. The clinical hold order will identify the studies under the IND to which the hold applies, and will briefly explain the basis for the action. The clinical hold order will be made by or on behalf of the Division Director with responsibility for review of the IND. As soon as possible, and no more than 30 days after imposition of the clinical hold, the Division Director will provide the sponsor a written explanation of the basis for the hold.

(e) *Resumption of clinical investigations.* An investigation may only resume after FDA (usually the Division Director, or the Director's designee, with responsibility for review of the IND) has notified the sponsor that the investigation may proceed. Resumption of the affected investigation(s) will be authorized when the sponsor corrects the deficiency(ies) previously cited or otherwise satisfies the agency that the investigation(s) can proceed. FDA may notify a sponsor of its determination regarding the clinical hold by telephone or other means of rapid communication. If a sponsor of an IND that has been placed on clinical hold requests in writing that the clinical hold be removed and submits a complete response to the issue(s) identified in the clinical hold order, FDA shall respond in writing to the sponsor within 30-calendar days of receipt of the request and the complete response. FDA's response will either remove or maintain the clinical hold, and will state the reasons for such determination. Notwithstanding the 30-calendar day response time, a sponsor may not proceed with a clinical trial on which a clinical hold has been imposed until the sponsor has been notified by FDA that the hold has been lifted.

(f) *Appeal.* If the sponsor disagrees with the reasons cited for the clinical hold, the sponsor may request reconsideration of the decision in accordance with §312.48.

(g) *Conversion of* IND *on clinical hold to inactive status.* If all investigations covered by an IND remain on clinical hold for 1 year or more, the IND may be placed on inactive status by FDA under §312.45.

[52 FR 8831, Mar. 19, 1987, as amended at 52 FR 19477, May 22, 1987; 57 FR 13249, Apr. 15, 1992; 61 FR 51530, Oct. 2, 1996; 63 FR 68678, Dec. 14, 1998; 64 FR 54189, Oct. 5, 1999; 65 FR 34971, June 1, 2000]

## §312.44 Termination.

(a) *General.* This section describes the procedures under which FDA may terminate an IND. If an IND is terminated, the sponsor shall end all clinical investigations conducted under the IND and recall or otherwise provide for the disposition of all unused supplies of the drug. A termination action may be based on deficiencies in the IND or in the conduct of an investigation under an IND. Except as provided in paragraph (d) of this section, a termination shall be preceded by a proposal to terminate by FDA and an opportunity for the sponsor to respond. FDA will, in general, only initiate an action under this section after first attempting to resolve differences informally or, when appropriate, through the clinical hold procedures described in §312.42.

(b) *Grounds for termination*—(1) *Phase 1.* FDA may propose to terminate an IND during Phase 1 if it finds that:

(i) Human subjects would be exposed to an unreasonable and significant risk of illness or unjury.

(ii) The IND does not contain sufficient information required under §312.23 to assess the safety to subjects of the clinical investigations.

(iii) The methods, facilities, and controls used for the manufacturing, processing, and packing of the investigational drug are inadequate to establish and maintain appropriate standards of identity, strength, quality, and purity as needed for subject safety.

(iv) The clinical investigations are being conducted in a manner substantially different than that described in the protocols submitted in the IND.

(v) The drug is being promoted or distributed for commercial purposes not justified by the requirements of the investigation or permitted by §312.7.

(vi) The IND, or any amendment or report to the IND, contains an untrue statement of a material fact or omits material information required by this part.

(vii) The sponsor fails promptly to investigate and inform the Food and Drug Administration and all investigators of serious and unexpected adverse experiences in accordance with §312.32 or fails to make any other report required under this part.

(viii) The sponsor fails to submit an accurate annual report of the investigations in accordance with §312.33.

(ix) The sponsor fails to comply with any other applicable requirement of this part, part 50, or part 56.

(x) The IND has remained on inactive status for 5 years or more.

(xi) The sponsor fails to delay a proposed investigation under the IND or to suspend an ongoing investigation that has been placed on clinical hold under §312.42(b)(4).

(2) *Phase 2 or 3.* FDA may propose to terminate an IND during Phase 2 or Phase 3 if FDA finds that:

(i) Any of the conditions in paragraphs (b)(1)(i) through (b)(1)(xi) of this section apply; or

(ii) The investigational plan or protocol(s) is not reasonable as a bona fide scientific plan to determine whether or not the drug is safe and effective for use; or

(iii) There is convincing evidence that the drug is not effective for the purpose for which it is being investigated.

(3) FDA may propose to terminate a treatment IND if it finds that:

(i) Any of the conditions in paragraphs (b)(1)(i) through (x) of this section apply; or

(ii) Any of the conditions in §312.42(b)(3) apply.

(c) *Opportunity for sponsor response.* (1) If FDA proposes to terminate an IND, FDA will notify the sponsor in writing, and invite correction or explanation within a period of 30 days.

(2) On such notification, the sponsor may provide a written explanation or correction or may request a conference with FDA to provide the requested explanation or correction. If the sponsor does not respond to the notification within the allocated time, the IND shall be terminated.

(3) If the sponsor responds but FDA does not accept the explanation or correction submitted, FDA shall inform the sponsor in writing of the reason for the nonacceptance and provide the sponsor with an opportunity for a regulatory hearing before FDA under part 16 on the question of whether the IND should be terminated. The sponsor's request for a regulatory hearing must be made within 10 days of the sponsor's receipt of FDA's notification of nonacceptance.

(d) *Immediate termination of* IND. Notwithstanding paragraphs (a) through (c) of this section, if at any time FDA concludes that continuation of the investigation presents an immediate and substantial danger to the health of individuals, the agency shall immediately, by written notice to the sponsor from the Director of the Center for Drug Evaluation and Research or the Director of the Center for Biologics Evaluation and Research, terminate the IND. An IND so terminated is subject to reinstatement by the Director on the basis of additional submissions that eliminate such danger. If an IND is terminated under this paragraph, the agency will afford the sponsor an opportunity for a regulatory hearing under part 16 on the question of whether the IND should be reinstated.

[52 FR 8831, Mar. 19, 1987, as amended at 52 FR 23031, June 17, 1987; 55 FR 11579, Mar. 29, 1990; 57 FR 13249, Apr. 15, 1992; 67 FR 9586, Mar. 4, 2002]

§312.45 **Inactive status.**

(a) If no subjects are entered into clinical studies for a period of 2 years or more under an IND, or if all investigations under an IND remain on clinical hold for 1 year or more, the IND may be placed by FDA on inactive status. This action may be taken by FDA either on request of the sponsor or on FDA's own initiative. If FDA seeks to act on its own initiative under this section, it shall first notify the sponsor in writing of the proposed inactive status. Upon receipt of such notification, the sponsor shall have 30 days to respond as to why the IND should continue to remain active.

(b) If an IND is placed on inactive status, all investigators shall be so notified and all stocks of the drug shall be returned or otherwise disposed of in accordance with §312.59.

(c) A sponsor is not required to submit annual reports to an IND on inactive status. An inactive IND is, however, still in effect for purposes of the public disclosure of data and information under §312.130.

(d) A sponsor who intends to resume clinical investigation under an IND placed on inactive status shall submit a protocol amendment under §312.30 containing the proposed general investigational plan for the coming year and appropriate protocols. If the protocol amendment relies on information previously submitted, the plan shall reference such information. Additional information supporting the proposed investigation, if any, shall be submitted in an information amendment. Notwithstanding the provisions of §312.30, clinical investigations under an IND on inactive status may only resume (1) 30 days after FDA receives the protocol amendment, unless FDA notifies the sponsor that the investigations described in the amendment are subject to a clinical hold under §312.42, or (2) on earlier notification by FDA that the clinical investigations described in the protocol amendment may begin.

(e) An IND that remains on inactive status for 5 years or more may be terminated under §312.44.

[52 FR 8831, Mar. 19, 1987, as amended at 52 FR 23031, June 17, 1987; 67 FR 9586, Mar. 4, 2002]

## §312.47 Meetings.

(a) *General.* Meetings between a sponsor and the agency are frequently useful in resolving questions and issues raised during the course of a clinical investigation. FDA encourages such meetings to the extent that they aid in the evaluation of the drug and in the solution of scientific problems concerning the drug, to the extent that FDA's resources permit. The general principle underlying the conduct of such meetings is that there should be free, full, and open communication about any scientific or medical question that may arise during the clinical investigation. These meetings shall be conducted and documented in accordance with part 10.

(b) *"End-of-Phase 2" meetings and meetings held before submission of a marketing application.* At specific times during the drug investigation process, meetings between FDA and a sponsor can be especially helpful in minimizing wasteful expenditures of time and money and thus in speeding the drug development and evaluation process. In particular, FDA has found that meetings at the end of Phase 2 of an investigation (end-of-Phase 2 meetings) are of considerable assistance in planning later studies and that meetings held near completion of Phase 3 and before submission of a marketing application ("pre-NDA" meetings) are helpful in developing methods of presentation and submission of data in the marketing application that facilitate review and allow timely FDA response.

(1) *End-of-Phase 2 meetings*—(i) *Purpose.* The purpose of an end-of-phase 2 meeting is to determine the safety of proceeding to Phase 3, to evaluate the Phase 3 plan and protocols and the adequacy of current studies and plans to assess pediatric safety and effectiveness, and to identify any additional information necessary to support a marketing application for the uses under investigation.

(ii) *Eligibility for meeting.* While the end-of-Phase 2 meeting is designed primarily for IND's involving new molecular entities or major new uses of marketed drugs, a sponsor of any IND may request and obtain an end-of-Phase 2 meeting.

(iii) *Timing.* To be most useful to the sponsor, end-of-Phase 2 meetings should be held before major commitments of effort and resources to specific Phase 3 tests are made. The scheduling of an end-of-Phase 2 meeting is not, however, intended to delay the transition of an investigation from Phase 2 to Phase 3.

(iv) *Advance information.* At least 1 month in advance of an end-of-Phase 2 meeting, the sponsor should submit background information on the sponsor's plan for Phase 3, including summaries of the Phase 1 and 2 investigations, the specific protocols for Phase 3 clinical studies, plans for any additional nonclinical studies, plans for pediatric studies, including a time line for protocol finalization, enrollment, completion, and data analysis, or information to support any planned request for waiver or deferral of pediatric studies, and, if available, tentative labeling for the drug. The recommended contents of such a submission are described more fully in FDA Staff Manual Guide 4850.7 that is publicly available under FDA's public information regulations in part 20.

(v) *Conduct of meeting.* Arrangements for an end-of-Phase 2 meeting are to be made with the division in FDA's Center for Drug Evaluation and Research or the Center for Biologics Evaluation and Research which is responsible for review of the IND. The meeting will be scheduled by FDA at a time convenient to both FDA and the sponsor. Both the sponsor and FDA may bring consultants to the meeting. The meeting should be directed primarily at establishing agreement between FDA and the sponsor of the overall plan for Phase 3 and the objectives and design of particular studies. The adequacy of the technical information to support Phase 3 studies and/or a marketing application may also be discussed. FDA will also provide its best judgment, at that time, of the pediatric studies that will be required for the drug product and whether their submission will be deferred until after approval. Agreements reached at the meeting on these matters will be recorded in minutes of the conference that will be taken by FDA in accordance with §10.65 and provided to the sponsor. The minutes along with any other written material provided to the sponsor will serve as a permanent record of any agreements reached. Barring a significant scientific development that requires otherwise, studies conducted in accordance with the agreement shall be presumed to be sufficient in objective and design for the purpose of obtaining marketing approval for the drug.

(2) *"Pre-NDA" and "pre-BLA" meetings.* FDA has found that delays associated with the initial review of a marketing application may be reduced by

exchanges of information about a proposed marketing application. The primary purpose of this kind of exchange is to uncover any major unresolved problems, to identify those studies that the sponsor is relying on as adequate and well-controlled to establish the drug's effectiveness, to identify the status of ongoing or needed studies adequate to assess pediatric safety and effectiveness, to acquaint FDA reviewers with the general information to be submitted in the marketing application (including technical information), to discuss appropriate methods for statistical analysis of the data, and to discuss the best approach to the presentation and formatting of data in the marketing application. Arrangements for such a meeting are to be initiated by the sponsor with the division responsible for review of the IND. To permit FDA to provide the sponsor with the most useful advice on preparing a marketing application, the sponsor should submit to FDA's reviewing division at least 1 month in advance of the meeting the following information:

(i) A brief summary of the clinical studies to be submitted in the application.

(ii) A proposed format for organizing the submission, including methods for presenting the data.

(iii) Information on the status of needed or ongoing pediatric studies.

(iv) Any other information for discussion at the meeting.

[52 FR 8831, Mar. 19, 1987, as amended at 52 FR 23031, June 17, 1987; 55 FR 11580, Mar. 29, 1990; 63 FR 66669, Dec. 2, 1998; 67 FR 9586, Mar. 4, 2002]

## §312.48 Dispute resolution.

(a) *General.* The Food and Drug Administration is committed to resolving differences between sponsors and FDA reviewing divisions with respect to requirements for IND's as quickly and amicably as possible through the cooperative exchange of information and views.

(b) *Administrative and procedural issues.* When administrative or procedural disputes arise, the sponsor should first attempt to resolve the matter with the division in FDA's Center for Drug Evaluation and Research or Center for Biologics Evaluation and Research which is responsible for review of the IND, beginning with the consumer safety officer assigned to the application. If the dispute is not resolved, the sponsor may raise the matter with the person designated as ombudsman, whose function shall be to investigate what has happened and to facilitate a timely and equitable resolution. Appropriate issues to raise with the ombudsman include resolving difficulties in scheduling meetings and obtaining timely replies to inquiries. Further details on this procedure are contained in FDA Staff Manual Guide 4820.7

that is publicly available under FDA's public information regulations in part 20.

(c) *Scientific and medical disputes.* (1) When scientific or medical disputes arise during the drug investigation process, sponsors should discuss the matter directly with the responsible reviewing officials. If necessary, sponsors may request a meeting with the appropriate reviewing officials and management representatives in order to seek a resolution. Requests for such meetings shall be directed to the director of the division in FDA's Center for Drug Evaluation and Research or Center for Biologics Evaluation and Research which is responsible for review of the IND. FDA will make every attempt to grant requests for meetings that involve important issues and that can be scheduled at mutually convenient times.

(2) The "end-of-Phase 2" and "pre-NDA" meetings described in §312.47(b) will also provide a timely forum for discussing and resolving scientific and medical issues on which the sponsor disagrees with the agency.

(3) In requesting a meeting designed to resolve a scientific or medical dispute, applicants may suggest that FDA seek the advice of outside experts, in which case FDA may, in its discretion, invite to the meeting one or more of its advisory committee members or other consultants, as designated by the agency. Applicants may rely on, and may bring to any meeting, their own consultants. For major scientific and medical policy issues not resolved by informal meetings, FDA may refer the matter to one of its standing advisory committees for its consideration and recommendations.

[52 FR 8831, Mar. 19, 1987, as amended at 55 FR 11580, Mar. 29, 1990]

## Subpart D—Responsibilities of Sponsors and Investigators

### §312.50 General responsibilities of sponsors.

Sponsors are responsibile for selecting qualified investigators, providing them with the information they need to conduct an investigation properly, ensuring proper monitoring of the investigation(s), ensuring that the investigation(s) is conducted in accordance with the general investigational plan and protocols contained in the IND, maintaining an effective IND with respect to the investigations, and ensuring that FDA and all participating investigators are promptly informed of significant new adverse effects or risks with respect to the drug. Additional specific responsibilities of sponsors are described elsewhere in this part.

## §312.52 Transfer of obligations to a contract research organization.

(a) A sponsor may transfer responsibility for any or all of the obligations set forth in this part to a contract research organization. Any such transfer shall be described in writing. If not all obligations are transferred, the writing is required to describe each of the obligations being assumed by the contract research organization. If all obligations are transferred, a general statement that all obligations have been transferred is acceptable. Any obligation not covered by the written description shall be deemed not to have been transferred.

(b) A contract research organization that assumes any obligation of a sponsor shall comply with the specific regulations in this chapter applicable to this obligation and shall be subject to the same regulatory action as a sponsor for failure to comply with any obligation assumed under these regulations. Thus, all references to "sponsor" in this part apply to a contract research organization to the extent that it assumes one or more obligations of the sponsor.

## §312.53 Selecting investigators and monitors.

(a) *Selecting investigators.* A sponsor shall select only investigators qualified by training and experience as appropriate experts to investigate the drug.

(b) *Control of drug.* A sponsor shall ship investigational new drugs only to investigators participating in the investigation.

(c) *Obtaining information from the investigator.* Before permitting an investigator to begin participation in an investigation, the sponsor shall obtain the following:

(1) A signed investigator statement (Form FDA-1572) containing:
(i) The name and address of the investigator;

(ii) The name and code number, if any, of the protocol(s) in the IND identifying the study(ies) to be conducted by the investigator;

(iii) The name and address of any medical school, hospital, or other research facility where the clinical investigation(s) will be conducted;

(iv) The name and address of any clinical laboratory facilities to be used in the study;

(v) The name and address of the IRB that is responsible for review and approval of the study(ies);

(vi) A commitment by the investigator that he or she:

(a ) Will conduct the study(ies) in accordance with the relevant, current protocol(s) and will only make changes in a protocol after notifying the sponsor, except when necessary to protect the safety, the rights, or welfare of subjects;

(b ) Will comply with all requirements regarding the obligations of clinical investigators and all other pertinent requirements in this part;

(c) Will personally conduct or supervise the described investigation(s);

(d ) Will inform any potential subjects that the drugs are being used for investigational purposes and will ensure that the requirements relating to obtaining informed consent (21 CFR part 50) and institutional review board review and approval (21 CFR part 56) are met;

(e) Will report to the sponsor adverse experiences that occur in the course of the investigation(s) in accordance with §312.64;

(f ) Has read and understands the information in the investigator's brochure, including the potential risks and side effects of the drug; and

(g ) Will ensure that all associates, colleagues, and employees assisting in the conduct of the study(ies) are informed about their obligations in meeting the above commitments.

(vii) A commitment by the investigator that, for an investigation subject to an institutional review requirement under part 56, an IRB that complies with the requirements of that part will be responsible for the initial and continuing review and approval of the clinical investigation and that the investigator will promptly report to the IRB all changes in the research activity and all unanticipated problems involving risks to human subjects or others, and will not make any changes in the research without IRB approval, except where necessary to eliminate apparent immediate hazards to the human subjects.

(viii) A list of the names of the subinvestigators (e.g., research fellows, residents) who will be assisting the investigator in the conduct of the investigation(s).

(2) *Curriculum vitae.* A curriculum vitae or other statement of qualifications of the investigator showing the education, training, and experience that qualifies the investigator as an expert in the clinical investigation of the drug for the use under investigation.

(3) *Clinical protocol.* (i) For Phase 1 investigations, a general outline of the planned investigation including the estimated duration of the study and the maximum number of subjects that will be involved.

(ii) For Phase 2 or 3 investigations, an outline of the study protocol including an approximation of the number of subjects to be treated with the drug and the number to be employed as controls, if any; the clinical uses to be investigated; characteristics of subjects by age, sex, and condition; the kind of clinical observations and laboratory tests to be conducted; the estimated duration of the study; and copies or a description of case report forms to be used.

(4) *Financial disclosure information.* Sufficient accurate financial information to allow the sponsor to submit complete and accurate certification or disclosure statements required under part 54 of this chapter. The sponsor shall obtain a commitment from the clinical investigator to promptly update this information if any relevant changes occur during the course of the investigation and for 1 year following the completion of the study.

(d) *Selecting monitors.* A sponsor shall select a monitor qualified by training and experience to monitor the progress of the investigation.

[52 FR 8831, Mar. 19, 1987, as amended at 52 FR 23031, June 17, 1987; 61 FR 57280, Nov. 5, 1996; 63 FR 5252, Feb. 2, 1998; 67 FR 9586, Mar. 4, 2002]

## §312.54 Emergency research under 50.24 of this chapter.

(a) The sponsor shall monitor the progress of all investigations involving an exception from informed consent under 50.24 of this chapter. When the sponsor receives from the IRB information concerning the public disclosures required by 50.24(a)(7)(ii) and (a)(7)(iii) of this chapter, the sponsor promptly shall submit to the IND file and to Docket Number 95S-0158 in the Division of Dockets Management (HFA-305), Food and Drug Administration, 5630 Fishers Lane, rm. 1061, Rockville, MD 20852, copies of the information that was disclosed, identified by the IND number.

(b) The sponsor also shall monitor such investigations to identify when an IRB determines that it cannot approve the research because it does not meet the criteria in the exception in 50.24(a) of this chapter or because of other relevant ethical concerns. The sponsor promptly shall provide this information in writing to FDA, investigators who are asked to participate in this or a substantially equivalent clinical investigation, and other IRB's that are asked to review this or a substantially equivalent investigation.

[61 FR 51530, Oct. 2, 1996, as amended at 68 FR 24879, May 9, 2003]

## §312.55 Informing investigators.

(a) Before the investigation begins, a sponsor (other than a sponsor-investigator) shall give each participating clinical investigator an investigator brochure containing the information described in §312.23(a)(5).

(b) The sponsor shall, as the overall investigation proceeds, keep each participating investigator informed of new observations discovered by or reported to the sponsor on the drug, particularly with respect to adverse effects and safe use. Such information may be distributed to investigators by means of periodically revised investigator brochures, reprints or published studies, reports or letters to clinical investigators, or other appropriate means. Important safety information is required to be relayed to investigators in accordance with §312.32.

[52 FR 8831, Mar. 19, 1987, as amended at 52 FR 23031, June 17, 1987; 67 FR 9586, Mr. 4, 2002]

## §312.56 Review of ongoing investigations.

(a) The sponsor shall monitor the progress of all clinical investigations being conducted under its IND.

(b) A sponsor who discovers that an investigator is not complying with the signed agreement (Form FDA-1572), the general investigational plan, or the requirements of this part or other applicable parts shall promptly either secure compliance or discontinue shipments of the investigational new drug to the investigator and end the investigator's participation in the investigation. If the investigator's participation in the investigation is ended, the sponsor shall require that the investigator dispose of or return the investigational drug in accordance with the requirements of §312.59 and shall notify FDA.

(c) The sponsor shall review and evaluate the evidence relating to the safety and effectiveness of the drug as it is obtained from the investigator. The sponsors shall make such reports to FDA regarding information relevant to the safety of the drug as are required under §312.32. The sponsor shall make annual reports on the progress of the investigation in accordance with §312.33.

(d) A sponsor who determines that its investigational drug presents an unreasonable and significant risk to subjects shall discontinue those investigations that present the risk, notify FDA, all institutional review boards, and all investigators who have at any time participated in the investigation of the discontinuance, assure the disposition of all stocks of the drug outstanding as required by §312.59, and furnish FDA with a full report of the sponsor's actions. The sponsor shall discontinue the investigation as soon as possible, and in no event later than 5 working days after making the determination that the investigation should be discontinued. Upon request, FDA will confer with a sponsor on the need to discontinue an investigation.

[52 FR 8831, Mar. 19, 1987, as amended at 52 FR 23031, June 17, 1987; 67 FR 9586, Mar. 4, 2002]

## §312.57 Recordkeeping and record retention.

(a) A sponsor shall maintain adequate records showing the receipt, shipment, or other disposition of the investigational drug. These records are required to include, as appropriate, the name of the investigator to whom the drug is shipped, and the date, quantity, and batch or code mark of each such shipment.

(b) A sponsor shall maintain complete and accurate records showing any financial interest in §54.4(a)(3)(i), (a)(3)(ii), (a)(3)(iii), and (a)(3)(iv) of this chapter paid to clinical investigators by the sponsor of the covered study. A sponsor shall also maintain complete and accurate records concerning all other financial interests of investigators subject to part 54 of this chapter.

(c) A sponsor shall retain the records and reports required by this part for 2 years after a marketing application is approved for the drug; or, if an application is not approved for the drug, until 2 years after shipment and delivery of the drug for investigational use is discontinued and FDA has been so notified.

(d) A sponsor shall retain reserve samples of any test article and reference standard identified in, and used in any of the bioequivalence or bioavailability studies described in, §320.38 or §320.63 of this chapter, and release the reserve samples to FDA upon request, in accordance with, and for the period specified in §320.38.
[52 FR 8831, Mar. 19, 1987, as amended at 52 FR 23031, June 17, 1987; 58 FR 25926, Apr. 28, 1993; 63 FR 5252, Feb. 2, 1998; 67 FR 9586, Mar. 4, 2002]

## §312.58 Inspection of sponsor's records and reports.

(a) *FDA inspection.* A sponsor shall upon request from any properly authorized officer or employee of the Food and Drug Administration, at reasonable times, permit such officer or employee to have access to and copy and verify any records and reports relating to a clinical investigation conducted under this part. Upon written request by FDA, the sponsor shall submit the records or reports (or copies of them) to FDA. The sponsor shall discontinue shipments of the drug to any investigator who has failed to maintain or make available records or reports of the investigation as required by this part.

(b) *Controlled substances.* If an investigational new drug is a substance listed in any schedule of the Controlled Substances Act (21 U.S.C. 801; 21 CFR part 1308), records concerning shipment, delivery, receipt, and disposition of the drug, which are required to be kept under this part or other applicable parts of this chapter shall, upon the request of a properly authorized employee of the Drug Enforcement Administration of the U.S. Department of Justice, be made available by the investigator or sponsor to whom the request is made, for inspection and copying. In addition, the sponsor shall assure that adequate precautions are taken, including storage of the investigational drug in a securely locked, substantially constructed cabinet, or other securely locked, substantially constructed enclosure, access to which is limited, to prevent theft or diversion of the substance into illegal channels of distribution.

### §312.59 Disposition of unused supply of investigational drug.

The sponsor shall assure the return of all unused supplies of the investigational drug from each individual investigator whose participation in the investigation is discontinued or terminated. The sponsor may authorize alternative disposition of unused supplies of the investigational drug provided this alternative disposition does not expose humans to risks from the drug. The sponsor shall maintain written records of any disposition of the drug in accordance with §312.57.

[52 FR 8831, Mar. 19, 1987, as amended at 52 FR 23031, June 17, 1987; 67 FR 9586, Mar. 4, 2002]

### §312.60 General responsibilities of investigators.

An investigator is responsible for ensuring that an investigation is conducted according to the signed investigator statement, the investigational plan, and applicable regulations; for protecting the rights, safety, and welfare of subjects under the investigator's care; and for the control of drugs under investigation. An investigator shall, in accordance with the provisions of part 50 of this chapter, obtain the informed consent of each human subject to whom the drug is administered, except as provided in §§50.23 or 50.24 of this chapter. Additional specific responsibilities of clinical investigators are set forth in this part and in parts 50 and 56 of this chapter.

[52 FR 8831, Mar. 19, 1987, as amended at 61 FR 51530, Oct. 2, 1996]

### §312.61 Control of the investigational drug.

An investigator shall administer the drug only to subjects under the investigator's personal supervision or under the supervision of a subinvestigator responsible to the investigator. The investigator shall not supply the investigational drug to any person not authorized under this part to receive it.

## §312.62 Investigator recordkeeping and record retention.

(a) *Disposition of drug.* An investigator is required to maintain adequate records of the disposition of the drug, including dates, quantity, and use by subjects. If the investigation is terminated, suspended, discontinued, or completed, the investigator shall return the unused supplies of the drug to the sponsor, or otherwise provide for disposition of the unused supplies of the drug under §312.59.

(b) *Case histories.* An investigator is required to prepare and maintain adequate and accurate case histories that record all observations and other data pertinent to the investigation on each individual administered the investigational drug or employed as a control in the investigation. Case histories include the case report forms and supporting data including, for example, signed and dated consent forms and medical records including, for example, progress notes of the physician, the individual's hospital chart(s), and the nurses' notes. The case history for each individual shall document that informed consent was obtained prior to participation in the study.

(c) *Record retention.* An investigator shall retain records required to be maintained under this part for a period of 2 years following the date a marketing application is approved for the drug for the indication for which it is being investigated; or, if no application is to be filed or if the application is not approved for such indication, until 2 years after the investigation is discontinued and FDA is notified.

[52 FR 8831, Mar. 19, 1987, as amended at 52 FR 23031, June 17, 1987; 61 FR 57280, Nov. 5, 1996; 67 FR 9586, Mar. 4, 2002]

## §312.64 Investigator reports.

(a) *Progress reports.* The investigator shall furnish all reports to the sponsor of the drug who is responsible for collecting and evaluating the results obtained. The sponsor is required under §312.33 to submit annual reports to FDA on the progress of the clinical investigations.

(b) *Safety reports.* An investigator shall promptly report to the sponsor any adverse effect that may reasonably be regarded as caused by, or probably caused by, the drug. If the adverse effect is alarming, the investigator shall report the adverse effect immediately.

(c) *Final report.* An investigator shall provide the sponsor with an adequate report shortly after completion of the investigator's participation in the investigation.

(d) *Financial disclosure reports.* The clinical investigator shall provide the sponsor with sufficient accurate financial information to allow an applicant to submit complete and accurate certification or disclosure statements as required under part 54 of this chapter. The clinical investigator shall promptly update this information if any relevant changes occur during the course of the investigation and for 1 year following the completion of the study.

[52 FR 8831, Mar. 19, 1987, as amended at 52 FR 23031, June 17, 1987; 63 FR 5252, Feb. 2, 1998; 67 FR 9586, Mar. 4, 2002]

### §312.66 Assurance of IRB review.

An investigator shall assure that an IRB that complies with the requirements set forth in part 56 will be responsible for the initial and continuing review and approval of the proposed clinical study. The investigator shall also assure that he or she will promptly report to the IRB all changes in the research activity and all unanticipated problems involving risk to human subjects or others, and that he or she will not make any changes in the research without IRB approval, except where necessary to eliminate apparent immediate hazards to human subjects.

[52 FR 8831, Mar. 19, 1987, as amended at 52 FR 23031, June 17, 1987; 67 FR 9586, Mar. 4, 2002]

### §312.68 Inspection of investigator's records and reports.

An investigator shall upon request from any properly authorized officer or employee of FDA, at reasonable times, permit such officer or employee to have access to, and copy and verify any records or reports made by the investigator pursuant to §312.62. The investigator is not required to divulge subject names unless the records of particular individuals require a more detailed study of the cases, or unless there is reason to believe that the records do not represent actual case studies, or do not represent actual results obtained.

### §312.69 Handling of controlled substances.

If the investigational drug is subject to the Controlled Substances Act, the investigator shall take adequate precautions, including storage of the investigational drug in a securely locked, substantially constructed cabinet, or other securely locked, substantially constructed enclosure, access to which is limited, to prevent theft or diversion of the substance into illegal channels of distribution.

## §312.70 Disqualification of a clinical investigator.

(a) If FDA has information indicating that an investigator (including a sponsor-investigator) has repeatedly or deliberately failed to comply with the requirements of this part, part 50, or part 56 of this chapter, or has submitted to FDA or to the sponsor false information in any required report, the Center for Drug Evaluation and Research or the Center for Biologics Evaluation and Research will furnish the investigator written notice of the matter complained of and offer the investigator an opportunity to explain the matter in writing, or, at the option of the investigator, in an informal conference. If an explanation is offered but not accepted by the Center for Drug Evaluation and Research or the Center for Biologics Evaluation and Research, the investigator will be given an opportunity for a regulatory hearing under part 16 on the question of whether the investigator is entitled to receive investigational new drugs.

(b) After evaluating all available information, including any explanation presented by the investigator, if the Commissioner determines that the investigator has repeatedly or deliberately failed to comply with the requirements of this part, part 50, or part 56 of this chapter, or has deliberately or repeatedly submitted false information to FDA or to the sponsor in any required report, the Commissioner will notify the investigator and the sponsor of any investigation in which the investigator has been named as a participant that the investigator is not entitled to receive investigational drugs. The notification will provide a statement of basis for such determination.

(c) Each IND and each approved application submitted under part 314 containing data reported by an investigator who has been determined to be ineligible to receive investigational drugs will be examined to determine whether the investigator has submitted unreliable data that are essential to the continuation of the investigation or essential to the approval of any marketing application.

(d) If the Commissioner determines, after the unreliable data submitted by the investigator are eliminated from consideration, that the data remaining are inadequate to support a conclusion that it is reasonably safe to continue the investigation, the Commissioner will notify the sponsor who shall have an opportunity for a regulatory hearing under part 16. If a danger to the public health exists, however, the Commissioner shall terminate the IND immediately and notify the sponsor of the determination. In such case, the sponsor shall have an opportunity for a regulatory hearing before FDA under part 16 on the question of whether the IND should be reinstated.

(e) If the Commissioner determines, after the unreliable data submitted by the investigator are eliminated from consideration, that the continued approval of the drug product for which the data were submitted cannot be justified, the Commissioner will proceed to withdraw approval of the drug product in accordance with the applicable provisions of the act.

(f) An investigator who has been determined to be ineligible to receive investigational drugs may be reinstated as eligible when the Commissioner determines that the investigator has presented adequate assurances that the investigator will employ investigatioal drugs solely in compliance with the provisions of this part and of parts 50 and 56.

[52 FR 8831, Mar. 19, 1987, as amended at 52 FR 23031, June 17, 1987; 55 FR 11580, Mar. 29, 1990; 62 FR 46876, Sept. 5, 1997; 67 FR 9586, Mar. 4, 2002]

## Subpart E—Drugs Intended to Treat Life-threatening and Severely-debilitating Illnesses

Authority: 21 U.S.C. 351, 352, 353, 355, 371; 42 U.S.C. 262.
Source: 53 FR 41523, Oct. 21, 1988, unless otherwise noted.

### §312.80 Purpose.

The purpose of this section is to establish procedures designed to expedite the development, evaluation, and marketing of new therapies intended to treat persons with life-threatening and severely-debilitating illnesses, especially where no satisfactory alternative therapy exists. As stated §314.105(c) of this chapter, while the statutory standards of safety and effectiveness apply to all drugs, the many kinds of drugs that are subject to them, and the wide range of uses for those drugs, demand flexibility in applying the standards. The Food and Drug Administration (FDA) has determined that it is appropriate to exercise the broadest flexibility in applying the statutory standards, while preserving appropriate guarantees for safety and effectiveness. These procedures reflect the recognition that physicians and patients are generally willing to accept greater risks or side effects from products that treat life-threatening and severely-debilitating illnesses, than they would accept from products that treat less serious illnesses. These procedures also reflect the recognition that the benefits of the drug need to be evaluated in light of the severity of the disease being treated. The procedure outlined in this section should be interpreted consistent with that purpose.

### §312.81 Scope.

This section applies to new drug and biological products that are being studied for their safety and effectiveness in treating life-threatening or severely-debilitating diseases.
(a) For purposes of this section, the term "life-threatening" means:

(1) Diseases or conditions where the likelihood of death is high unless the course of the disease is interrupted; and

(2) Diseases or conditions with potentially fatal outcomes, where the end point of clinical trial analysis is survival.

(b) For purposes of this section, the term "severely debilitating" means diseases or conditions that cause major irreversible morbidity.

(c) Sponsors are encouraged to consult with FDA on the applicability of these procedures to specific products.

[53 FR 41523, Oct. 21, 1988, as amended at 64 FR 401, Jan. 5, 1999]
§312.82 Early consultation.

For products intended to treat life-threatening or severely-debilitating illnesses, sponsors may request to meet with FDA-reviewing officials early in the drug development process to review and reach agreement on the design of necessary preclinical and clinical studies. Where appropriate, FDA will invite to such meetings one or more outside expert scientific consultants or advisory committee members. To the extent FDA resources permit, agency reviewing officials will honor requests for such meetings

(a) *Pre-investigational new drug (IND) meetings.* Prior to the submission of the initial IND, the sponsor may request a meeting with FDA-reviewing officials. The primary purpose of this meeting is to review and reach agreement on the design of animal studies needed to initiate human testing. The meeting may also provide an opportunity for discussing the scope and design of phase 1 testing, plans for studying the drug product in pediatric populations, and the best approach for presentation and formatting of data in the IND.

(b) *End-of-phase 1 meetings.* When data from phase 1 clinical testing are available, the sponsor may again request a meeting with FDA-reviewing officials. The primary purpose of this meeting is to review and reach agreement on the design of phase 2 controlled clinical trials, with the goal that such testing will be adequate to provide sufficient data on the drug's safety and effectiveness to support a decision on its approvability for marketing, and to discuss the need for, as well as the design and timing of, studies of the drug in pediatric patients. For drugs for life-threatening diseases, FDA will provide its best judgment, at that time, whether pediatric studies will be required and whether their submission will be deferred until after approval. The procedures outlined in §312.47(b)(1) with respect to end-of-phase 2 conferences, including documentation of agreements reached, would also be used for end-of-phase 1 meetings.

[53 FR 41523, Oct. 21, 1988, as amended at 63 FR 66669, Dec. 2, 1998]

**§312.83 Treatment protocols.**

If the preliminary analysis of phase 2 test results appears promising, FDA may ask the sponsor to submit a treatment protocol to be reviewed under the procedures and criteria listed in §§312.34 and 312.35. Such a treatment protocol, if requested and granted, would normally remain in effect while the complete data necessary for a marketing application are being assembled by the sponsor and reviewed by FDA (unless grounds exist for clinical hold of ongoing protocols, as provided in §312.42(b)(3)(ii)).

**§312.84 Risk-benefit analysis in review of marketing applications for drugs to treat life-threatening and severely-debilitating illnesses.**

(a) FDA's application of the statutory standards for marketing approval shall recognize the need for a medical risk-benefit judgment in making the final decision on approvability. As part of this evaluation, consistent with the statement of purpose in §312.80, FDA will consider whether the benefits of the drug outweigh the known and potential risks of the drug and the need to answer remaining questions about risks and benefits of the drug, taking into consideration the severity of the disease and the absence of satisfactory alternative therapy.

(b) In making decisions on whether to grant marketing approval for products that have been the subject of an end-of-phase 1 meeting under §312.82, FDA will usually seek the advice of outside expert scientific consultants or advisory committees. Upon the filing of such a marketing application under §314.101 or part 601 of this chapter, FDA will notify the members of the relevant standing advisory committee of the application's filing and its availability for review.

(c) If FDA concludes that the data presented are not sufficient for marketing approval, FDA will issue (for a drug) a not approvable letter pursuant to §314.120 of this chapter, or (for a biologic) a deficiencies letter consistent with the biological product licensing procedures. Such letter, in describing the deficiencies in the application, will address why the results of the research design agreed to under §312.82, or in subsequent meetings, have not provided sufficient evidence for marketing approval. Such letter will also describe any recommendations made by the advisory committee regarding the application.

(d) Marketing applications submitted under the procedures contained in this section will be subject to the requirements and procedures contained in part 314 or part 600 of this chapter, as well as those in this subpart.

## §312.85 Phase 4 studies.

Concurrent with marketing approval, FDA may seek agreement from the sponsor to conduct certain postmarketing (phase 4) studies to delineate additional information about the drug's risks, benefits, and optimal use. These studies could include, but would not be limited to, studying different doses or schedules of administration than were used in phase 2 studies, use of the drug in other patient populations or other stages of the disease, or use of the drug over a longer period of time.

## §312.86 Focused FDA regulatory research.

At the discretion of the agency, FDA may undertake focused regulatory research on critical rate-limiting aspects of the preclinical, chemical/manufacturing, and clinical phases of drug development and evaluation. When initiated, FDA will undertake such research efforts as a means for meeting a public health need in facilitating the development of therapies to treat life-threatening or severely debilitating illnesses.

## §312.87 Active monitoring of conduct and evaluation of clinical trials.

For drugs covered under this section, the Commissioner and other agency officials will monitor the progress of the conduct and evaluation of clinical trials and be involved in facilitating their appropriate progress.

## §312.88 Safeguards for patient safety.

All of the safeguards incorporated within parts 50, 56, 312, 314, and 600 of this chapter designed to ensure the safety of clinical testing and the safety of products following marketing approval apply to drugs covered by this section. This includes the requirements for informed consent (part 50 of this chapter) and institutional review boards (part 56 of this chapter). These safeguards further include the review of animal studies prior to initial human testing (§312.23), and the monitoring of adverse drug experiences through the requirements of IND safety reports (§312.32), safety update reports during agency review of a marketing application (§314.50 of this chapter), and postmarketing adverse reaction reporting (§314.80 of this chapter).

### Subpart F—Miscellaneous

## §312.110 Import and export requirements.

(a) Imports. An investigational new drug offered for import into the United States complies with the requirements of this part if it is subject to an IND that is in effect for it under 312.40 and: (1) The consignee in the United States is the sponsor of the IND; (2) the consignee is a qualified investigator named in the IND; or (3) the consignee is the domestic agent of a foreign sponsor, is responsible for the control and distribution of the investigational drug, and the IND identifies the consignee and describes what, if any, actions the consignee will take with respect to the investigational drug.

(b) Exports . An investigational new drug may be exported from the United States for use in a clinical investigation under any of the following conditions:

(1) An IND is in effect for the drug under 312.40, the drug complies with the laws of the country to which it is being exported, and each person who receives the drug is an investigator in a study submitted to and allowed to proceed under the IND; or

(2) The drug has valid marketing authorization in Australia, Canada, Israel, Japan, New Zealand, Switzerland, South Africa, or in any country in the European Union or the European Economic Area, and complies with the laws of the country to which it is being exported, section 802(b)(1)(A), (f), and (g) of the act, and 1.101 of this chapter; or

(3) The drug is being exported to Australia, Canada, Israel, Japan, New Zealand, Switzerland, South Africa, or to any country in the European Union or the European Economic Area, and complies with the laws of the country to which it is being exported, the applicable provisions of section 802(c), (f), and (g) of the act, and 1.101 of this chapter. Drugs exported under this paragraph that are not the subject of an IND are exempt from the label requirement in 312.6(a); or

(4) Except as provided in paragraph (b)(5) of this section, the person exporting the drug sends a written certification to the Office of International Programs (HFG-1), Food and Drug Administration, 5600 Fishers Lane, Rockville, MD 20857, at the time the drug is first exported and maintains records documenting compliance with this paragraph. The certification shall describe the drug that is to be exported (i.e., trade name (if any), generic name, and dosage form), identify the country or countries to which the drug is to be exported, and affirm that:

(i) The drug is intended for export;

(ii) The drug is intended for investigational use in a foreign country;

(iii) The drug meets the foreign purchaser's or consignee's specifications;

(iv) The drug is not in conflict with the importing country's laws;

(v) The outer shipping package is labeled to show that the package is intended for export from the United States;

(vi) The drug is not sold or offered for sale in the United States;

(vii) The clinical investigation will be conducted in accordance with 312.120;

(viii) The drug is manufactured, processed, packaged, and held in substantial conformity with current good manufacturing practices;

(ix) The drug is not adulterated within the meaning of section 501(a)(1), (a)(2)(A), (a)(3), (c), or (d) of the act;

(x) The drug does not present an imminent hazard to public health, either in the United States, if the drug were to be reimported, or in the foreign country; and

(xi) The drug is labeled in accordance with the foreign country's laws.

(5) In the event of a national emergency in a foreign country, where the national emergency necessitates exportation of an investigational new drug, the requirements in paragraph (b)(4) of this section apply as follows:

(i) Situations where the investigational new drug is to be stockpiled in anticipation of a national emergency . There may be instances where exportation of an investigational new drug is needed so that the drug may be stockpiled and made available for use by the importing country if and when a national emergency arises. In such cases:

(A) A person may export an investigational new drug under paragraph (b)(4) of this section without making an affirmation with respect to any one or more of paragraphs (b)(4)(i), (b)(4)(iv), (b)(4)(vi), (b)(4)(vii), (b)(4)(viii), and/or (b)(4)(ix) of this section, provided that he or she:

( 1 ) Provides a written statement explaining why compliance with each such paragraph is not feasible or is contrary to the best interests of the individuals who may receive the investigational new drug;

( 2 ) Provides a written statement from an authorized official of the importing country's government. The statement must attest that the official agrees with the exporter's statement made under paragraph (b)(5)(i)(A)( 1 ) of this section; explain that the drug is to be stockpiled solely for use of the importing country in a national emergency; and describe the potential national emergency that warrants exportation of the investigational new drug under this provision; and

( 3 ) Provides a written statement showing that the Secretary of Health and Human Services (the Secretary), or his or her designee, agrees with the findings of the authorized official of the importing country's government. Persons who wish to obtain a written statement from the Secretary should direct their requests to Secretary's Operations Center, Office of Emergency Operations and Security Programs, Office of Public Health Emergency Preparedness, Office of the Secretary, Department of Health and Human Services, 200 Independence Ave. SW., Washington, DC 20201. Requests may be also be sent by FAX: 202-619-7870 or by e-mail: HHS.SOC@hhs.gov .

(B) Exportation may not proceed until FDA has authorized exportation of the investigational new drug. FDA may deny authorization if the statements provided under paragraphs (b)(5)(i)(A)( 1 ) or (b)(5)(i)(A)( 2 ) of this section are inadequate or if exportation is contrary to public health.

(ii) Situations where the investigational new drug is to be used for a sudden and immediate national emergency . There may be instances where exportation of an investigational new drug is needed so that the drug may be used in a sudden and immediate national emergency that has developed or is developing. In such cases:

(A) A person may export an investigational new drug under paragraph (b)(4) of this section without making an affirmation with respect to any one or more of paragraphs (b)(4)(i), (b)(4)(iv), (b)(4)(v), (b)(4)(vi), (b)(4)(vii), (b)(4)(viii), (b)(4)(ix), and/or (b)(4)(xi), provided that he or she:

( 1 ) Provides a written statement explaining why compliance with each such paragraph is not feasible or is contrary to the best interests of the individuals who are expected to receive the investigational new drug and

( 2 ) Provides sufficient information from an authorized official of the importing country's government to enable the Secretary, or his or her designee, to decide whether a national emergency has developed or is developing in the importing country, whether the investigational new drug will be used solely for that national emergency, and whether prompt exportation of the investigational new drug is necessary. Persons who wish to obtain a determination from the Secretary should direct their requests to Secretary's Operations Center, Office of Emergency Operations and Security Programs, Office of Public Health Emergency Preparedness, Office of the Secretary, Department of Health and Human Services, 200 Independence Ave. SW., Washington, DC 20201. Requests may be also be sent by FAX: 202-619-7870 or by e-mail: *HHS.SOC@hhs.gov* .

(B) Exportation may proceed without prior FDA authorization.

(c) Limitations . Exportation under paragraph (b) of this section may not occur if:

(1) For drugs exported under paragraph (b)(1) of this section, the IND pertaining to the clinical investigation is no longer in effect;

(2) For drugs exported under paragraph (b)(2) of this section, the requirements in section 802(b)(1), (f), or (g) of the act are no longer met;

(3) For drugs exported under paragraph (b)(3) of this section, the requirements in section 802(c), (f), or (g) of the act are no longer met;

(4) For drugs exported under paragraph (b)(4) of this section, the conditions underlying the certification or the statements submitted under paragraph (b)(5) of this section are no longer met; or

(5) For any investigational new drugs under this section, the drug no longer complies with the laws of the importing country.

(d) Insulin and antibiotics . New insulin and antibiotic drug products may be exported for investigational use in accordance with section 801(e)(1) of the act without complying with this section.

[52 FR 8831, Mar. 19, 1987, as amended at 52 FR 23031, June 17, 1987; 64 FR 401, Jan. 5, 1999; 67 FR 9586, Mar. 4, 2002; 70 FR 70729, Nov. 23, 2005]

## §312.120 Foreign clinical studies not conducted under an IND.

(a) *Introduction.* This section describes the criteria for acceptance by FDA of foreign clinical studies not conducted under an IND. In general, FDA accepts such studies provided they are well designed, well conducted, performed by qualified investigators, and conducted in accordance with ethical principles acceptable to the world community. Studies meeting these criteria may be utilized to support clinical investigations in the United States and/or marketing approval. Marketing approval of a new drug based solely on foreign clinical data is governed by §314.106.

(b) *Data submissions.* A sponsor who wishes to rely on a foreign clinical study to support an IND or to support an application for marketing approval shall submit to FDA the following information:

(1) A description of the investigator's qualifications;

(2) A description of the research facilities;

(3) A detailed summary of the protocol and results of the study, and, should FDA request, case records maintained by the investigator or additional background data such as hospital or other institutional records;

(4) A description of the drug substance and drug product used in the study, including a description of components, formulation, specifications, and bioavailability of the specific drug product used in the clinical study, if available; and

(5) If the study is intended to support the effectiveness of a drug product, information showing that the study is adequate and well controlled under §314.126.

(c) *Conformance with ethical principles.* (1) Foreign clinical research is required to have been conducted in accordance with the ethical principles stated in the "Declaration of Helsinki" (see paragraph (c)(4) of this section) or the laws and regulations of the country in which the research was conducted, whichever represents the greater protection of the individual.

(2) For each foreign clinical study submitted under this section, the sponsor shall explain how the research conformed to the ethical principles contained in the "Declaration of Helsinki" or the foreign country's standards, whichever were used. If the foreign country's standards were used, the sponsor shall explain in detail how those standards differ from the "Declaration of Helsinki" and how they offer greater protection.

(3) When the research has been approved by an independent review committee, the sponsor shall submit to FDA documentation of such review and approval, including the names and qualifications of the members of the committee. In this regard, a "review committee" means a committee composed of scientists and, where practicable, individuals who are otherwise qualified (e.g., other health professionals or laymen). The investigator may not vote on any aspect of the review of his or her protocol by a review committee.

(4) The "Declaration of Helsinki" states as follows:

## RECOMMENDATIONS GUIDING PHYSICIANS IN BIOMEDICAL RESEARCH INVOLVING HUMAN SUBJECTS

### Introduction
It is the mission of the physician to safeguard the health of the people. His or her knowledge and conscience are dedicated to the fulfillment of this mission.

    The Declaration of Geneva of the World Medical Association binds the physician with the words, "The health of my patient will be my first consideration," and the International Code of Medical Ethics declares that, "A physician shall act only in the patient's interest when providing medical care which might have the effect of weakening the physical and mental condition of the patient."

The purpose of biomedical research involving human subjects must be to improve diagnostic, therapeutic and prophylactic procedures and the understanding of the aetiology and pathogenesis of disease.

In current medical practice most diagnostic, therapeutic or prophylactic procedures involve hazards. This applies especially to biomedical research.

Medical progress is based on research which ultimately must rest in part on experimentation involving human subjects.

In the field of biomedical research a fundamental distinction must be recognized between medical research in which the aim is essentially diagnostic or therapeutic for a patient, and medical research, the essential object of which is purely scientific and without implying direct diagnostic or therapeutic value to the person subjected to the research.

Special caution must be exercised in the conduct of research which may affect the environment, and the welfare of animals used for research must be respected.

Because it is essential that the results of laboratory experiments be applied to human beings to further scientific knowledge and to help suffering humanity, the World Medical Association has prepared the following recommendations as a guide to every physician in biomedical research involving human subjects. They should be kept under review in the future. It must be stressed that the standards as drafted are only a guide to physicians all over the world. Physicians are not relieved from criminal, civil and ethical responsibilities under the laws of their own countries.

### I. Basic Principles

1. Biomedical research involving human subjects must conform to generally accepted scientific principles and should be based on adequately performed laboratory and animal experimentation and on a thorough knowledge of the scientific literature.

2. The design and performance of each experimental procedure involving human subjects should be clearly formulated in an experimental protocol which should be transmitted for consideration, comment and guidance to a specially appointed committee independent of the investigator and the sponsor provided that this independent committee is in conformity with the laws and regulations of the country in which the research experiment is performed.

3. Biomedical research involving human subjects should be conducted only by scientifically qualified persons and under the supervision of a

clinically competent medical person. The responsibility for the human subject must always rest with a medically qualified person and never rest on the subject of the research, even though the subject has given his or her consent.

4. Biomedical research involving human subjects cannot legitimately be carried out unless the importance of the objective is in proportion to the inherent risk to the subject.

5. Every biomedical research project involving human subjects should be preceded by careful assessment of predictable risks in comparison with foreseeable benefits to the subject or to others. Concern for the interests of the subject must always prevail over the interests of science and society.

6. The right of the research subject to safeguard his or her integrity must always be respected. Every precaution should be taken to respect the privacy of the subject and to minimize the impact of the study on the subject's physical and mental integrity and on the personality of the subject.

7. Physicians should abstain from engaging in research projects involving human subjects unless they are satisfied that the hazards involved are believed to be predictable. Physicians should cease any investigation if the hazards are found to outweigh the potential benefits.

8. In publication of the results of his or her research, the physician is obliged to preserve the accuracy of the results. Reports of experimentation not in accordance with the principles laid down in this Declaration should not be accepted for publication.

9. In any research on human beings, each potential subject must be adequately informed of the aims, methods, anticipated benefits and potential hazards of the study and the discomfort it may entail. He or she should be informed that he or she is at liberty to abstain from participation in the study and that he or she is free to withdraw his or her consent to participation at any time. The physician should then obtain the subject's freely-given informed consent, preferably in writing.

10. When obtaining informed consent for the research project the physician should be particularly cautious if the subject is in a dependent relationship to him or her or may consent under duress. In that case the informed consent should be obtained by a physician who is not engaged in the investigation and who is completely independent of this official relationship.

11. In case of legal incompetence, informed consent should be obtained from the legal guardian in accordance with national legislation. Where

physical or mental incapacity makes it impossible to obtain informed consent, or when the subject is a minor, permission from the responsible relative replaces that of the subject in accordance with national legislation.

Whenever the minor child is in fact able to give a consent, the minor's consent must be obtained in addition to the consent of the minor's legal guardian.

12. The research protocol should always contain a statement of the ethical considerations involved and should indicate that the principles enunciated in the present Declaration are complied with.

## II. Medical Research Combined with Professional Care (Clinical Research)

1. In the treatment of the sick person, the physician must be free to use a new diagnostic and therapeutic measure, if in his or her judgment it offers hope of saving life, reestablishing health or alleviating suffering.

2. The potential benefits, hazards and discomfort of a new method should be weighed against the advantages of the best current diagnostic and therapeutic methods.

3. In any medical study, every patient—including those of a control group, if any—should be assured of the best proven diagnostic and therapeutic method.

4. The refusal of the patient to participate in a study must never interfere with the physician-patient relationship.

5. If the physician considers it essential not to obtain informed consent, the specific reasons for this proposal should be stated in the experimental protocol for transmission to the independent committee (I, 2).

6. The physician can combine medical research with professional care, the objective being the acquisition of new medical knowledge, only to the extent that medical research is justified by its potential diagnostic or therapeutic value for the patient.

## III. Non-Therapeutic Biomedical Research Involving Human Subjects (Non-Clinical Biomedical Research)

1. In the purely scientific application of medical research carried out on a human being, it is the duty of the physician to remain the protector of the life and health of that person on whom biomedical research is being carried out.

2. The subjects should be volunteers—either healthy persons or patients for whom the experimental design is not related to the patient's illness.

3. The investigator or the investigating team should discontinue the research if in his/her or their judgment it may, if continued, be harmful to the individual.

4. In research on man, the interest of science and society should never take precedence over considerations related to the well-being of the subject.

[52 FR 8831, Mar. 19, 1987, as amended at 52 FR 23031, June 17, 1987; 56 FR 22113, May 14, 1991; 64 FR 401, Jan. 5, 1999; 67 FR 9586, Mar. 4, 2002]

**§312.130 Availability for public disclosure of data and information in an IND.**

(a) The existence of an investigational new drug application will not be disclosed by FDA unless it has previously been publicly disclosed or acknowledged.

(b) The availability for public disclosure of all data and information in an investigational new drug application for a new drug will be handled in accordance with the provisions established in 314.430 for the confidentiality of data and information in applications submitted in part 314. The availability for public disclosure of all data and information in an investigational new drug application for a biological product will be governed by the provisions of 601.50 and 601.51.

(c) Notwithstanding the provisions of 314.430, FDA shall disclose upon request to an individual to whom an investigational new drug has been given a copy of any IND safety report relating to the use in the individual.

(d) The availability of information required to be publicly disclosed for investigations involving an exception from informed consent under 50.24 of this chapter will be handled as follows: Persons wishing to request the publicly disclosable information in the IND that was required to be filed in Docket Number 95S-0158 in the Division of Dockets Management (HFA-305), Food and Drug Administration, 5630 Fishers Lane, rm. 1061, Rockville, MD 20852, shall submit a request under the Freedom of Information Act.

[52 FR 8831, Mar. 19, 1987. Redesignated at 53 FR 41523, Oct. 21, 1988, as amended at 61 FR 51530, Oct. 2, 1996; 64 FR 401, Jan. 5, 1999; 68 FR 24879, May 9, 2003]

### §312.140 Address for correspondence.

(a) A sponsor must send an initial IND submission to the Center for Drug Evaluation and Research (CDER) or to the Center for Biologics Evaluation and Research (CBER), depending on the Center responsible for regulating the product as follows:

(1) For drug products regulated by CDER . Send the IND submission to the Central Document Room, Center for Drug Evaluation and Research, Food and Drug Administration, 5901-B Ammendale Rd., Beltsville, MD 20705-1266.

(2) For biological products regulated by CDER. Send the IND submission to the CDER Therapeutic Biological Products Document Room, Center for Drug Evaluation and Research, Food and Drug Administration, 12229 Wilkins Ave., Rockville, MD 20852.

(3) For biological products regulated by CBER . Send the IND submission to the Document Control Center (HFM-99), Center for Biologics Evaluation and Research, Food and Drug Administration, 1401 Rockville Pike, suite 200N, Rockville, MD 20852-1448.

(b) On receiving the IND, the responsible Center will inform the sponsor which one of the divisions in CDER or CBER is responsible for the IND. Amendments, reports, and other correspondence relating to matters covered by the IND should be directed to the appropriate Center and division. The outside wrapper of each submission shall state what is contained in the submission, for example, "IND Application", "Protocol Amendment", etc.

(c) All correspondence relating to export of an investigational drug under 312.110(b)(2) shall be submitted to the International Affairs Staff (HFY-50), Office of Health Affairs, Food and Drug Administration, 5600 Fishers Lane, Rockville, MD 20857.

[70 FR 14981, Mar. 24, 2005]

### §312.145 Guidance documents.

(a) FDA has made available guidance documents under §10.115 of this chapter to help you to comply with certain requirements of this part.

(b) The Center for Drug Evaluation and Research (CDER) and the Center for Biologics Evaluation and Research (CBER) maintain lists of guidance documents that apply to the centers' regulations. The lists are maintained on the Internet and are published annually in the FEDERAL REGISTER. A request for a copy of the CDER list should be directed to the Office of

Training and Communications, Division of Communications Management, Drug Information Branch (HFD-210), Center for Drug Evaluation and Research, Food and Drug Administration, 5600 Fishers Lane, Rockville, MD 20857. A request for a copy of the CBER list should be directed to the Office of Communication, Training, and Manufacturers Assistance (HFM-40), Center for Biologics Evaluation and Research, Food and Drug Administration, 1401 Rockville Pike, Rockville, MD 20852-1448.

[65 FR 56479, Sept. 19, 2000]

## Subpart G—Drugs for Investigational Use in Laboratory Research Animals or In Vitro Tests

§312.160 Drugs for investigational use in laboratory research animals or in vitro tests.

(a) *Authorization to ship.* (1)(i) A person may ship a drug intended solely for tests in vitro or in animals used only for laboratory research purposes if it is labeled as follows:

CAUTION: Contains a new drug for investigational use only in laboratory research animals, or for tests in vitro. Not for use in humans.

(ii) A person may ship a biological product for investigational in vitro diagnostic use that is listed in §312.2(b)(2)(ii) if it is labeled as follows:

CAUTION: Contains a biological product for investigational in vitro diagnostic tests only.

(2) A person shipping a drug under paragraph (a) of this section shall use due diligence to assure that the consignee is regularly engaged in conducting such tests and that the shipment of the new drug will actually be used for tests in vitro or in animals used only for laboratory research.

(3) A person who ships a drug under paragraph (a) of this section shall maintain adequate records showing the name and post office address of the expert to whom the drug is shipped and the date, quantity, and batch or code mark of each shipment and delivery. Records of shipments under paragraph (a)(1)(i) of this section are to be maintained for a period of 2 years after the shipment. Records and reports of data and shipments under paragraph (a)(1)(ii) of this section are to be maintained in accordance with §312.57(b). The person who ships the drug shall upon request from any properly authorized officer or employee of the Food and Drug Administration, at reasonable times, permit such officer or employee to have access to and copy and verify records required to be maintained under this section.

(b) *Termination of authorization to ship.* FDA may terminate authorization to ship a drug under this section if it finds that:

(1) The sponsor of the investigation has failed to comply with any of the conditions for shipment established under this section; or

(2) The continuance of the investigation is unsafe or otherwise contrary to the public interest or the drug is used for purposes other than bona fide scientific investigation. FDA will notify the person shipping the drug of its finding and invite immediate correction. If correction is not immediately made, the person shall have an opportunity for a regulatory hearing before FDA pursuant to part 16.

(c) *Disposition of unused drug.* The person who ships the drug under paragraph (a) of this section shall assure the return of all unused supplies of the drug from individual investigators whenever the investigation discontinues or the investigation is terminated. The person who ships the drug may authorize in writing alternative disposition of unused supplies of the drug provided this alternative disposition does not expose humans to risks from the drug, either directly or indirectly (e.g., through food-producing animals). The shipper shall maintain records of any alternative disposition.

[52 FR 8831, Mar. 19, 1987, as amended at 52 FR 23031, June 17, 1987. Redesignated at 53 FR 41523, Oct. 21, 1988; 67 FR 9586, Mar. 4, 2002]

## Form FDA 1572

| DEPARTMENT OF HEALTH AND HUMAN SERVICES<br>PUBLIC HEALTH SERVICE<br>FOOD AND DRUG ADMINISTRATION<br>**STATEMENT OF INVESTIGATOR**<br>*TITLE 21, CODE OF FEDERAL REGULATIONS (CFR) Part 312*<br>(See instructions on reverse side.) | Form Approved: OMB No. 0910-004<br>Expiration Date: June 30, 1992<br>*See OMB Statement on Reverse.* |
|---|---|
| | Note: No investigator may participate in an investigation until her/she provides the sponsor with a completed, signed Statement of investigator. Form FDA 1572 (21 CFR 312.53)). |

1. NAME AND ADDRESS OF INVESTIGATOR.

2. EDUCATION, TRAINING AND EXPERIENCE THAT QUALIFIES THE INVESTIGATOR AS AN EXPERT IN THE CLINICAL INVESTIGATION OF THE DRUG FOR TH USE UNDER INVESTIGATION. ONE OF THE FOLLOWING IS ATTACHED:

   ☐ CURRICULUM VITAE          ☐ OTHER STATEMENT OF QUALIFICATIONS

3. NAME AND ADDRESS OF ANY MEDICAL SCHOOL, HOSPITAL OR OTHER RESEARCH FACILITY WHERE THE CLINICAL INVESTIGATION(S) WILL BE CONDUCTED.

4. NAME AND ADDRESS OF ANY CLINICAL LABORATORY FACILITIES TO BE USED IN THE STUDY.

5. NAME AND ADDRESS OF THE INSTITUTIONAL REVIEW BOARD (IRB) THAT IS RESPONSIBLE FOR REVIEW AND APPROVAL OF THE STUDY(IES).

6. NAME(S) OF THE SUBINVESTIGATORS (e.g. research fellows, residents, associates) WHO WILL BE ASSISTING THE INVESTIGATOR IN THE CONDUCT OF THE INVESTIGATION(S).

7. NAME AND CODE NUMBER, IF ANY, OF THE PROTOCOL(S) IN THE IND FOR THE STUDY(IES) TO BE CONDUCTED BY THE INVESTIGATOR.

FORM FDA 1572 (12/91)          PREVIOUS EDITION IS OBSOLETE.

435

8. ATTACH THE FOLLOWING CLINICAL PROTOCOL INFORMATION:

Ν FOR PHASE 1 INVESTIGATIONS, A GENERAL OUTLINE OF THE PLANNED INVESTIGATION INCLUDING THE ESTIMATED DURATION OF THE STUDY AND THE MAXIMUM NUMBER OF SUBJECTS THAT WILL BE INVOLVED.

Ν FOR PHASE 2 OR 3 INVESTIGATIONS, AN OUTLINE OF THE STUDY PROTOCOL INCLUDING AN APPROXIMATION OF THE NUMBER OF SUBJECTS TO BE TREATED WITH THE DRUG AND THE NUMBER TO BE EMPLOYED AS CONTROLS IF ANY: THE CLINICAL USES TO BE INVESTIGATED: CHARACTERISTICS OF SUBJECTS BY AGE, SEX AND CONDITION; THE KIND OF CLINICAL OBSERVATIONS AND LABORATORY TESTS TO BE CONDUCTED: THE ESTIMATED DURATION OF THE STUDY; AND COPIES OR A DESCRIPTION OF CASE REPORT FORMS TO BE USED.

9. COMMITMENTS:

I agree to conduct the study(ies) in accordance with the relevant, current protocol(s) and will only make changes in a protocol after notifying the sponsor, except when necessary to protect the safety, rights, or welfare of subjects.

I agree to personally conduct or supervise the described investigation(s).

I agree to inform any patients, or any persons used as controls, that the drugs are being used for investigational purposes and I will ensure that the requirements relating to obtaining informed consent in 21 CFR Part 50 and institutional review board (IRB) review and approval in 21 CFR Part 56 are met.

I agree to report to the sponsor adverse experiences that occur in the course of the investigation(s) in accordance with 21 CFR 312.64.

I have read and understand the information in the investigator's brochure, including the potential risks and side effects of the drug.

I agree to ensure that all associates, colleagues, and employees assisting in the conduct of the study(ies) are informed about their obligations in meeting the above commitments.

I agree to maintain adequate and accurate records in accordance with 21 CFR 312 62 and to make those records available for inspection in accordance with 21 CFR 312 68.

I will ensure that an IRB that complies with the requirements of 21 CFR Part 56 will be responsible for the initial and continuing review and approval of the clinical investigation. I also agree to promptly report to the IRB all changes in the research activity and all unanticipated problems involving risks to human subjects or others. Additionally, I will not make any changes in the research without IRB approval, except where necessary to eliminate apparent immediate hazards to human subjects.

I agree to comply with all other requirements regarding the obligations of clinical investigators and all other pertinent requirements in 21 CFR Part 312.

## INSTRUCTIONS FOR COMPLETING FORM FDA 1572
## STATEMENT OF INVESTIGATOR:

1. Complete all sections. Attach a separate page if additional space is needed.

2. Attach curriculum vitae or other statement of qualifications as described in Section 2.

3. Attach protocol outline as described in Section 8.

4. Sign and date below.

5. FORWARD THE COMPLETED FORM AND ATTACHMENTS TO THE SPONSOR. The sponsor will incorporate this information along with other technical data into an Investigational New Drug Application (IND). INVESTIGATORS SHOULD NOT SEND THIS FORM DIRECTLY TO THE FOOD AND DRUG ADMINISTRATION.

| 10. SIGNATURE OF INVESTIGATOR | 11. DATE |
|---|---|
| | |

# A B O U T  C E N T E R W A T C H

---

Founded in 1994, CenterWatch is a trusted source and global destination of clinical trials information for both professionals and patients. CenterWatch provides a wide variety of information services including grant leads for investigative sites; business development leads for contract service providers; postings of career opportunities; listings of clinical trials actively seeking patients; advertising and promotional opportunities; and proprietary business analysis and data about the global clinical trials industry.

As a pioneer in publishing clinical trials information, CenterWatch was the first Internet site to publish detailed information about active clinical trials that could be accessed by patients and their advocates. Today, we have one of the largest databases of clinical trials actively seeking patients on the Internet.

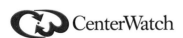 CenterWatch

100 North Washington Street, Suite 301
Boston, MA 02114
www.centerwatch.com

## Industry News

### *The CenterWatch Monthly*

*The CenterWatch Monthly*, our flagship publication, is a premier industry resource providing in-depth, authoritative business coverage for the clinical trials community, including the latest developments from around the industry as well as competitive intelligence on grant opportunities and new drug therapies—all in one comprehensive publication designed to assist professionals in conducting and managing their clinical research activities more effectively.

### *CWWeekly*

*CWWeekly* is a leading news source covering top stories and breaking news in the clinical trials industry. Every Monday morning, subscribers start their week with the most current business headlines and trends, financial news and market intelligence they need to stay a step ahead.

### *Research Practitioner*

This bi-monthly journal is a valuable, educational and career advancement resource that provides readers with timely and informative articles on regulatory developments and trends, protocol design and implementation, ethical issues in human research, and practical clinical research management tools. Subscribers can earn up to 18 CNE credits per year.

## Clinical Research Training Guides

CenterWatch's training guides offer effective and practical tools for those interested in clinical research as well as seasoned professionals seeking to better understand their roles and improve the management of their clinical trials operations in a safe and ethical manner. Titles in this series include:

- *A Guide to Patient Recruitment and Retention*
- *Becoming a Successful Clinical Research Investigator*
- *Protecting Study Volunteers in Research (CE credits)*
- *The CRA's Guide to Monitoring Clinical Research*
- *The CRC's Guide to Coordinating Clinical Research*

## Jobs in Clinical Research

### *JobWatch*

*JobWatch*, located on www.centerwatch.com, and the monthly *JobWatch e-Publication* are key clinical research recruitment and career resources. Both provide job listings, upcoming industry events, educational programs, company profiles and more. Registered seekers can also manage resumes, setup e-mail alerts and apply directly for positions online while employers can review resumes, post and manage current openings and maximize exposure with a variety of recruitment and advertising opportunities both online and in the monthly e-Publication.

## Information Solutions and Content Licensing

### Drugs in Clinical Trials Database

With more than 4,000 new investigational treatments in clinical trials worldwide, this database is updated weekly and helpful for monitoring the performance of drugs in clinical trials, tracking competitors' development activity and identifying development partners and clinical grant opportunities. Detailed drug profiles are completely searchable and include indications for use, current trial results, study phase status and manufacturer contact information.

### Content License Services

CenterWatch offers licensing of our database-driven and static-text content to provide companies with the latest in scientific clinical trial activity and drug development information using market intelligence and knowledge resources. Content can be offered as data feeds and co-branded to seamlessly integrate with a company's web site or Intranet. Our offerings include:

- *Clinical Trials Listing Service™*
- *Drugs in Clinical Trials Database*
- *Recently Approved Drugs by the FDA*
- *New Medical Therapies™*
- *Patient Education*
- *Publication Content Portal*

### Market Research Services

CenterWatch provides a wide range of quantitative and qualitative market intelligence services focusing on all aspects of the clinical trials industry, including outsourcing and vendor information, research and examination of new industry technologies, targeted site surveys that measure and improve company performance and relationships and more. Our experienced market research team works directly with companies to provide mission-critical information and detailed market analysis their organizations need to make more effective business decisions. Our services are completely customizable to meet our client's budget, level of analysis and deadlines.

## Grant Notification and Site Identification Services

### TrialWatch for Sites

*TrialWatch for Sites* is a complimentary grant notification service designed to help research centers easily connect with sponsors and CROs seeking qualified investigators for upcoming trials. Sites complete a brief online profile that is stored in a database and then matched against grant requests from sponsors and CROs. When a match is found, the site information is forwarded to the requesting company for consideration. Site profiles can be completed at www.centerwatch.com/ trialwatch_signup.

### TrialWatch for Sponsors and CROs

*TrialWatch for Sponsors and CROs* is a complimentary site identification service that helps companies quickly and effectively identify active and qualified investigative sites worldwide to conduct upcoming and active phase I through phase IV clinical trials. Confidential requests can be submitted online at www.centerwatch.com/ clinical-trials/trialwatch.

### Research Center Profile Pages

*Research Center Profile Pages* are an easy and cost-effective way for sites to showcase detailed information online about their site offerings and expertise to secure clinical research grants and contracts, increase their site's exposure and reach a captive and targeted audience. Profile Pages are completely customizable and can include images, video presentations, links to company documents, trial listings and more.

## Patient Recruitment

### The CenterWatch *Clinical Trials Listing Service™*

CenterWatch's *Clinical Trials Listing Service™* is one of the largest and most comprehensive online listings of industry-funded, global clinical trials. This searchable database allows patients to easily find and connect with ongoing trials actively seeking study volunteers and receives over a million unique visitors annually making it a proven and effective forum for online patient recruitment.

## Regulatory Compliance

### Standard Operating Procedures for the Conduct of Clinical Research

This SOP was developed to help clinical research sites meet the challenge of maintaining rigorous standards in a world of diminishing resources. This template has been expanded to include more procedures to assess study feasibility, recruit subjects and ensure regulatory compliance and is based on the Code of Federal Regulations and GCP Consolidated Guidelines.

### Policies and Standard Operating Procedures for the Institutional Review Board

This SOP is an easy way for IRBs to document policies and procedures that reflect their organization's philosophies, standards and innovations while continuing to comply with federal regulations. This template is based on the Code of Federal Regulations, guidance and ICH/GCP Consolidated Guideline and the Association for the Accreditation of Human Research Protection Program's (AAHRPP) standards for human subject protection.

### Standard Operating Procedures for Good Clinical Practice
### by Sponsors of Clinical Trials

This SOP was created to help pharmaceutical and biotechnology companies maintain the quality performance and ethical conduct of clinical trials while adhering to U.S. federal regulations. This template contains 30 procedures addressing all Good Clinical Practice requirements and is based on FDA regulations and ICH guidelines.

### Standard Operating Procedures for Good Clinical Practice
### by Sponsors of Medical Device Clinical Trials

This SOP provides detailed procedures that address specific requirements for medical device research practices while adhering to a discrete set of FDA regulations and guidance. Organizations that sponsor clinical research on new medical devices must implement procedures that comply with both Good Clinical Practice guidelines and federal regulations.

## Business Development Resources

### Industry Provider Profile Pages

*Industry Provider Profile Pages,* located on www.centerwatch.com, create visibility for contract service providers to showcase their products and services online to the clinical trials community making it a useful and cost-effective way for providers to generate new business leads, increase exposure and reach a captive and targeted audience.

## Patient Education Resources

### Volunteering For a Clinical Trial

*Volunteering for a Clinical Trial* is an easy-to-read, IRB-approved pamphlet designed as a quick reference guide for potential volunteers interested in participating in a research study. It includes an overview of the clinical trials process and answers some of the most commonly asked questions about volunteering for a clinical trial.

### Understanding the Informed Consent Process

*Understanding the Informed Consent Process* is a comprehensive, IRB-approved brochure providing study volunteers with important information regarding the informed consent process, including facts and information about the volunteer's "Bill of Rights."

For a complete list of CenterWatch's publications and services, please visit our web site at www.centerwatch.com.

## About the Authors

### Dr. Karen Woodin

Dr. Karen Woodin is currently a consultant/trainer to the pharmaceutical industry in the areas of clinical operations, GCPs, SOPs, IRBs and site monitoring.

Karen received an M.S. in applied statistics from Western Michigan University. Her Ph.D. is in epidemiology from the School of Public Health at the University of Massachusetts in Amherst. She has 25 years of experience in the pharmaceutical industry, primarily at The Upjohn Company, where she worked as a biostatistician, a CRA, CRA manager, and director, corporate pharmacovigilance. Dr. Woodin was very involved in implementing Total Quality Management and reengineering programs within the clinical research and safety surveillance areas.

Karen also served as vice president of clinical monitoring for a large CRO. Dr. Woodin is actively involved in the Drug Information Association (DIA), serving as faculty/chairperson for the CRA training course, as well as chairing workshops relevant to clinical trial management activities. She served five years on the DIA Board of Directors and a two-year term as Chairperson of the Steering Committee for the Americas, and has received the DIA's Outstanding Service Award. Karen has been instrumental in developing postgraduate courses in clinical research administration at Eastern

Michigan University and Western Michigan University, where she is currently an adjunct professor.

**John C. ("JC") Schneider**

After receiving a B.S. in zoology from Michigan State University, JC was employed by the Upjohn Company. His tenure at Upjohn included seven years as a biologist, 13 years as a medical research associate and 12 years in management before "retiring" in 1994.

After retirement from Upjohn, JC was a senior clinical consultant for a large consulting company where he directed their clinical consulting operations. JC helped develop a postgraduate course in clinical research administration at Eastern Michigan University and Western Michigan University, where he currently teaches. He is now an independent consultant/trainer to the pharmaceutical industry in the areas of GCPs, SOPs and site monitoring.

JC had a 30-year career in the Army Reserve as a Medical Service Corps officer that included command of a 1500-bed hospital and seven years at the Clinical Investigation Division of the Army's Health Services Command at Brooke Army Medical Center in San Antonio, Texas. He holds the rank of Colonel.

He is a long time member of the Drug Information Association (DIA) and the Association of Clinical Research Professionals (ACRP). JC helped revise DIA's Entry Level CRA Course, which he has taught for several years in addition to conducting numerous tutorials during the DIA Annual Meeting. He was a member of the Steering Committee of the Americas and is the recipient of DIA's Outstanding Service Award.